7 Times a Woman

Ancient Wisdom on Health & Beauty for Every Stage of Your Life

by Dr. Lia G. Andrews, DAOM, L.Ac.

Alcyone Press
San Diego

Published by Alcyone Press
10432 Reserve Dr, Ste 111
San Diego, CA 92127
www.AlcyonePress.com

ISBN-10: 0989326004
ISBN-13: 978-0-9893260-0-1

This book is intended to be informational and should not be considered a substitute for advice from a medical professional, whom the reader should consult before beginning any diet or exercise regimen, and before taking any dietary supplements or other medications. The author and publisher expressly disclaim responsibility for any adverse effects arising from the use or application of the information in this book.

For more information please see www.7TimesAWoman.com

For information on Dr. Andrews' clinic in San Diego, please see www.CinnabarAcupuncture.com

For rights and permission inquiries please contact 7TimesAWoman@gmail.com

Editor: Anita Edmondson
Layout Design: Miya Uchida
Cover Design: Lia Andrews
Author Photograph: Judith Andrews
Illustrations: Lia Andrews

Dedication

To Dr. Judith Andrews,

my mom, friend, and business partner.

and

To Natalie Jean and Kitana Stephanie Bernth,

two powerful little goddesses who helped me get my voice back.

Contents

Acknowledgements

I have heard authors say this, but it is true: this book wrote me. I have been the listener and student all my life until this book decided it was time to come through me. She brought people into my life without which this book would not have been possible.

I want to thank Miya Uchida for being a dear friend and teacher. She designed the inside of this book.. She patiently tutored me in InDesign and Illustrator. Her ingenuity, work ethic, and attention to detail were necessary for the creation of this book. Special thanks to Jenny Yoshida Park for consulting on the design.

Thank you to Dr. Jiang Zheng who gave me a copy of Dr. Shuqi Zhuang's book on postpartum care for me to translate while I was in my doctoral program, which was the basis for my capstone, and eventually inspired this book. Dr. Lily Chang was so generous in her time and talent to verify my translation.

I want to thank my mom, Dr. Judith Andrews, for her constant support and technical insights. Special thanks to Jen Leong for her guidance and emotional support on publishing. I also want to thank those for their insightful feedback of my initial scrawls that helped transform them into the finished product: Amanda Langley, Dr. Judith Andrews, Justin Scott, Tyler Smith, Matt Wuchner, and KC Carnine. Many thanks to Carissa Schumacher for helping me to heal during this process.

A big thank you to my teachers who influenced my practice in unique ways: Master Huaching Ni, Dr. Maoshing Ni, Dr. Daoshing Ni, Dr. Yueying Li, Dr. Huabing Wen, Dr. David Cohen, Dr. Jiling Hu, Dr. Shaoting Jing, Dr. Biao Lu, Dr. John Chen, Patrician McCarthy, Dr. David King, Michael Redmond, Dr. Giovanni Maciocia, Dr. Alex Tiberi, Dr. Mikio Sankey, Master Mantak Chia, and others who are too numerous to mention here. I want to thank my human, plant, and animal friends, my family, and my patients for believing in me more than I believed in myself and for the Divine guidance I have received.

And I want to thank my high school English teacher, Ms. Todd, who, many years ago, said I would publish one day.

My Story

I want to share the knowledge that changed my life in the hopes that it will change yours as well. Sometimes the greatest gifts come to us in the façade of tragedy, for when things do not go as planned we are forced to do things differently from the way we were doing them or the way others around us do.

When I was a little girl I was in tune with the energy of plants and animals. I was deeply affected by the energies of people and non-people. I remembered being an adult before. I remembered times and lands I had never seen. Very early I realized that this kept me from relating with others and I consciously shut it down.

I had always been physically healthy until puberty, when suddenly my body became unpredictable. I began to suffer from a litany of seemingly unrelated symptoms. I had joint pain, debilitating headaches, severe acne, and dizzy spells. My menstrual periods were completely erratic. I was diagnosed with Polycystic Ovarian Syndrome (PCOS) and migraine headaches. Over the years I became depressed and hopeless about my condition. One day my mom, out of desperation, took me to a naturopathic doctor who diagnosed me with a pituitary tumor. This was confirmed by a subsequent MRI. I felt relief that finally there was a physical answer to explain my symptoms. My allopathic doctor wanted to perform laser surgery to remove the tumor. There was a chance of damaging my pituitary gland, whereby I would be on hormones for the rest of my life.

My mom, who carried the weight of this illness more than I did, received a sign; in one week three people told her about a particular acupuncturist. We decided to see Chuck Hipple, who practiced in an old Victorian house in Charlotte, NC. It was in his office that I felt heard for the first time by a doctor and where I had my first of many transformative experiences with acupuncture. After that first treatment my relationship with my health shifted. I became conscious of the effects of my diet and lifestyle on my body. My mom and I began to read and study everything we could on the subject of Traditional Chinese Medicine (TCM) and alternative health. We slowly began to change our lives. We attended Science of Mind, read Louise Hays, Wayne Dyer, Christiane Northrup, and Deepak Chopra, and learned Reiki. Within three months of treatment, I had a normal period for the first time in my life. Within one year an MRI showed no tumor.

Both my life and my mom's life had changed forever. After I finished college, we decided to move to California and attend acupuncture school together. We attended a small lineage-based, Daoist school called Yo San University. I remember during our orientation Dr. Daoshing Ni said that as an acupuncturist our job was to heal ourselves first and to "become the medicine" that would heal others. This stood at such opposition to what I had been taught.

At Yo San we learned much more than Chinese herbology, acupuncture theory and practice, and sciences. We had qigong class every semester. We had classes on classical texts and Daoist theory. My education on the power of thought begun in my teenage years was deepened by these Daoist and TCM teachings.

My mom and I graduated together and opened our clinic, Cinnabar Acupuncture Clinic & Spa. We also went on to pursue our doctorates in acupuncture and oriental medicine at Pacific College of Oriental Medicine in San Diego. Through all these experiences, as both a student and practitioner, my concept of health has continued to expand for myself and for my patients. Every day I learn a new lesson.

I am forever grateful for that illness for three reasons: 1.) it saved me from an unconscious life, 2.) it brought me into a deeper relationship with my mom, and 3.) it gave me my life's purpose. Though it comes from a distant time and place, Traditional Chinese Medicine is my medicine. It continues to teach me who I am. I hope it does the same for you.

Introduction

The Yellow Emperor's Inner Canon is presented as a dialogue where the mythical Yellow Emperor asks the sage Qi Bo questions about how to live. This book, written at least 2,500 years ago, is the first work on Daoism and the basis for Traditional Chinese Medicine (TCM). In the first chapter, Qi Bo describes the 7 Cycles of Jing (Essence) in women and 8 Cycles of Jing in men.

It was the Introduction to TCM class in my first year of acupuncture school. I swear my teacher had a smirk on her face when she dropped this passage like a bomb on our class. At first we laughed at the descriptions. Then we were consumed with doom. It struck at the heart of all our unspoken fears about aging; that it was a slow, hellish, process where we watch everything we value fall away. A fierce debate erupted as we tried to reason ourselves out of this prediction for our future: "This was about starving people 2,000 years ago." "This was some crazy Chinese man." "I know plenty of men over 64 who still have their teeth." "Such and such actress is over 49 and she still looks hot." And yet, the truth was, the essence of what Qi Bo described was just as relevant today; that most people lose their vitality long before they are ready to die.

Later, when I actually read the Yellow Emperor's Inner Canon, I realized that it was a lament of how people abuse their bodies out of ignorance. It was both a warning and a wake-up call to live life differently. Immediately after this passage on the Cycles, Qi Bo went on to explain that there were various groups of people (immortals, sages, and naturalists) who had transcended these Cycles because they had learned to live in tune with Nature. The rest of the Canon is a guide on how people can live in accordance with universal laws and change their future.

This book was the first hint of an answer to the question I had asked myself as a teenager: "How can I change the state of my health?" I have spent the last 13 years of my life compiling what that transcendence, described in the Yellow Emperor's Inner Canon, looks like for women in our time. The conversation begins with understanding the concept of Jing. Understanding ourselves transforms us and our world. When we know the power of our own creative force, when we know how to cultivate our spiritual connection, when we know how to conserve our vitality, we become powerful, kind beings.

Jing is a challenging concept to grasp in the West. Jing is concentrated creative power that is passed to us from our ancestors and parents through the egg and sperm; through our DNA. Our Jing acts as our reserves of energy, and is related to our hormonal and reproductive functioning. The quantity and quality of our Jing dictates our ability to manifest in this world. Jing moves in a cyclical manner throughout our lives. By understanding these cycles we can maximize the potential for our lives.

I was inspired to write specifically on women's Cycles because even with all our advances, we as a collective are still confused as to the true nature and rightful place of the feminine. This has thrown modern people into disharmony, both with our environment and ourselves. In the Dao De Jing it states "Know masculinity, maintain femininity, and be a ravine for all under heaven."[1] This was a directive for all living creatures, and for both men and women. The masculine (Yang), acts on the outside world and drains its own energy in the process. The feminine principle (or Yin nature) is self-sustaining and internally governed. When we align ourselves with that mysterious Yin nature, when we surrender to it and allow it to embody us, we paradoxically grow in power, vitality, love, and awareness.

It is easier for us as women to align ourselves with the natural rhythms of the universe due to the physicality of our Cycles. These Cycles, outlined thousands of years ago in the first chapter of the Yellow Emperor's Inner Canon, offer insight into the natural cycles of energy, which we can use to optimize our own health. They are also a reminder to the ego that it is not in control. Women's cycles are often inconvenient for modern life, because they tie us to a natural life.

When we as women deny our Cycles it leads to a loss of identity, disconnection with the natural world, vanity, propensity to abuse of power, and all the sicknesses of modern society. Understanding these Cycles is the key to understanding ourselves and bringing ourselves back into balance with the natural order. Our loved ones and eventually the world will follow.

Before delving into the Cycles, I will review some basic principles in Traditional Chinese Medicine (TCM) in the next section, including foundational philosophies and concepts, basic disease patterns, and herbal medicine.

---

1. Huaching Ni, trans. *The Complete Works of Lao Tzu; Tao Teh Ching & Hua Hu Ching.* (Santa Monica: Seven Star Communications, 1979).

Guide to Reading this Book

Table FM.1. Guide to the 7 Cycles in this Book

Cycle	Age Range	Special Considerations	Challenges & Health Topics
Prologue	0-6	Our Constitutional Inheritance	Digestion & Immunity
1	7-13	Building a Strong Foundation Strengthen the Kidneys	Identity and Boundaries Building a Healthy Foundation: Diet, Exercises
2	14-20	Menarche Strengthen the Kidneys	Menstrual Care Fertility Gynecological Disorders, Safe Sex
3	21-27	Step into Womanhood Balance the Liver	Sex & Self-Cultivation, Inner Alchemy Spiritual Abuse Healing Trauma Transmuting Shadow Addictions Physical Development
4	28-34	Full Maturity Balance the Liver	Pregnancy Postpartum Care
5	35-41	Begin Rejuvenating Prepare for Menopause Balance the Liver	Rejuvenation (Boost Hormones)
6	42-48	Prepare for Menopause Balance the Liver	Detoxification
7	49-55	Treat Menopausal Symptoms Balance the Liver Strengthen the Spleen	Menopausal Disorders Death
Epilogue	56+	Post-Menopause Strengthen the Spleen	Post-Menopausal Care Rebirth

Each chapter begins with a discussion on one of the seven year Cycles. This is followed by a discussion on a general topic that is particularly pertinent to that Cycle, yet relevant to every age. The prologue and epilogue explain what happens before the beginning of the first Cycle at age 7, and after the end of the last at age 56. Regardless of your age or what Cycle you are approaching or are in currently, read the entire book. Daoist philosophy is about preparation and knowing where you are in reference to the bigger picture. When we are prepared, what could have been a major trauma becomes a minor bump or even a gift. Additionally, every chapter contains universal topics that were placed in a specific Cycle because it seemed most relevant. The Cycles also represent the stages of growth in all areas of our lives.

Attempts were made to accommodate a wider audience of students, practitioners, and the general public. The first section on Traditional Chinese Medicine: 2500 Years in a Nutshell, in the beginning of the book and glossary of terminology in the appendix section seek to educate laypeople on the fundamentals of this medicine. Parentheses and footnotes are included throughout to clarify technical or historical significance. Shaded areas are used to give a visual cue for sections geared towards acupuncturists and practicing students.

Chinese herbs are listed in Mandarin pin yin followed by the common English name in parentheses. Appendix A at the end of the book lists the herbs with their pharmaceutical and botanical names as well. The Resources section guides you where to find them. Traditional Chinese Medical terms are capitalized to make them visually distinct. Common words are capitalized when they are used in a Traditional Chinese Medical context. For example, "Spleen" is capitalized when referring to the organ system in charge of transforming and transporting food, etc. If the biological functioning of the spleen organ was intended, then "spleen" would be in lower case.

I want to clarify the term Traditional Chinese Medicine (TCM) as used in this book. TCM is often used to describe only the standardized traditional medicine of China created by post-revolutionary China and devoid of all local variations and possible destabilizing concepts. My exposure to the traditional medicine of China is broader. I went to a lineage-based Daoist school and learned from teachers with varied backgrounds. I also include in this book Taiwanese traditions that were not influenced by post-revolutionary mainland China. I choose to use the term TCM to include all the traditional Chinese medical practices and modern global evolution of this medicine.

From the Yellow Emperor's Inner Canon

(circa 500 B.C.)

a girl age 7. The Kidney energy becomes abundant, her baby teeth are replaced by permanent ones, and the hair grows.

女子七岁。 肾气盛，齿更发长；（7岁）

2 x 7, The dew of Heaven arrives (menstruation), the Ren channel begins to flow, the Chong channel is flourishing, the periods come regularly, and she can conceive.

二七，而天癸至，任脉通，太冲脉盛，月事以时下，故有子；（14岁）

3 x 7, Kidney Essence peaks, the wisdom teeth come out, and growth is at its utmost.

三七，肾气平均，故真牙生而长极；（21岁）

4 x 7, Tendons and bones become strong, the hair grows longest, and the body is strong and flourishing.

四七，筋骨坚，发长极，身体盛壮；（28岁）

5 x 7, The Yang-ming channels begin to weaken, the complexion starts to wither, and the hair begins to fall.

五七，阳明脉衰，面始焦，发始堕；（35岁）

6 x 7, The three Yang channels are weak, the face darkens, and the hair begins to turn gray.

六七，三阳脉衰于上，面皆焦，发始白；（42岁）

7 x 7 , The Ren channel is empty, the Chong channel depleted, the dew of Heaven dries up, the Earth Passage (uterus) is not open, so weakness and infertility set in.

七七，任脉虚，太冲脉衰少，天癸竭，地道不通，故形坏而无子也。（49岁）

Traditional Chinese Medicine

2,500 Years in a Nutshell

Beijing traffic, to my untrained eye, was pure chaos. It was a wild sea of cars, buses, bicycles, carts, and pedestrians, all acting independently of traffic signals and police cars. Upon further observation I noticed two things: first, how few accidents there were; and second, the absolute lack of aggression. It was a marvel how the movement of so many people could be so harmonious. It taught me a great deal about the way Chinese culture responds to a problem. Rather than seeking to directly control an uncontrollable amount of people, the city dwellers worked with the chaos to create harmony.

Traditional Chinese Medicine (TCM) emerged from a quest to achieve immortality. This quest drove much of China's early expansion in search of new medicinals and practices. TCM is more than preventive medicine, it is the study and practice of optimizing vitality and longevity.

Much like Beijing traffic, life is a complicated and contradictory creature. TCM, in seeking to optimize life, is predicated on paradox. It takes a chaotic mess of opposites and uses them to create balance. This requires the philosophies and practice of TCM to hold opposites. TCM demands that its practitioners engage both the intellect and intuition. TCM practice makes use of any modalities that will work, traditional or modern. It has taken ideas from various sources: shamanic, scientific, and cross-cultural influence, and tested these ideas with observation and analysis. These were systematically repeated, recorded, and adjusted by Chinese practitioners over millennia. So foreign a concept – that multiple and contradictory patterns can present in a single person and that these patterns can be treated multiple ways, successfully, by different practitioners. These contradictions, TCM's simplicity and intricacy, are what have kept its practice elusive to the Western mind. To understand this medicine, one needs to enter a different world.

Philosophic Foundation of TCM

The three major religions of ancient China – Daoism, Confucianism, and Buddhism – shaped TCM philosophy.[1] In American society it is more comfortable to call these "philosophies" rather than religions, as religions are thought to require exclusivity; that is, if you are a member of one religion you cannot be faithful to another. In cultures formed by multiple traditions, however, multiple religions often overlap; one filling in the spaces left by another. China is one such place. For example, adherents of Daoism or Confucianism are often also Buddhist. Each religion has contributed to Traditional Chinese Medicine in a fundamental way.

Daoism originated 2,500 years ago or more in China. It concerns itself with the study of Nature in an effort to achieve balance in this world. Happiness comes from following the "Dao" or "way" by living in harmony with natural laws. The principles of compassion, moderation, and humility are paramount. The goal is to live a natural life. Rather than be enslaved by human rules, the ideal is to live in accordance with natural divine order. Once a Daoist has developed him/herself through alchemical practices, he/she becomes naturally virtuous.

Daoism is the most colorful of the three religions. It retains China's shamanic, mystical past, and its temples are adorned with fantastical figures. Daoism prefers to deify great scholars, leaders, and healers who have passed on, similar to saints in the Catholic religion, rather than worship a creator God. Most of the foundational principles of TCM come from Daoism, including the 5 Elements, Yin and Yang, the 12 Earthly Branches and the 10 Heavenly Stems,[2] wu wei[3], and early qigong[4] practice. Medicine and Daoism are strongly intertwined and many Daoist monks are herbalists. Famous TCM doctors Zhang Zhong Jing, Sun Simiao, and Hua Tuo, for example, are all deified. The quest for immortality and internal alchemy are Daoist principles that drove the evolution of Traditional Chinese Medicine. The Yellow Emperor's Inner Canon (Huangdi Neijing) and Laozi's Dao De Jing are the most famous Daoist works. The I Ching, at once a book on philosophy and divination, is fundamental to both Daoism and Confucianism.

Like Daoism, Confucianism originated some 2,500 years ago in China. Confucianism was founded by Confucius (Kong Qiu) and centers on an impersonal creator God and ancestor worship. Again, noble people who have passed on are deified and worshiped, though they are far fewer in number; most notably, Confucius and Mencius.

In stark contrast to Daoism, Confucianism centers on rules. It stresses human conduct and provides specific parameters of how humans should coexist without emphasis on Nature, spirits, or even

1. I refer to them as religions here. Philosophy, religion, and cult are often used to define the same practice based on the point of view of the speaker.
2. Better known as the 12 animals and Yin and Yang aspects of the 5 Elements used in the Chinese calendar system and astrology. The Chinese calendar runs on two concurrently running cycles that match up differently each day, similar to the Mayan Calendar, that were used for predicting marriage compatibility, auspicious times for business deals, and planting schedules.
3. Wu wei is the concept of non-action or effortless action.
4. Qigong literally means "Qi exercise." Like yoga in India, qigong encompasses a wide variety of meditation, breathing, and movement practices used to cultivate the mind, body and spirit in ancient and modern China..

God. People achieve harmony through their adherence to a set hierarchy. Power and decisions come from the top down, while reverence and obedience run from the bottom up. God rules the universe, though It does not interact directly with humans. Amongst people, government rules the people, men rule their wives, parents rule their children, and elders rule younger members. Rules of conduct enforce this hierarchy in daily life.

Confucianism strives to create out of its adherents noble and scholarly gentlemen.[5] The virtues of honesty, righteousness, benevolence, loyalty, etiquette, and love between parents and children are the crux of the religion. The mores of Confucianism are challenging to the modern mind, however, its rigidity organizes and balances more chaotic forces. In TCM, Confucianism shows itself in the hierarchy of herb categorization and formula creation. It is apparent in the observance of ritual and technique, as well as the deference shown to teachers. Confucianism also lends a sense of social responsibility and integrity that is crucial to any healing practice. It teaches us that we have a moral obligation to make our society and our world a better place through our actions; that good is increased in the world by our daily choice to live virtuously. The "Analects of Confucius and Mencius" and the "Doctrine of Mean" are key Confucianist writings.

While Daoism and Confucianism concern themselves with the current world, Buddhism focuses on the attainment of enlightenment. Buddhism originated 2,500 years ago in Nepal and arrived in China in the 4th century C.E. In Buddhism, happiness comes from letting go of desires. Buddhism is non-theistic, meaning it does not claim or deny the existence of a creator God. Like the other two religions, adherents worship numerous deities who were once living people, in this case Gautama Buddha and various other buddhas.

Buddhist breathing and meditation practices influenced the evolution of qigong. Buddhist thought also had a great impact on the psychological aspect of Traditional Chinese Medicine. The focus on purifying the mind is present in the Buddhist scriptures, including the "Sutras," "Pali" canon, and "Tipitaka,"

The three major religions influenced the evolution of TCM. In addition to the major religions, China's empire also included Muslims, Christians, and shamanic influences from smaller groups that likely impacted the local practice of TCM. The traditional medicine of China was historically a lineage-based, eclectic practice that varied from family to family, and from region to region.

Additionally, ancient Chinese culture exalted the ideal of a Renaissance man; someone who was adept at interdisciplinary scholastics, including science, the arts, history, and mathematics. This concept led to TCM's inclusion of both intellectual and intuitive mastery. It also influenced its openness to different modalities of treatment and harmonization with other forms of medicine.

During the political upheaval of the last century in China, TCM fell in and out of favor, severely impacting its modern practice. At first, key officials and Mao Zedong attempted to eradicate the "backwards" old medicine of China in favor of Western medicine and new standards of hygiene.

---

5. Women's virtue is in observing their proper place.

When it became advantageous to do so, Mao Zedong reversed his stance and created a new standardized TCM, influenced by Western allopathic medicine and stripped of its religious and imperialistic flavor. TCM enjoyed acceptance until the Cultural Revolution (1966-1976). During the anti-intellectual fervor in China in that period TCM practitioners were again vilified.

The current usage of the term Traditional Chinese Medicine is confusing. Many intend TCM to mean Mao's standardized medicine that has been stripped of spirituality and variation. I prefer to use TCM as an umbrella term for the varied traditional medicine that emerged from ancient and contemporary China, as practiced around the world. The current practice of TCM was greatly influenced by, but not limited to, Mao's reforms. There are notable teachers and practitioners of TCM who escaped communist China with their lineage-based medicine intact.[(6)] Additionally, scholars and doctors continue to evolve TCM practice.

TCM practices exported to Western countries continue to transform in accordance with changing values and tastes. For example, the use of animal-based medicinals and the unequal status accorded to women in pre-communist teachings are widely rejected in the West; whereas Buddhist and Daoist philosophical influences are readily embraced by Western practitioners and patients alike.

Currently TCM in the U.S. finds itself in a time of great change. As it becomes increasingly mainstream it moves into the cross hairs of the corruptive influence of the corporate medical machine. My grandfather, who was an OB-GYN, used to practice similarly as I do today. He spent time with his patients and treated generations within families. It was how Western allopathic medicine used to be. The corporatization of medicine by insurance companies, major medical centers, and pharmaceutical companies dehumanizes both practitioners and patients. Becoming a part of this corporate model threatens to remove the benefits of TCM, providing individualized care and disease prevention. Acupuncturists who accept insurance are under the same pressure as other health care providers to create assembly line-style patient care. There is a push to be "scientifically proven" to standards that do not take into account the unique aspects of TCM. Part of gaining mainstream acceptance is the minimization of artistic, intuitive, and personal aspects of TCM.

6. Such as the founder of Yo San University, Master Huaching Ni.

Yin and Yang, and the Birth of the 10,000 Things

The first stirrings in the universe were the primordial Yin Qi and Yang Qi. The feminine and masculine existed in equal balance. When they danced, they gave birth to the 5 Elements, which in turn gave birth to the 10,000 things. Yin and Yang are the origin of all manifestation. Understanding the interplay of duality offers key insight into understanding Eastern philosophy and Traditional Chinese Medicine.

Yin and Yang are not static entities. They are relative terms. For example, men as a group are relatively Yang compared to women as a group, and older people are Yin compared to younger people. However, an otherwise very Yin old woman will become extremely Yang in the defense of her grandchild. An otherwise extremely Yang young man will become Yin after orgasm. An individual older person may present as more Yang than an individual younger person. In addition, every individual has both Yin and Yang aspects.

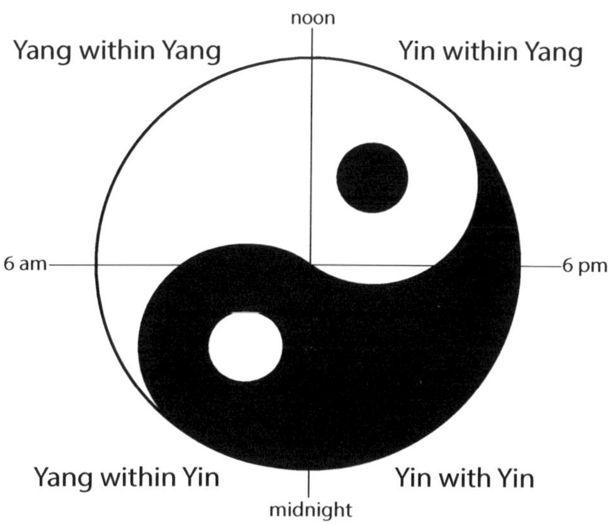

Figure 0.1. Yin and Yang

This understanding removes the tendency to label either Yin or Yang as better or worse. Rather, Yin and Yang theory teaches that there is no innate good and evil. "Good" is a product of balance and appropriateness. "Evil" is a product of imbalance and inappropriateness. Balance itself changes with the ebb and flow of different variables.

The concept of Yin and Yang can be used to describe all phenomena. It is used for TCM diagnosis and personal cultivation. Like the Western concept of Divine Marriage within the self, Daoist cultivation seeks to marry the internal opposite forces of Yin and Yang. Women are encouraged to take on traditionally masculine roles and men to embrace feminine characteristics. This can be done in an exterior fashion, as in engaging in a particular hobby, or internally, through meditation and visualization. Meditating on embodying the archetypal masculine and archetypal feminine is very healing. It highlights the wounds and deficiencies in our own Yin and Yang polarity. Whatever your gender, it is important to work with both, especially the one that is least comfortable. This is simple to do and powerful in its effect.

Both men and women have Yin and Yang energies at their disposal and can learn to alter these energies to best suit a particular situation. If you believe in reincarnation, everyone has had feminine and masculine bodies, and can access those memories. Ideally, our doing (masculine) nature is in service to our spiritual (feminine) nature.[7] When this occurs, our personality is united in service with our soul.

The Internal Alchemy of harmonizing Yin and Yang is a process of integration. Most people are a compilation of personalities; a result of traumas and unresolved issues. Once these have been thoroughly worked through, a single, sane, kind presence becomes the primary actor within us. When our whole being can set a single intention it is extremely powerful and literally dissolves the problems in our lives.

HOW YIN AND YANG INTERACT

Stand in opposition: They represent opposites. Yang is energy, excitement, restless, hot, acute, back of the body, sun, light. Yin is calm, introspective, quiet, chronic, front of the body, moon, dark.

Inter-dependent: Yin and Yang cannot exist without the other. "existence and nonexistence give birth to each other. Difficult and easy define each other...".[1] Pure Yang is the unmanifest seed of pure consciousness. Without Yin it is constantly searching and never manifests. Pure Yin is ceaseless, chaotic manifestation. Without Yang, manifestation will not have direction or order.

Inter-consuming: Yin and Yang consume one another. When we are hot (Yang) we sweat, depleting fluids (Yin). When we act heroically under extreme danger (Yang) we use up our Kidney Jing (adrenals, Yin).

Inter-transforming: Yin and Yang change into one another. Night turns into day. Extreme activity turns to collapse. Extreme repression turns to violence.

Further Division: Yin and Yang aspect can be divided infinitely into Yin and Yang. Cold is Yin and hot is Yang. Very cold is Yin and moderately cold is relatively Yang.

1. Huaching Ni. *The Complete Works of Lao Tzu: Tao Teh Ching & Hua Hu Ching.* (Santa Monica: Sevenstar Communications, 1995), 8.

7. This is the symbolism behind chivalric imagery and artwork, which represent internal alchemical practices.

Meditation: Pure Yang and Pure Yin

This exercise connects us with our own duality; our internal Yin and Yang aspects. Practicing these meditations integrates the dualistic aspects of our nature.

1. Sit or lie comfortably.
2. Become aware of your body.
3. **Yang Exercise:** Begin to feel yourself as the ultimate masculine embodiment. Feel your jaw, brows, features become massive. Feel your shoulders broaden and your chest tighten like armor. Feel the protection and vulnerability of your heart. Feel a massive, solid energy move down your arms, back, abdomen. Feel your hips narrow and your center of gravity rise slightly. Feel what it is like to have your genitals and sexual energy protrude out from your body. Feel the power and vulnerability of this. Feel the grounded power of your legs down to your wide, solid feet. Notice how your vision is different. Notice how your sight becomes penetrating, projecting, and outward focused, rather than receptive. Feel your readiness to act upon the outside world. Notice feelings of protectiveness, honor, and pride. Notice less pleasant urges such as predatory tendencies or the drive for power. Play with this for a while. How would you be received walking around in public? How would you interact with others? Notice the subtleties of your strengths and vulnerabilities in this body. You may decide to spend an extended period embodying your Yang energy.
4. **Yin Exercise:** Begin to feel yourself as the ultimate feminine embodiment. Feel the delicateness of your features, the fleshiness of your lips and cheeks, the softness of your hair and skin. Your body is covered by a layer of softness and delicacy that senses every detail of the world around you. Feel your shoulders narrow. The softness of your breasts extend out from your open heart into the world, penetrating it with your love. Feel the natural curves narrow into your waist then widen into powerful, sensual hips. Feel what it is like to have your genitals travel deep into your body connecting to your heart. Feel both the vulnerability and strength of this. Feel the fleshiness of your buttocks, thighs, and calves, down to your dainty feet. Notice how your eyes widen to take in the world. It is like you can see the depth of another's soul through the depth of yours. You sense the constant change of the world but your center stays still. You feel little motive to act. Rather, the perfect opportunities effortlessly appear. Notice feelings of compassion, playfulness, and creativity. Notice less pleasant urges such as the desire to manipulate others or vanity. Play with this for a while. How would you be received walking around in public? How would you interact with others? Notice the subtleties of your strengths and vulnerabilities in this body. You may decide to spend an extended period embodying your Yin energy.

The 5 Elements

The 5 Elements are the next categorization of primordial building blocks, after Yin and Yang. They include: Wood, Fire, Earth, Metal, and Water. The 5 Elements are also translated as the 5 Phases. Neither of these translations is perfect. The term "elements" ties the concept to Western 4 element theory (Earth, Water, Air, and Fire) and the 5 elements used in Ayurvedic (Hindu) tradition (Earth, Water, Fire, Wind, and Aether). While the term "phases" captures their moving quality; I use these terms interchangeably throughout this book. They were a mnemonic device used to describe and predict interactions in diverse disciplines, including: medicine, martial arts, Feng Shui, Chinese face reading, military strategy, and music.

The 5 Phases serve as a tool to understand the movement of energy through different phenomenon. For example, they can be used to describe the overarching cycles of a person's life. Childhood is a Wood period; a time of great expansion and growth. In puberty, children enter the Fire phase. Women reach their full height at age 21 and enter the Earth cycle until they are 35 years old. Then Earth declines and goes into Metal, when women go inward and question core beliefs (midlife crisis). At 49, women enter the depths of the Water cycle. After the menopausal period is over, the cycle can begin anew.

The 5 Elements can also be used to describe the phases of romantic love and relationship.[8] The initial pursuit and courtship is Wood. This is followed by the passionate, idealistic Fire phase. As a couple settles into real intimacy and companionship, the relationship has entered the Earth phase. In the Metal phase there is analysis, the unearthing of gold, or perhaps something less desirable. Finally, in the Water phase there is a pulling away and individual introspection. In a healthy relationship the cycle begins anew.

Table 0.1. Table of 5 Phase Associations

	Wood	**Fire**	**Earth**	**Metal**	**Water**
Virtues, Value	Compassion, Benevolence, Passion	Love, Joy, Humility	Faith, Trust	Purity, Justice, Idealism, Rectitude	Wisdom, Truth
Unbalanced Emotion	Anger, Depression, Repression	Mania, Scatteredness, Overstimulation	Worry, Rumination	Grief, Rigidity	Fear
Negative Drive[i]	Hostility	Greed	Ambition	Stubbornness	Desire
Corrupting Agent[ii]	Competition	Sex	Mind (over thinking)	Money	Alcohol

8.Patrician McCarthy's adaptation of Elaine Hatfield. *Love, Sex, and Intimacy: Their Psychology, Biology, and History.* (Harper Collins College Publ., 1993).

	Wood	Fire	Earth	Metal	Water
Needs from Others	To be Admired, Idolized as a Hero	Attention, to be Adored & Cherished	To be Needed & Liked, to be of Accepted	To be Respected, a Certain Level of Conduct	Depth, to be Sexually Desirable, to be Protected
Romantic Relationships	Conquest and Challenge	Novelty and Romance	Security and Nurturing	Fulfill a Social Role or a Romantic Ideal	Mystery and Romance
Sex	Goal-oriented, as in techniques to produce bigger orgasms	Connection, Excitement, and Attention	Pure Carnal Pleasure	Ideal of Purity or Deviant,"dirty" Behavior	Sensual Experience
Bonds	Direction, Assertion	Passion for Union	Holding & Maturing bonds; Loyalty, Dependability	Letting Go of the old and taking in the new	Power, Will, Courage for Bonding
Delusional About	Level of Mastery	Love	Loyalties	Credentials	List of Admirers
Spirit	Hun, "Ethereal soul" or "Soul"	Shen, "Spirit", "Mind" or "Consciousnes"	Yi, "Intellect" or "Intention"	Po, "Corporeal soul" or "Instinct"	Zhi, "Willpower" or "Soul's Purpose"
Sense	Sight	Taste	Touch	Smell	Hearing
Flavor	Sour	Bitter	Sweet	Pungent	Salty
Climate	Wind	Heat	Humidity	Dryness	Cold
Season	Spring	Summer	Indian Summer, transition between seasons	Autumn	Winter
Color	Green, or Blue-Green	Red	Yellow	White	Black or Indigo
Body Tissue	Tendons, Ligaments, Nerves, Nails	Blood	Muscles	Skin, Body Hair	Bones, Brain, Spinal Cord, Head & Pubic Hair
Orifice	Eyes	Tongue	Lips, Mouth	Nose, Mucous Membranes	Urethra, Anus, Ears
Fluid	Tears, Bile	Blood, Perspiration	Saliva, Lymph	Mucous Secretions	Sexual Secretions
Natural Rhythm	Renewal & Cleansing	Rapid Expansion & Contraction	Fruition	Slower Expansion & Contraction	Generation

	Wood	Fire	Earth	Metal	Water
Identity[iii]	Rejection of what aren't: No, I'm not	Positive Assertion of what are: Yes, I am	Boundaries of "I am"	Incorporation of internal authority into "I am"	I am One with God
Organs with their Time of Day	Liver 1-3am Gallbladder 11pm-1am	Heart 11am- 1pm Small Intestine 1-3pm Pericardium 7-9pm San Jiao 9-11pm	Stomach 7-9 am Spleen 9-11am	Lung 3-5am Large Intestine 5-7am	Urinary Bladder 3-5pm Kidney 5-7pm

i. Huaching Ni. *Tao; the Subtle Universal Law and the Integral Way of Life.* (Santa Monica: Seven Star Communications, 1979), 16.
ii. Ni, *Tao*, 16.
iii. Leon Hammer. *Dragon Rises, Red Bird Flies: Psychology & Chinese Medicine.* (Seattle: Eastland Press, 2005).

5 Elements & Personality

The 5 Phases are no more than abstract concepts until they come alive in the world around us. The 5 Elements come to life most vividly as they appear in the personality. When learning about the Elements beware the temptation to develop Element prejudice. Each Phase has its gifts and challenges. Like Yin and Yang, everyone has all 5 Elements within each of themselves. Some people are very balanced in all the Phases. Others show a predominance of one or two Elements. People who are weak in a particular Element will naturally be attracted to people with a predominance of that same Element in order to balance themselves. You can also cultivate a specific Element in yourself to make yourself more balanced.

The 5 Elements manifest in the personality are used in diagnosis of physical disease. When there is a dysfunction in an organ system, a person will exhibit negative behavior patterns of that Element. For example, when toxins build up in the Liver, a person might become depressed, irritable, or hostile. A person with a healthy Liver and Gallbladder will exhibit positive Wood traits, as in courage and decisiveness. This understanding allows you to observe where you are strong or weak in an Element and a way to balance it.(9) Figure 0.3 shows the appearance of each Element predominance.

Some people are afraid that face reading will reveal their secrets. Chinese face reading is not necessary for this. Everyone has the ability to sense, when they are talking to a person, if that person

9. This section on the 5 Elements are my experience and interpretation, the foundation of which came from the teachings of Patrician McCarthy and David Cohen.

INTERACTION OF THE 5 ELEMENTS

The 5 Phases interact in four ways: two ways constructively, and two ways destructively (Figure 0.2).

Constructively

They **generate** or create one another (the outer circle of arrows). Fire burns and becomes Earth. Earth consolidates into Metal. Metal generates Water. Water nurtures the growth of Wood. Wood feeds Fire.

They **control** or keep each other in check (the inner circle of arrows). The warmth of Fire melts Metal that has become too rigid and cold. Earth dams up destructive Water. Metal cuts down overgrown Wood. Water quells erratic Fire. Wood moves stuck Earth.

Destructively or Pathologically

They **over control** each other (the inner circle of arrows in excess). Fire melts away healthy Metal boundaries. Earth muddies up Water so it cannot flow. Metal cuts Wood down to the stump. Water extinguishes Fire. Wood restricts Earth.

They can **insult** each other (the inner circle of arrows in the opposite direction). Metal insults Fire. Water insults Earth. Wood insults Metal. Fire insults Water. Earth insults Wood.

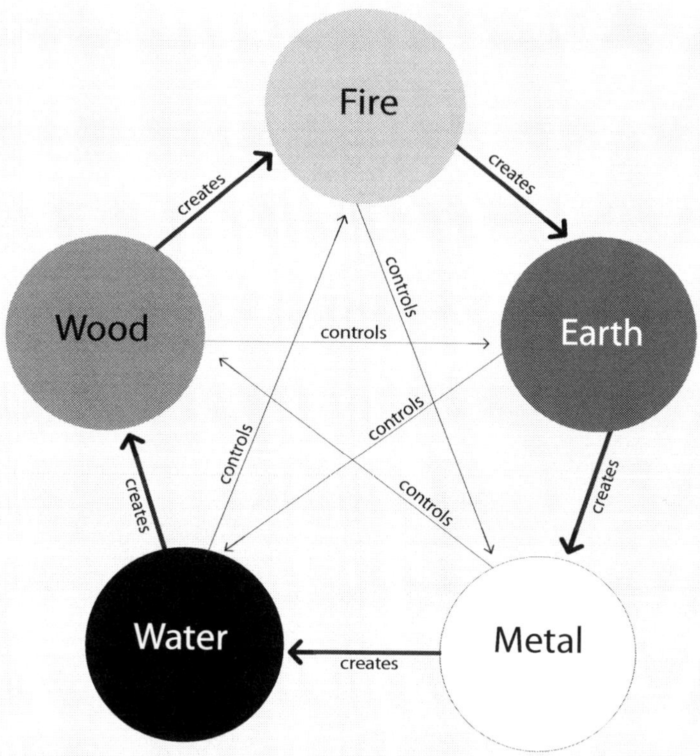

Figure 0.2 Interaction of the 5 Elements

is being deceptive. It will be a subtle feeling in your gut that their voice, words, mannerisms, and energy are not all in alignment. People are deceived because they either have not learned to trust this instinct or because they have a strong motive to want to believe. A predominance of a certain Element will not make you good or bad, though it will influence how you act out good or bad behavior.

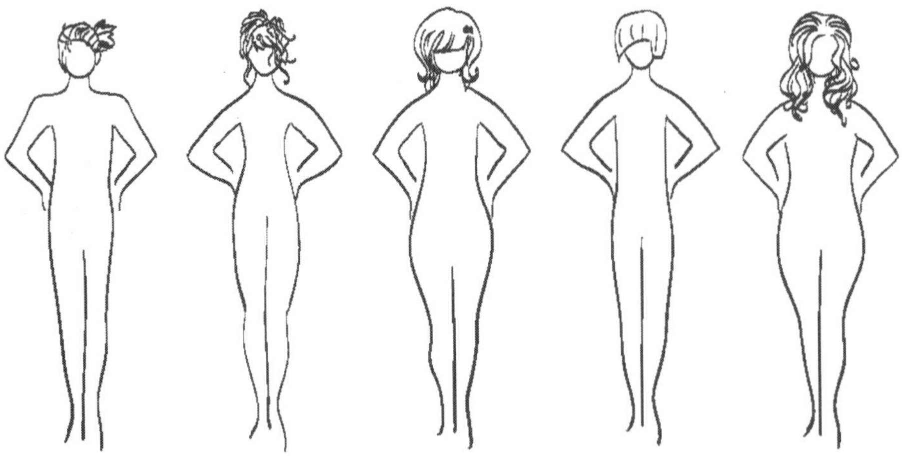

Figure 0.3

The Wood Phase

Physical Characteristics of Wood Predominance: Wood comes in tree and shrub forms. Tree Wood people are like basketball players: tall, tree-like structures, with broad shoulders and sinewy muscles. Shrub Wood people are like gymnasts: little, solid, and ready to explode into action. The Wood face is rectangular and long. Prominent eyebrows, an intense gaze, and a strong chin are common. Energy tends to get stuck in the shoulders. There is tense affect. The hands are knobby, lined, and proportional.

Gifts and Challenges of Wood Predominance

When it comes to 5 Element personalities, Wood is the Element everyone loves to hate. Everyone has at least some Wood, and it is often the aspect ourselves that creates the most challenge. Wood is associated with both the positive and negative aspects of the ego. It relates to the survival instincts that keep us alive and the arrogance that gets us in trouble.

The positive aspects of Wood are highly revered in our society. Wood, like a large tree, is constantly moving upward, growing, and expanding. Wood is the entrepreneur and pioneer. It stirs things up, initiates, and instigates. Wood tames the wilderness. It seeks challenge and is impelled to push its limits. Wood is a courageous fighter and athlete. It is protective of the weak and rescuer of those in distress. Wood excels under pressure and thrives with competition. Wood is at its best when it is in service to a greater good. Wood needs the acclaim and acknowledgment that it has done a good job. It likes to be the first, best, and only in everything. Wood loves action and admires speed and skill.

Wood gone rotten is impossible to ignore. This is because Wood asserts itself onto the world. Unbalanced Wood is hypersensitive to its own boundaries and oblivious to anyone else's. In fact, it sees exterior boundaries as a challenge that must be obliterated. This makes Wood gone bad the most destructive of the unbalanced elements. These are the bullies, criminals, corrupt cops, and predators. Whereas balanced Wood takes pride in protecting, unbalanced Wood proudly destroys. Wood can also take its bragging and shameless self-promotion to the heights of arrogance and narcissism. It imagines itself to be a great master after a weekend course. Wood can vacillate between impulsivity and extreme discipline. It can be intolerant, impatient, and emotionally volatile. Hypocrisy can be a big Wood handicap.

Wood Organs and Their Roles

Each Element has a Yin organ and Yang organ pair. Yin organs are full and hold vital essences. Yang organs are empty (with the exception of the Gallbladder which holds bile). The Yin and Yang organs of the Wood Element are:

Liver (Yin organ) – The Liver is the General of the body. It is in charge of directing the flow of Qi (life energy), particularly in regards to defense of the body. The Liver is the organ hardest hit by environmental and emotional toxicity.

Gallbladder (Yang organ) – The Gallbladder stores the bile. Emotionally, a strong or big Gallbladder relates to courage. A weak Gallbladder is associated with timidity.

Health of Wood

When you find yourself exhibiting Wood personality traits, it is a direct reflection of the strength and weakness of your Wood organ system. Positive traits indicate a healthy Liver and Gallbladder system. Negative traits indicate an imbalance in these organ systems.

PMS, depression, muscle spasms (especially of the upper back and neck), headaches, high blood pressure, and inflammatory nerve conditions are common Wood imbalance symptoms. Wood imbalance can cause or be caused by stimulant, drug, and alcohol addiction (this includes prescription painkillers, diet or energy drinks, coffee, and processed foods). In terms of health, Wood has a strong constitution. It is always "fine." When in discomfort Wood-predominant people are either highly stoic or violent whiners. When Wood does get sick, however, it the worst sprain, infection, etc., ever. There will be an intense struggle, where the best doctor, who also treats professional athletes, was at first bewildered, then performs a heroic surgery. This is accompanied with a dramatic story of recovery, achieved in record time, as never seen before. They tend to become advocates, after the fact, to raise awareness.

Spiritual & Psychological Aspect of Wood

The spirit of the Liver is the Hun or "Ethereal Soul." The Hun is the aspect of the soul that connects us to the Universal mind and archetypes. It enters the body three days after birth and leaves the body at death. It is responsible for our psychic abilities, life dreams, and artistic inspiration. As the Yang aspect of the soul, the Hun concerns itself with movement. It is the part of us that travels during dreams, it reaches towards other people in relationships, and it carries us along our life purpose and goals. The Hun keeps the balance between too much and too little movement of emotions. It pushes out to connect and empathize with people.

The Hun is an aspect of spirit shared by all living things. There are three kinds of Hun: Shuang Ling (Clear Spirit) that exists in plants, animals, and humans, Tai Guang (Brilliant Light) that exists in animals and humans, and You Jing (Dark Essence) that exists only in humans.

The Hun is rooted in Liver Blood and Yin. When these are deficient, the Hun becomes ungrounded and is said to wander, leading to insomnia and excessive or exhausting dreams. During the day the Hun sees through the eyes, at night it resides in the Liver and dreams, and on a psychic level it receives visions and insight. The Hun, when the Liver Blood is strong, gives us courage. When the Liver Blood is deficient, the Hun becomes cowardly, timid, and indecisive.[10]

Psychologically, Liver Yin relates to the ability to withdraw, in which the ego surrenders for a greater purpose. In Liver Yin deficiency, retreat is impossible. Retreat, even if strategic, is associated with failure and humiliation. In Liver Yin excess, there is constant withdrawing, which manifests as extreme pacifism.

Liver Yang is the means to assert; the ability to advance and act. Liver Yang deficiency, when due to toxicity of the Liver, produces underachievers who are unable to move visions into action.[11] In cases where Wood energy is stifled in early childhood, it results in passive-aggressive behavior. In these instances, excessive authority squashes the child's ability to assert their identity. The individual is never allowed to be themselves around others and struggles to share his/her gifts with the world. In Liver Yang excess there is unremitting aggression and a determination to always get his/her way, oblivious to the needs of others. This is what is referred to as the "Livery person" and the one that gives the Wood element a bad name. Wood relates to the ability to assert ourselves appropriately to get what we want. It must be tempered with strong Kidney Yin (Divine Love) and Earth (self-esteem).[12]

---

10. Giovanni Maciocia. *The Psyche in Chinese Medicine; Treatment of Emotional and Mental Disharmonies with Acupuncture and Chinese Herbs.* (Nanjing: Churchill Livingstone, 2009), 25-35.

11. Dr. Leon Hammer observes this occurs with habitual marijuana use.

12. Leon Hammer. *Dragon Rises Red Bird Flies; Psychology and Chinese Medicine.* (Barrytown: Station Hill Press, 1990), 153-165.

Wood Meditation

Doing this meditation will strength your connection with the Wood Element within yourself and your surroundings. It benefits the Liver and Gallbladder organ systems and fosters positive Wood personality traits such as courage and growth.

1. Sit in front of a tree. A big tree in the middle of an old forest is ideal, but a sapling or bonsai will do. You want to feel the energy of a type of tree that gets big because independent of its age or size, its self-concept is already a huge tree. This teaches us an important lesson about the Wood element; this plan of expansion and knowing its own greatness.
2. Close your eyes. Imagine your own roots going down deep into the Earth.
3. Imagine drawing up the cool water through these roots and through the channels of your body. Imagine your branches reaching up towards the Heavens, interacting with the sunlight or starlight, bringing it into you. Feel yourself as a tree. With patience, the tree may open up to you.

Things That Cut Down Wood

1. Criticism and biting comments.
2. Routine and excessive structure.

Activities to Increase Your Wood Element

1. Formulate a plan of action for one of your goals.
2. Challenge yourself in a sport or physical exercise.
3. Go on a hike with Wood people.
4. Take direct action.
5. Express your anger appropriately.

The Fire Phase

Physical Characteristics of Fire Predominance: Fire predominance shows as a heart or diamond-shaped face. Points on ear tips, eyebrows, nose, and other facial features are also indicators. Fire has long legs in relation to their torsos. The hair tends to be red or unruly. The fingers have pointed tips. The energy of the body is focused in the heart area.

Gifts and Challenges of Fire Predominance

The nature of Fire is to radiate outwards in all directions. Healthy Fire is witty, joyous, entertaining, loving, and artistic. Fire is open-hearted and this comes with great vulnerability. Intimacy, creative intuition, and empathy are all attributes of Fire. Fire needs romance and to feel loved. Out of control giggling, playful flirting, and spontaneity are all expressions of Fire. Fire likes to be vibrant and bright. It wants to entertain and lift the spirits of others. Fire will retreat when sad or if its heart is wounded. Fire predominant people "love" their friends, their car, their house, etc. Love is Fire's primary value; its virtue and addiction.

Fire craves attention and novelty and this leads to a darker aspect. Fire gone bad has issues with intimacy. It becomes obsessed with excitement, gets over-stimulated, and develops many superficial connections. It grows scattered, erratic, and manic. Fire will misuse its charisma. Sex and love addiction and drug abuse (particularly ecstasy and cocaine) can occur. Fire is attracted to bright shiny things and people, which can lead to trouble. Fire also takes EVERYTHING personally. Fire can become self-centered and cruel.

Fire Organs and Their Roles

Each element has a Yin organ and Yang organ pair. Fire is unique in that it has two pairs. Yin organs are full and hold vital essences, while Yang organs are empty.

Aligning with Inspiration

The process of downloading artistic inspiration is similar to, or perhaps the same as, channeling and receiving spiritual insights. People who depend on inspiration to make a living such as artists and writers often feel frustrated when inspiration and the ability to record in a way people can understand don't match up. Every creative person has experienced periods when the inspiration simply would not flow. This can be punctuated by times when the inspiration comes out of nowhere, but it is too much, too fast so that your logical mind cannot keep up. The nature of inspiration is that the ego and its time lines cannot control it. Though we cannot control it, we can learn to align ourselves with it in such a way that the process becomes effortless and joyous.

First connect your Heart Yin and Yang with your Source of inspiration:

1. Stop and still yourself.
2. Focus on the higher message of your project. See the Divine Spirit behind this project. Feel how Divine Spirit loves and supports you in finishing this project. She has chosen you to work through. Connect with Her with your heart. Allow yourself to feel the inspiration without worry about how it will get done. Feel how this relaxes you and raises your vibration.
3. The more you can stay in this state, the easier the creative process. As you relax, Divine Spirit works through you at a pace you can work with.
4. Now feel the world around you supporting your project. People and experiences will be drawn to you to move the project along in Divine right timing.

If you remember that creativity is an act of surrender and trust, it will always flow through you. If you are in a place of self-loathing and frustration, inspiration will come through in a frustrating manner. You need to get out of your own way and allow the higher part of you flow through you.

Heart (Yin organ) – The Heart is the Emperor of the body. This is where the Shen[13] of the body resides. It is the seat of consciousness and awareness and is responsible for circulating the Blood in the vessels. The Blood houses the Mind.

Small Intestine (Yang organ) – The Small Intestine separates the clear from the turbid. It is responsible for clarity and sound judgment.

Pericardium (Yin organ) – Also known as the "heart protector," its main function. The Pericardium is responsible for appropriateness.

San Jiao or "Triple warmer" (Yang organ) – The San Jiao relates to the movement between the upper, middle, and lower zones of the trunk. It is responsible for metabolism.

Health of Fire

When you find yourself exhibiting Fire traits, it is a direct reflection on the strength and weakness of your Fire organ system. Positive traits indicate a healthy Heart, Pericardium, and Small Intestine systems. Negative traits indicate an imbalance in these organ systems.

There may be physical heart abnormalities, palpitations, or in extreme cases, heart attack. Emotions deeply affect the health of the Fire Element. Fire predominant types seem capable of dying of heartbreak or deep rejection. Anxiety, insomnia, and mental problems are common Fire imbalance symptoms. These can escalate to agitation, frenzy, and personality disorders.

Spiritual & Psychological Aspect of Fire

The spirit of the Heart is the Shen. Shen has three meanings and is often translated as "spirit" or "mind." Shen, as "mind," refers to mental functioning, such as memory, consciousness, and integration of information taken in by the senses.

Shen as "spirit" refers to the small spirit of the Heart that expands outward to connect with the outside world. The Shen in the Heart is responsible for resonance. Resonance is a process whereby we attune our frequency with the frequency of another living thing. At this level of connection we can truly empathize; literally feeling what another feels. Great healing and wisdom can occur with this level of connection when used in clinical practice or for communion with plant spirits. Resonance allows us to connect on a deeper level with friends, family, and lovers. (For more, please see "Entering Into Resonance" on page 151).

Shen as "Spirit" is an umbrella for the spirits of the other four organ systems. All emotions and spiritual issues relating to the other organs filter through the big spirit, or Shen, of the Heart. For this reason, mental and emotional problems are referred to as Shen Disturbance, and involve a disorder of the Heart system. The spirits of the Spleen (Yi-Intellect) and Kidney (Zhi-Willpower) function in

13. Includes the overarching spirit and mental functioning. The word for heart, "xin", in Chinese means both heart and mind.

Fire Meditation

Doing this meditation will strength your connection with the Fire Element within yourself and your surroundings. It benefits the Heart, Pericardium, Small Intestine, and San Jiao organ systems and fosters positive Fire personality traits such as love and spontaneity.

1. Build a fire. To do this, form a triangular, tepee-like shape with logs or thick branches and place the kindling (leaves, pine cones, twigs) underneath. This will keep you from getting a face-full of smoke and accentuate the shape of Fire. Then light it.
2. Sit before it. Notice its bright colors: blues, reds, oranges. Feel its warmth. Notice how it radiates out and how it does all of this for you. Connect to the fire within your heart. Feel gratitude for it: for keeping us warm, for cooking our food, and for bringing us together to laugh and tell stories.

a fully integrated manner with the Shen. The spirits of the Lung (Po) and Liver (Hun) represent Yin and Yang aspects of the soul, respectively, and work with the Shen in an independent fashion.[14]

Psychologically, Heart Yin relates to Divine Inspiration and Divine Creative Love. This is connected to Kidney Yin, which is Divine Love. Through the Heart Yin, Divine Love is allowed consciousness and expression. In Heart Yin deficiency patterns, there is a lack of warmth, spontaneity, and inspiration. In Heart Yin excess, which exists solely as a psychological pattern, there are too many ideas for the body to handle leading to agitation and restlessness.

Heart Yang is the organizing principle necessary to execute an inspired idea into being; what Dr. Hammer refers to as Divine Intelligence. In Heart Yang deficiency there is not enough Qi to execute to completion the inspiration that comes through. There will also be an inability to express the love and feelings experienced. In Heart Yang excess, which exists solely as a psychological pattern, there is an excessive drive to express, with or without substance.[15]

Things that Extinguish Fire

1. Heartbreak, betrayal, abuse, and isolation.
2. The Fire Element can irritate certain people. Being around these people will extinguish our own Fire. Note: sometimes the Fire Element does need to be reined in.

Activities to Increase Fire

1. Connect with people/animals/ nature with your heart and with humor. (Improv groups and comedy clubs are especially helpful).

14. Giovanni Maciocia. *The Psyche in Chinese Medicine; Treatment of Emotional and Mental Disharmonies with Acupuncture and Chinese Herbs*. (Nanjing: Churchill Livingstone, 2009), 15-22.

15. Leon Hammer. *Dragon Rises Red Bird Flies; Psychology and Chinese Medicine*. (Barrytown: Station Hill Press, 1990), 174-176.

2. Listen and speak from your heart.
3. Give unconditionally.
4. Immerse yourself in love poems or a romantic comedy.
5. Do something silly and spontaneous with a Fire person.
6. Burn lots of candles.

The Earth Phase

Physical Characteristics of Earth Predominance: The face is round (features may be bunched close together) or there is a double chin. The body is fleshy even when thin, with a propensity towards obesity. The legs are short and the torso long. The body's energy is very grounded, as if it would be difficult to unbalance them. The fingers are short with large palms.

Gifts and Challenges of Earth Predominance

The original 5 Element pictures placed the Earth Element in the center surrounded by the other four Elements. Though the Earth Element is now shown in the outer circle, it remains the link between all the Phases. It is the glue that holds everything together. There can be no communities, families, or long-term relationships without the steady nurturing of the Earth Phase. The archetype of Motherhood and the developmental stage of bonding are part of this Element, independent of gender. Mother wounds cause imbalances in this Phase in the body. At its best, Earth is solid and loyal. It nurtures and builds. Harmony is a high value. Earth's need to be liked makes it very accommodating. There is warmth and softness to Earth-types in their voice, affect, and body, even when they are thin. Earth needs loyalty, routine, security, and predictability. Earth is very practical and has a common-sense approach. Earth loves its physical comforts and takes care to maintain financial security.

When it goes bad, Earth frets and worries. Trust, boundaries, and self-worth are issues for Earth. This is why Earth needs predictability and hates change. It needs to be involved and needed. Earth likes to be in charge but is often not confident enough to be in the limelight. Clinginess can become an issue. It tends towards unrealistic expectations leading to subsequent disappointments. Earth is the master of guilt trips. Earth can bring new meaning to the word stubborn. When it digs in its heels, it is literally immovable. Earth can also be quite the hedonist, particularly when it comes to good food and wine.

Earth Organs and Their Roles

Spleen (Yin organ) – The Spleen is the Official of the Granary (food reserves). The Spleen is a key organ in TCM, unlike the secondary status it holds in Western allopathic medicine. It oversees the entire digestive process, and the transformation and transportation of all food that is consumed. It is about much more than digestion. The healthy Spleen keeps the muscles strong, the skin tight, and the breasts and face lifted. It keeps the Blood in the vessels. It is the basis of the body's immunity. Spiritually, the Spleen takes in and processes energy on a spiritual level. It is in charge of digesting the experiences of everyday life.

Stomach (Yang organ) – The Stomach begins the rotting and ripening process of digestion.

Health of Earth

When you find yourself exhibiting Earth traits, it is a direct reflection on the strength and weakness of your Earth organ system. Positive traits indicate a healthy Spleen and Stomach system. Negative traits indicate an imbalance in these organ systems.

Digestive problems are often the first sign of Earth imbalance: nausea, excessive hunger, poor absorption, Irritable Bowel Disease, colitis, etc. Excess weight is often an issue. This may result from food addiction because they do not feel nurtured. It is common for unbalanced Earth to lead people

Earth Meditation

Doing this meditation will strength your connection with the Earth Element within yourself and your surroundings. It benefits the Spleen and Stomach organ systems and fosters positive Earth personality traits such as groundedness and connection.

1. Take your shoes off and stand on bare earth. Wiggle your toes in it.
2. Widen your stance to more than hip width apart, tuck your tailbone under, and slightly bend your knees. You want to feel your quadriceps muscles activate and your buttocks and hamstrings relax. Bring your arms to a little below shoulder height and hold a ball of energy. Make minor adjustments until you find the point you can relax into it.
3. Feel the energy coming up from the center of the Earth, through your feet and up your body. If you can, touch the tip of your tongue to the roof of your mouth and slightly tense your PC muscles.(For an explanation of the PC muscles see page 143).
4. You will want to stand here for at least 20 min. (I recommend using a timer.) This will give you time to work through the natural desire to flee. Standing in this posture will make you feel grounded and earth-bound, which will be very uncomfortable to those who are not grounded. The more grounded you are, the higher you can go without losing touch with reality.

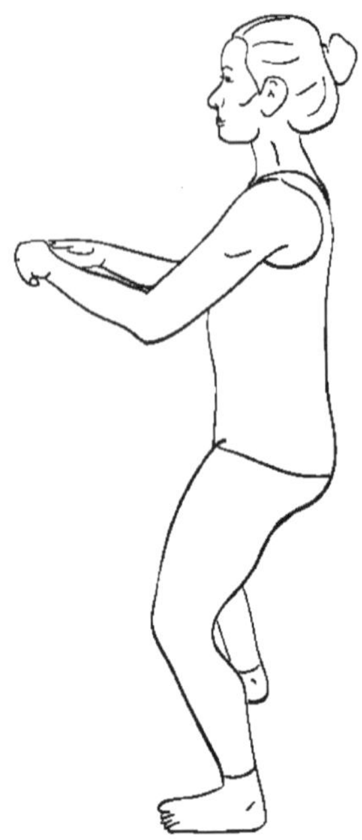

Figure 0.4

into situations beyond their capacity, resulting in Chronic Fatigue. Autoimmune disease, organ prolapse, low energy, cold limbs, and hypothyroidism are other common maladies. People with a predominance of Earth will take care of others excessively in the ways they secretly hope to be taken care of. They can be long suffering and silent about their needs. Alternately, they may complain and then absolutely refuse care.

Spiritual & Psychological Aspect of Earth

The Spirit of Spleen is the Yi or "intellect". The Yi relates to the functioning of the mind involving studying, focus, intention, and memorization of information. This is why tonifying the Spleen and clearing Phlegm-Damp increases cognitive functioning. The Yi functions under the direction of the Shen (Spirit and Mind).

Psychologically, Spleen energy relates to the ability to handle everyday life in a calm, practical, and easy manner. Trust and self-worth develop through initial bonding with the mother. Issues with maternal bonding or physical Spleen deficiencies create dysfunction in bonding, boundaries, and trust. People who are weak in Earth develop a need to be liked and obsessive worry.[16]

Things That Deplete Earth

1. Eating food you do not enjoy; dieting.
2. Inconsistency, unpredictability, extreme change, or not having a home.
3. Lack of fulfilling, nurturing, long-term relationships. Abuse.

Activities to Increase Your Earth

1. Grow your own food.
2. Nurture others, i.e. tend to a sick friend, take care of children and pets.
3. Engage in baking, volunteering, or gardening (get your hands in the dirt) with Earth people.
4. Be reliable and consistent. Be aware of how you feel.

The Metal Phase

Physical Characteristics of Metal Predominance: The face has points or bony protuberances, such as high cheekbones and highly arched brows. The skin has a distinctive sheen to it. The skin and body look delicate. The body is thin, especially around the chest. The chest is often concave (indicating childhood lung issues). The fingers are long and thin.

16. Leon Hammer. *Dragon Rises Red Bird Flies; Psychology and Chinese Medicine*, 225-227.

Gifts and Challenges of Metal Predominance

Metal is the element of "hidden treasure" and the most Yin of the elements. You may be around a Metal predominant person for a while before they let you in. The archetype of Father, external authority, and rites of passage are present in this element and father issues tend to show as Metal imbalance in the body. Metal tends to be aloof, elegant, and also hyper aware of boundaries; both others' and its own need for respectful space. Metal concerns itself with what is proper, fair, and right. It creates containers of respect and fairness in the world around it. Metal is very sensitive to its environment: physically, emotionally, aesthetically, and energetically. It notices every detail. This can make Metal types master craftsman, designers, artists, and organizers. Refinement, artistry, intellectualism, beauty, and perfection are highly valued. There are rules that must be obeyed and lines that should not be crossed. Japanese, Korean, French, and German cultures are highly Metal in their own ways. There is both a reverence for the past and a passion for the newest technology.

Metal gone bad has a distinct cutting quality. Metal hurts and is hurt with words. Biting comments, aloofness, and cold calculating maneuvers are all Metal weapons. Metal holds itself and others to the highest standards and it will cut others off when they do not live up to these ideals. Metal can cut itself off from the rest of the world with thick energetic walls or a formal, unnatural affect. Metal's sensitivity to its environment can make it paranoid about being contaminated by it; unable to keep out the lower element. They can also be quite cruel should they decide to use their sensitivity to do harm to others. Metal needs to keep up appearances. Their facade of purity and propriety can mask dark shadow aspects that are "dirty" related to hidden addictions, sexual deviousness, and cruelty.

Metal Organs and Their Roles

Lung (Yin organ) – The Lung is the Prime Minister to the Emperor (Heart). The pure, white canopy of the Lungs protects the Heart. The Lung assists in the creation of Zong (Post-Heaven) Qi and descends and disperses this Qi throughout the body. It is the first line of defense against pathogenic invasion and is associated with the Wei (Protective) Qi.

Large Intestine (Yang organ) – The Large Intestine is where the body salvages what is useful and discards what is not. It is also where the body holds onto things that need to be let go of. The Large Intestine is easily affected by grief and worry.

Health of Metal

When you find yourself exhibiting Metal traits, it is a direct reflection on the strength and weakness of your Metal organ systems. Positive traits indicate a healthy Lung and Large Intestine system. Negative traits indicate an imbalance in these organ systems.

Lung issues such as asthma, chronic cough, sinus congestion, shallow breathing, and chronic infections are typical examples of Metal imbalance. Stiff joints and muscles, sensitivity to climate, skin conditions, and dry skin and hair can also occur. Those with a Metal predominance have a delicate constitution, often beginning with lung issues in childhood. Due to this tendency, Metal types can develop endless rules and rituals around health.

Spiritual & Psychological Aspect of Metal

The spirit of the Lungs is the Po or "Corporeal Soul." The Po is the aspect of the soul tied to the physical senses and disintegrates with the body at death, going back to the Earth. It enters the body on the third day after conception and orchestrates the building of the material body using the Jing (Essence) of the parents.

The Po is the Yin aspect of the soul, while the Hun (spirit of the Liver) is the Yang aspect. The Po guides the movement and functioning of the Essence in the body. The Po is affected by unconscious feelings, particularly grief. Weeping or other emotional expression is important to release these emotions, and their constriction of the Po. The skin relates to the Po and it is through the Po that physical pain is felt. The Po connects to animal instinct and intuition felt physically in the body, such as the hair standing up on the back of the neck upon sensing danger. The Po is responsible for breathing. Thus, breathing techniques and meditation directly affect and still the Po, which then

Metal Meditation

Doing this meditation will strength your connection with the Metal Element within yourself and your surroundings. It benefits the Lung and Large Intestine organ systems and fosters positive Metal personality traits such as integrity and purity.

1. Set up your meditation space meticulously and beautifully; shut out all distractions. Sit on something with nice fabric. Place a freshly cut flower and a glass of water near you. Finally, set before you a beautiful crystal.
2. Close your eyes and begin to breathe deeply. Back is straight, hands gracefully on your lap. Begin to focus on your Lungs.
3. Breathe energy into your Lungs. Imagine a circle of angelic white Light surrounding you. Feel its exact boundary. Its slight coolness. Feel it containing you.
4. Now open your eyes and look at the crystal. Mentally ask permission to connect.Then do so with the greatest reverence and respect. This means that your energy and gaze gently meet the crystal rather than overwhelm it. (Sitting in reverence and consuming with your gaze are very different activities.)
5. Notice every detail. Notice how perfect every striation is. Notice things that were at first hidden.
6. Now imagine a gentle connection of Light between the white light around you and the crystal. Sit here for a moment. Allow the beauty and purity to overwhelm you.
7. Thank the crystal. Then gently let go of the connection.

calms the mind, leaving the Hun free to connect with the Divine. Po also constricts, separates, and gives us individuality.[17]

Psychologically, the Yin of the Metal Element relates to the energetic threads or cords that connect people to each other (as well as to animals, places, concepts, etc.). When these cords are cut, it creates feelings of grief. Yin Metal deficiency relates to an inability to create the threads of attachment necessary to form relationships. Yin Metal excess creates a domineering and possessive personality that attaches its cords too strongly.

The Yang of Metal relates to letting go and moving on. It relates to the elation of adventure and newfound freedom. In Yang Metal deficiency there is insufficient energy to let go and move on to the next stage in a timely fashion. There is clinging to old relationships, patterns, and ideas that no longer serve. Yang Metal excess produces a drifter who floats constantly (from person to person, idea to idea), effortlessly letting go of deep bonds it has just made, often leaving pain in its wake. This is distinct from a driving sense of conquest or novelty, but rather originates from an overactive action of cutting ties.[18]

Things That Melt Metal

1. Disorder, dirt, and clutter.
2. Rough, rude behavior and shoddy workmanship.

Activities to Increase Your Metal

1. Practice restraint.
2. Act with integrity.
3. Take up an artistic project. Be detail-oriented in its completion.
4. Work on a project with Metal people.
5. Avoid crowds.

The Water Phase

Physical Characteristics of Water Predominance: Water naturally takes on the form of its surroundings making it the most difficult Element to pinpoint. Its identification is often when all other Elements have been eliminated. The Water face does not have a specific, identifiable shape. The body is voluptuous, fleshy, or curvaceous. Energy floats and undulates in the middle of the body, particularly the lower abdomen. The hands are square with flat fingernails.

---

17. Giovanni Maciocia. *The Psyche in Chinese Medicine; Treatment of Emotional and Mental Disharmonies with Acupuncture and Chinese Herbs*. (Nanjing: Churchill Livingstone, 2009), 47-59.

18. Leon Hammer. *Dragon Rises Red Bird Flies; Psychology and Chinese Medicine*. (Barrytown: Station Hill Press, 1990), 261-279.

Gifts and Challenges of Water

Water can float into any situation remaining self-contained and self-sufficient. It is all depth with no fixed form, maintaining its integrity in any container. Often misread by others, it is easy to see in Water a mirror reflection of ourselves. It likes to remain hidden. Water relates to mystery, spirituality, and sensuality. There is a languid, sensual, spiritual nature to its people. Unlike Metal, Water welcomes us in with its large, dreamy, hypnotic eyes and yet remains an utter enigma. Water loves to explore and is determined in its goals. Yet, unlike Wood, who makes a beeline and ruffles a few feathers on the way, Water meanders and gets around things effortlessly.[19] Water's ultimate goal is Truth. It is clever and introspective. Water gets lost in a world of ideas (consider Albert Einstein), in communion with nature, or in the timelessness of making love. Water seems to live in a state of perpetuity; it ages slowly, and has no sense of time. In fact, Water is never on time. This can give Water the reputation of being lazy or not caring. It also has no concept of a straight line or rigidity.

Water gone bad has escaped into an altered state of reality. It is critical of others while oblivious to its own faults. When crossed, it can be tactless and unforgiving. Water can become quite delusional, inflating its seductive abilities and imagining a long list of admirers. It dresses inappropriately for its shape. Water can be the height of divadom and drama. Water is prone to excessive emotionality, phobias, and paranoia. Where Wood is a narcissist, Water is a histrionic. Fear is an issue with Water, especially concerning bodies of water. When it overcomes its struggles with fears, Water can become the opposite extreme: a reckless daredevil. Water's self-sufficient nature can turn to isolation, emotional inaccessibility, and loneliness.

Water Organs and Their Roles

Kidney (Yin organ) – The Kidney is the Sage secluded in the mountains. It is where the Jing (Essence) is stored as well as the seat of willpower. The Kidney relates to hormonal functioning, the condition of the brain, and governs the rate of aging.

Urinary Bladder (Yang organ) – The Urinary Bladder stores the urine.

Health of Water

When you find yourself exhibiting Water personality traits, it is a direct reflection on the strength and weakness of your Water organ system. Positive traits indicate a healthy Kidney and Urinary Bladder system. Negative traits indicate an imbalance in these organ systems.

Diseases of the urinary and reproductive organs often indicate a Water imbalance, such as: chronic urinary tract infections, impotence or frigidity, infertility, and fibroids. Edema, low back and knee issues, and teeth weakness are also concerns. In terms of health, Water can be a bit of a hypochondriac, and very dramatic in descriptions of how it is feeling.

19. I often think about Southern women as a good example of this.

Spiritual & Psychological Aspect of Water

The spirit of the Water Phase is the Zhi. The Zhi is usually translated as "Willpower." I also like to translate it as "Soul Purpose" as it does not refer to the ego's will, but rather the deepest will of one's being. The Zhi is our determination to fulfill our soul's purpose in this lifetime. To hear and know our soul's purpose requires "getting still enough to hear your bones" as one of my teachers would say. The Zhi is the marriage of the spiritual Kidney Yin and Yang energies.

The Zhi also concerns the long-term storage of memory. Memory loss with age is associated with decline in Kidney energy, and thus Zhi. Both the willpower and memory of the Zhi act in concert with the Shen. The consciousness of the Shen directs the power and drive of the Zhi.[20]

Psychologically, Kidney Qi is the Divine Spirit. Kidney Qi deficiency produces lack of faith. Kidney Qi excess creates rigid fanaticism for a cause or religion. Kidney Yin is the connection with Divine Love. It governs our ability to forgive and is associated with grace. It anchors the wayward ego (Liver Yang). The over-stimulation of modern life depletes Kidney Yin. Kidney Yin is rejuvenated by rest and contemplation. Kidney Yin deficiency relates to a brutal competitor who lives by the kill-or-be-killed philosophy. In Kidney Yin excess there is excessive pride in the superiority of the brain.

Kidney Yang is Divine Will and Divine Power. Kidney Yang provides the determination, single-mindedness, and motivation to pursue a goal. It acts and follows through to completion against all odds. In a spiritual sense this translates to the drive to connect to reality beyond the five senses and to transcend the obvious. It relates to intuitive wisdom. In Kidney Yang deficiency there is a lack of power to act, leading to laziness and procrastination. With Kidney Yang excess there is too much will and drive leading to excessive risk-taking. This produces burnout if Yin is deficient, or tyranny if there is sufficient Yin (and other people) to sustain it. This creates the "Power of God without the Love" and such individuals are charismatic, if destructive, leaders.[21]

When Divine Will and Divine Love are joined we arrive at our Soul's Purpose. True Power is found through this union with God. The Kidneys relate to inner Truth. Fear of the unknown, also associated with the Kidneys, blocks this progress.

Things That Muddy Water

1. Too much mundane responsibility.
2. Constant work and activity.

Activities to Increase Your Water

1. Spend a quiet, relaxing afternoon alone daydreaming.
2. Meditate without a goal.

---

20. Giovanni Maciocia. *The Psyche in Chinese Medicine; Treatment of Emotional and Mental Disharmonies with Acupuncture and Chinese Herbs*. (Nanjing: Churchill Livingstone, 2009), 67-69.

21. Leon Hammer. *Dragon Rises Red Bird Flies; Psychology and Chinese Medicine*, 103-145.

3. Spend time wandering near a quiet body of water.
4. Wear sensual clothes.
5. Spend time with a Water person.

Water Meditation

Doing this meditation will strength your connection with the Water Element within yourself and your surroundings. It benefits the Kidney and Urinary Bladder organ systems and fosters positive Water personality traits such as wisdom and spirituality.

There is something about being in or around water that merges the spirit world with our world. When the air is heavy with water, it acts as a physical medium for ideas and spirits to manifest. You will notice where there is higher humidity that the spirit world is closer to our world and creativity abounds.

1. Decide you want to sit in a pool, lake, or bath. It must be a calm body of water; preferably one where you can see the bottom. You want to feel safe and peaceful so you don't get distracted.
2. Slowly get in, feeling the silkiness of the water; its coolness. Let yourself merge with her and get lost in one thought after another. When your wandering thoughts find their way back to the present, you are done.

Major TCM Concepts

To make a diagnosis in Traditional Chinese Medicine, acupuncturists look at the tongue, feel the pulse in depth, look for signs of imbalance on the skin, hair, and nails, feel into the energy and affect of the patient, perform palpation, and listen at length to the patient's history and symptoms. All of this information is assimilated and used to categorize the patient's condition according to disease patterns. The process can be complicated and takes time for each acupuncturist to develop his/her style. The best way to start learning is to begin seeing these patterns in yourself and those around you. Here, I simplify the most important terms, concepts, and disease patterns in TCM. First we will cover the basics of our internal environment, followed by external influences.

Pre-Heaven Essence, Post-Heaven Essence, and Jing

Jing, like Qi, is a fundamental concept for which there is no direct translation in Western languages. Read the description below and do not get frustrated if it does not make sense immediately. Mastering its meaning will deepen over time. Many of our imbalances occur precisely because we do not understand our Jing and the purpose of this book is to explain it in a way that makes sense and can be applied in how you live your life.

Pre-Heaven Essence:
We are all born with a certain amount of Pre-Heaven Essence we inherit from the sexual energies of our parents. The health of our Pre-Heaven Essence is dependent upon their genetics, their health, and the conditions during our conception and gestation. Our Pre-Heaven Essence determines our constitution and uniqueness. There is debate about whether or not we can increase our Pre-Heaven Essence through self-cultivation and Inner Alchemy practice (see "Sex and Self-Cultivation" on page 134). It is clear, however, that we can conserve what we were given by practicing moderation, good nutrition, and breathing and meditation techniques. We can also squander our Jing by living out of sync with natural laws. This is why optimizing the general health of the parents is so important in fertility cases. It is at the stage of the parents that the constitution of the child is formed.

Post-Heaven Essence:
We amass Post-Heaven Essence, as the name implies, after we are born, from the food, drink, and air we take in from our environment. It is directly associated with Spleen, Stomach, and Lung functioning.

Jing (Essence):
Our Jing is the product of both our Pre- and Post-Heaven Essence. It is stored in the Kidneys but also circulates throughout the body. It is influenced by diet, lifestyle, and herbs. It relates to our constitution, which is possible, yet difficult to alter. Kidney Jing guides our maturation, development,

and reproduction. It is the slow, fluid movement of the Kidney Jing that is described in the 7-year Cycles women experience.[22]

Qi, Blood, and Body Fluids

Qi:
Qi is often translated as "vital energy." It is non-substantial. Qi shows itself in the functioning of the body. We can feel Qi and might be able to see it, but it does not have form. It is what enlivens the body; like electricity that lights up a house. Qi has six functions within the body: transforming, transporting, holding, raising, protecting, and warming. When describing the Qi of an organ we are referring to the function of the organ. For example, Spleen Qi deficiency is the lack of energy available to transport and transform food.

Blood:
Blood is the physical manifestation of Qi and is inseparable from it. Qi gives life to the Blood, while Blood gives Qi physical form. Blood is nourishing and moistening. The health of the Spleen, and a lesser extent Kidneys, Lungs, and Heart, are crucial for Blood production. Blood is ruled by the Heart and stored in the Liver.

Body Fluids:
Body fluids are derived from food and drink. The Spleen separates the pure fluids and sends them to the Lungs and Kidneys, sending the impure fluids to the Small Intestines.

Causes of Disease

There are six external causes of disease, called the **6 External Evils**, that can invade us from our environment. These are Wind, Cold, Fire, Summer-Heat, Damp, and Dryness. Their symptoms are described in the Table 0.3 on page 32.

There are seven internal causes of disease, called the **7 Emotions**, that are generated by our internal reaction to our environment. These are anger (ascends the Qi), joy (relaxes the Qi), worry and pensiveness (knots the Qi), grief (dissolves the Qi), fear (descends the Qi), and shock (scatters the Qi). The organ systems they affect were discussed in the section on 5 Elements.

Additional causes of disease are: constitution, over exertion, excessive sexual activity, improper diet, traumatic injury, parasites and poisons, and wrong treatment.

22. Men have cycles of 8 years.

8 Principle Differentiation

8 Principle Differentiation is a quick way to assess a condition that can be used by both practitioners and laypeople. You simply divide the condition into four major categories:

Is the condition Exterior or Interior in origin?
Disease can either originate as an invading pathogen from the outside or from an internal imbalance.(23) The primary indicator of an exterior pattern is an aversion or oversensitivity to Wind (drafts, windy weather, or air conditioning). Wind conditions are characterized by rapid movement. They begin suddenly, quickly change symptoms and location, and (hopefully) leave quickly. There may be fever, clamminess, stiff neck, and nose and sinus symptoms. In exterior conditions the pathogen needs to be escorted out the way it came i.e. through diaphoresis (sweating).

Is the condition Hot or Cold?
Hot conditions are characterized by redness, restlessness, constipation, dryness (heat consumes fluids), dark urine, and fever. Hot conditions are alleviated by cold. Pain that is alleviated with an ice pack, preference for cold drinks or cold weather, and sensitivity to heat are key indicators.

Cold conditions are characterized by pallor, malaise, loose stools, water retention, clear urine, and lack of thirst. Cold conditions are alleviated by heat. Pain that is alleviated by heat, preference for hot drinks or hot weather, and sensitivity to cold are key indicators.

Is the condition Excess or Deficient?
Excess symptoms include agitation, sturdiness, coarse breathing, distention or fullness in the chest and abdomen, pain worse with pressure, constipation, and dark urine. Excess conditions are treated by dispersing, clearing, and reducing modalities.

Deficiency symptoms include emaciation, listlessness, pallor, dislike of speaking, shortness of breath, palpitations, poor memory, spontaneous sweating, night sweats, nocturnal emission, nocturia (night urination), and pain alleviated by pressure. Deficient conditions are treated with tonifying and building modalities.

Is the condition Yin or Yang?
Yang conditions are Exterior, Hot, and Excess. Yin conditions are Interior, Cold, and Deficient.

Basic Patterns in TCM

Traditional Chinese Medicine is unique in that it classifies all pathologies in the body according to disease patterns. The following charts give the basic disease patterns. TCM further classifies disease according to the organs and channels affected, 5 Element theory, the 6 Stages of Shang Han Lun, the 4 Levels of Wen Bing, and the 3 Burners.

---

23. This can be complicated as imbalances in the internal environment makes us susceptible to certain pathogens.

Table 0.2. Interior Disease Patterns

Interior Disease Patterns	Typical Symptoms	Causes (Etiology)
Qi Deficiency (Spleen, Lung, Kidney, Heart, or local)	Abdominal distention. Poor appetite. Cravings for sweets. Borborygmus (gurgling in abdomen). Poor muscle tone. Fatigue. Low immunity. Spontaneous sweating. Weakness in the extremities. Pale menstrual blood and short cycles.	Can be constitutional, poor eating and sleeping habits, overwork, and stress.
(Liver) Qi Stagnation	Tension. Irritability. Depression. PMS. Irregular periods. Breast tenderness. Mood swings. Alternating constipation/diarrhea. Frequent sighing. Feeling trapped or bored.	Most often caused by emotional stress. Locally can occur due to trauma. Can also be due to Qi Deficiency.
Blood Deficiency (Heart, Liver)	Pallor. Fatigue. Emotionally and physically sensitive/vulnerable. Palpitations. Insomnia. Blurred vision. Pale and light menstrual bleeding with long cycles. Dry skin. Fear going to bed at night. Timidity/ lack of courage. Feeling of dissatisfaction. Craving for sweets and nurturing.	Can be caused by constitution, blood loss, Spleen Qi (digestive) deficiency, excessive caretaking, or emotional trauma. Liver Blood Deficiency is more relevant in gynecology.
Blood Stagnation	Stabbing, intense, fixed pain. Anything purple, visible dark veins, or blood clots indicates Blood Stagnation. Severe depression or insomnia years after physical or emotional trauma.	Common pattern after physical and/or emotional trauma. Long-term Qi Stagnation or Cold Invasion are common causes.
Yin Deficiency (with interior Heat) (Heart, Lung, Stomach, Kidney)	Blood Deficiency symptoms plus: Dryness (dry cough, throat, skin, vagina). Dizziness. Constipation. Poor memory. Heat worse at night. Night sweats, Thirst. Flushed cheeks. Dark urine. 5 Hearts Heat (in the palms, feet, and head). Insomnia. Tinnitus. Memory loss. Excess libido. Low back soreness. Ache in the bones. Bright red menstrual blood.	Can be constitutional, Heat or Fluid damage, chronic illness, excessive sexual activity, mental overwork, prolonged emotional distress, emotional trauma, or older age. Can relate to deficiency in estrogen.
Yang Deficiency (with interior Cold) (Heart, Spleen, or Kidney)	Qi Deficiency symptoms plus: Low back and knee weakness, soreness, and/or cold. Loose stools early in the morning (cock's crow diarrhea). Cold that isn't alleviated by covering up. Edema in lower body. Copious urination. Urinary or fecal incontinence. Nocturia (night urination).	Can be constitutional, after longstanding Qi Deficiency, Cold damage, physical overwork (includes excessive exercise), exhaustion. Can relate to deficiency in testosterone and/or progesterone.
Jing Deficiency	Both Yin and Yang of the Kidneys is deficient. Weak teeth. Softening of bones. Low back soreness. Hair loss. The natural decline of Jing with age signals the beginning of menopause. In younger people can present as developmental abnormalities, infertility, or constitutional weaknesses.	Aging. Constitution. Overwork. Excessive drug use, particularly methamphetamines, cause Jing deficiency.

Interior Disease Patterns	Typical Symptoms	Causes (Etiology)
Excess Heat or Fire (Internal) (Liver, Stomach)	Anger. Irritability. Red eyes. Headaches. Bitter taste in mouth. Excess hunger. Stomach ulcers. Restless sleep. Feels hot. Bad smell.	Constitution, emotional disturbance, long-term stress, heating diet, hot climate.
Deficiency Heat (Internal)	Associated with Yin deficiency.	
Cold (Internal) in the Uterus	Menstrual cramps can be severe. Menstrual clots. Pain alleviated with applications of heat. White vaginal discharge. Infertility.	Caused be Yang deficiency or external cold invasion (swimming, air conditioning/ wind exposure, cold food and drink during menstruation).
Deficiency Cold (Internal)	Associated with Yang deficiency.	
Food Stagnation	Belching. Bad breath. Abdominal bloating. No appetite. Foul smelling stools. Can cause insomnia.	Caused by inappropriate foods and/or weak digestion.
Phlegm-Dampness (Lungs, Spleen, Heart)	Brain fog. Fatigue. Soreness in joints. Edema, particularly in extremities. Heaviness. White vaginal discharge. Turbid urination. Frequent, urgent urination. Mental confusion.	Caused by Spleen Qi deficiency, and sometimes Kidney deficiency.
Damp-Heat (Liver,Gallbladder Urinary Bladder, Large Intestine, Lower Jiao)	Inability to digest fats. Abdominal bloating. Yellow vaginal discharge. Anger. Resentment. Indecisiveness. Thirst with inability to drink. Red, itchy, and weepy skin conditions.	Caused by long-standing Liver Qi Stagnation and Spleen Qi deficiency. Longstanding Phlegm-Damp. Consuming excess rich foods.
Phlegm-Heat (Lungs, Heart)	Chest oppression. Yellow or green mucous discharge. Rash behavior. Bitter taste. Uncontrolled laughing or crying. Tendency to hit or scold people. Insomnia. Dream disturbed sleep.	Caused by longstanding Liver Qi Stagnation and Spleen Qi deficiency. Long-standing Phlegm-Damp. Consuming excess rich foods.
Liver (Internal) Wind	Headaches. Tremors. Vertigo. Seizures. Convulsions.	Caused by a combination of Heat and Blood or Yin deficiency.

Table 0.3. Exterior Disease Patterns

Exterior Causes of Disease	Symptoms – sudden onset	Causes
Wind Cold	Aversion to cold. Chills. Clear, copious mucous. Neck stiffness and pain.	Often relates to colds of viral origin.
Wind Heat	Aversion to drafts. Yellow mucous. Sore throat. Chills. Fever. Thirst.	Often relates to colds of bacterial and fungal origin.

Exterior Causes of Disease	Symptoms – sudden onset	Causes
Cold	Joint or channel pain. Contraction of tendons. Chilled sensation in the body. Pain alleviated with application of heat.	Cold weather or environment.
Fire	Delirium. Constipation. Fever. Intense thirst. More damaging to fluids and mental functioning than Heat.	Hot weather or environment.
Dampness	Heaviness. Sticky, cloudy discharges in the nose, urine, vagina, and bowels. Joint pain. Eczema. Oozing skin conditions.	Caused by damp climate, wearing wet clothes, or sitting on damp ground.
Dryness	Dryness in the body. Dry throat. Dry skin. Dry stools. Scanty urination.	Caused by very dry weather or dry internal heating.
Summer-Heat	Aversion to heat. Sweating. Thirst. Malaise. Headache. Dark urine.	Occurs in summertime.

Specific to Women

There are additional principles specific to women's health. Under the age of 20, treatment should focus on the Kidneys. Hormonal imbalances at this stage are related to a developmental deficiency. Between the ages of 20 and 50, treatment should focus on the Liver. Monthly bleeding, caretaking, and stress all exhaust Liver Blood. Liver Qi Stagnation is often the culprit in hormonal imbalance at this stage. After age 50, treatment focuses on the Spleen. Imbalances at this stage are most often associated with poor absorption of nutrients, weight gain, and other Spleen issues. Other disease patterns and organ systems may be implicated at any age as well.(24)

There are three "Golden Opportunities"(25) that each woman encounters to dramatically alter the state of her health. These are times when the constitution of the body can either be renewed or devastated:

1. First Golden Opportunity: proper care and regulation of menstruation.
2. Second Golden Opportunity: proper postpartum care.
3. Third Golden Opportunity: proper care during menopause.

24. Shaoting Jing, "TCM Gynecology" (lecture, Yo San University, Los Angeles, CA, May 22, 2003).
25. Shuqi Zhuang. *Postpartum Recovery Program; a Manual of Rules and Recipes for the Postpartum Woman.* (Taiwan: Guang He Chu Ban She, 2005). ISBN 9578807015

TCM Approach to Treatment

Integration of Body, Mind, & Spirit

Qi is the thread that ties all levels of existence together. Qi disperses becoming spirit. Qi condenses becoming matter. Through the Qi, spirit, emotion, intellect, and body affect each other. Injury and healing can come from each of these levels of our being. Acupuncturists access the Qi directly through acupuncture, moxibustion,[26] and medical qigong. Through herbal medicine, diet therapy, qigong exercises, cupping,[27] gua sha,[28] and massage, acupuncturists are able to build the health of the body on multiple levels.

This connection extends outside the body as well. The time of day, season, weather, planetary alignment, political and social forces all interact with our internal environment. In order for treatment to be effective it must take into consideration numerous internal and external factors. The core philosophy of TCM is to learn how to work with Nature. When we try to go against Nature, we always lose in the end.

The Pursuit of Peace

Chaotic or unbalanced emotions are a major cause of disease. The Daoist prescription for a long, happy life is to live simply and nurture peace within ourselves. We often become habituated (and addicted) to dramatic ups and downs. It takes practice for us to make peace our default setting. This does not mean we should not feel.

A healthy person feels all the emotions. We remain healthy as long as we allow them to pass through us. When we become stuck in a certain emotion, for example feeling angry most of the time, it creates disease. Acupuncture, herbs, qigong, and diet therapy can assist in easing difficult emotions out of the body more gracefully. Inner Alchemy practices, discussed in Chapter 3, allow us to transform deep-seated emotional patterns.

Herbal Medicine

Traditional Chinese Medicine began as the pursuit of immortality and optimal vitality. It was not the

---

26. Moxibustion is the practice of using the herb Ai Ye (mugwort) and burning it directly or indirectly on specific points and channels. The smoke, essential oils, and ash from Ai Ye (mugwort) have special properties to penetrate, warm, and move Qi and Blood in the channels.

27. Cupping is the practice of using local suction with cups to increase Qi and Blood flow, relax the muscles, and to release Heat and Toxins.

28. Gua Sha is a practice involving scraping the skin with a spoon, coin, or special gua sha tool to move Qi and Blood, relax the muscles, clear Heat, and release Wind (colds and fever).

treatment of disease. This is a critical distinction. In TCM, the skilled physician kept patients healthy. TCM is more than preventive medicine. It gives us tools to improve our health infinitely. Once a level of vitality is reached, there is always potential for a better state. And so goes the advancement of the medicine.

Diet and lifestyle are the foundation for increasing health. Most diseases can be averted by simply living in accordance with natural laws, such as eating warming foods when it is cold. Herbal medicine, acupuncture, and moxibustion are considered more invasive interventions reserved for conditions diet and lifestyle cannot treat. This is the opposite view of Western medicine.

In TCM herbology, side effects are not acceptable save for a few exceptions. Herbs were originally classified into three categories: superior, common, and inferior.[29] Superior herbs were associated with Heaven. They were non-toxic and were used long-term to promote health and longevity. Think of them as angels who only do good. Examples included Ling Zhi (reishi), Ren Shen (ginseng), and Wu Wei Zi (schizandra). Common herbs were associated with the Human realm. These were non-toxic or slightly toxic. Common herbs both tonified the body and expelled "evil Qi" from the body and were used for limited periods of time. Think of them as people who can do both good and harm. Examples included Dang Gui (Chinese angelica) and Ma Huang (ephedra). Inferior herbs were associated with Earth. They were strong and toxic (produced side effects) and were used short-term for specific purposes to expel disease.[30] Think of them as surly characters you bring in to do the dirty work but do not want hanging around. Examples include Da Huang (rhubarb).

TCM views Western allopathic medicine[31] as being like an inferior herb, in that it is necessary for short-term use in serious cases where the benefits are worth the side effects. Food therapy, lifestyle, and herbs are used to mitigate the side effects and protect the body. After the allopathic intervention has served its purpose, the focus becomes restoring the health of the body. As integrative medicine is becoming more popular there is also a rise in antagonism by some allopathic practitioners. This antagonism blocks open communication. Because most allopathic practitioners do not fully understand nutrition or herbal medicine they tell patients not to use them, cheating patients out of optimum care.

29. Divine Farmer's Classic of Materia Medica (Shen Nong Ben Cao Jing 神農本草經) (circa 20-220 A.D.). This is the first surviving materia medica in TCM.

30. This bias against fierce or aggressive medicinals also kept more hallucinogenic herbs out of common use.

31. Allopathic medicine refers to what most would call Western medicine. I use the term allopathic medicine to differentiate it from other forms of Western medical traditions such as homeopathy, naturopathy, and Western herbalism.

Plants as Teachers

It is sunset and I am sitting on a big rock meditating. I face a tree I dearly love. She is a Jaboticaba tree. They can be huge shade trees, but this one is but a baby. She is my height. Already she has dark berries that sprout from her trunk. She sheds her dainty bark like a snake and she wears pieces of it furled into ringlets. My mind wanders and I sit in awe of her. I begin to feel her energy. Her leaves opening to receive the last rays of sun. The gentle yet determined flow of water from the earth flowing through her veins. I can feel the distinct coolness and heat she holds. It is as if I can feel her heartbeat. I feel so honored to be invited in. It humbles me.

There is a saying in the Afro-Brazilian religion, "without herbs there are no orixá (saints)." That is to say, plants are our connection with the Divine. The most fragile sapling stands perfectly as a conduit between Heaven and Earth and has more to teach us than the greatest Daoist sage.

Herbal medicine of any system is limited until we first form relationships with the plants we work with. All primitive cultures learned how to use plants by listening to them. This is difficult for many modern people to understand, as, increasingly for us, contact with Nature is a choice. If you have ever been in old growth forest and you are still, the conversations of the plant kingdom can be deafening. If your very survival depended on interacting with this environment you would become a good listener.

To construct and prescribe herbal formulas requires a deep knowing of each herb. The substances used in Traditional Chinese Medical formulas form synergistic and antagonistic interactions with each other as well with the body of the individual patient. An herbalist goes through a similar process in constructing a formula as a host does in developing a guest list or a natural perfumer does in making a perfume. When you have formed an intimate relationship with the herbs it is easier to pair them with patients and conditions.

If you intend to work with herbs, I recommend reading a book on plant spirit medicine[32] and growing plants. You develop relationships with plants just as you would with people or animals. You spend time with them. You speak to them as you water them. You smell their flowers.

There is a great deal we have to learn from plants. When we live in harmony with Nature, we thrive and are vibrant. When we live out of sync with Nature, we fall ill, we are unhappy, and life has no purpose. Humans are rejuvenated by being in a natural environment, as it reminds us of our own nature. As women, in serving nature we learn how we are to be honored. In following Her cycles it teaches us about our own. We have come to view our Life cycles as a great burden; as something backwards to be medicated. When we take this attitude we kill our own spirit. Honoring Nature and Her cycles is directly related to honoring ourselves as women.

Next we will visit the seven major Cycles of a woman's life with related topics. Read every chapter,

32.Please see Resources section.

even if it is not your age range. This is for two reasons: 1.) the information in this entire book is pertinent to women of all ages and 2.) understanding the entire Cycle helps you understand better where you are.

Note that some topics have been included in chapters where it was most crucial to that age range. For example, menstruation is covered in Chapter 2 (ages 14 through 20), because this is when girls traditionally began menstruating. However the information is relevant to all menstruating women so they can take proper care of themselves during this time. This information is important to all women, even those who no longer menstruate, as a key piece of their health history. The menstrual cycle is one of the best diagnostics of a woman's constitution.

When we can see the 7 Cycles in their entirety it helps us see where we have been and where we are going. This allows us to make adjustments and preparations along the way.

Let the Cycles begin…

Prologue

The Beginning

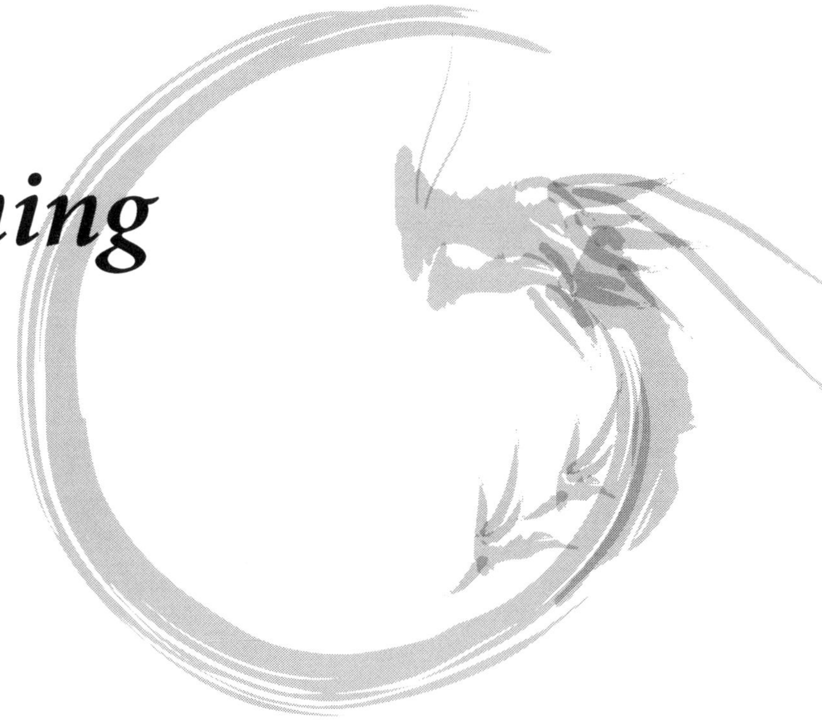

Before Conception

A great deal of our lives is spent in preparation for what we will become. Before our Jing, our Essence, can move through the 7 Cycles, it must first be cultivated carefully. During the 7 Cycles in the life of a woman we have many choices that will impact our health and the course of our lives. Before our own life even begins, our choices are made for us by our parents, our ancestors, the configuration of the Heavens, and the culture into which we are born. What happens at this stage lays the groundwork of our reserves that will carry us through the challenges of life.

We are not developed yet to become actors. If we are lucky, we will be blessed with healthy parents who nurture us through this stage. We will inherit enough Qi (energy) to carry us through mistakes and hardships later on in life. If we are less lucky, our parents have less to give us. As adults we will have to make good choices to maintain what we have. This is the time of our Pre-Heaven; our inheritance of Jing.

In the Womb

Conception

At conception, the Jing of each parent, in the form of egg and sperm, comes together to form the fetus. The Jing is the material made of the best and worst of the parents physically and psychologically: their genetics, the sum result of how they chose to live their lives, whether they came together in love or in lust, etc. Three to six months prior to conception, parents should optimize their physical health, as well as emotional and spiritual state, in order to give the best to their baby.(1)

In addition to optimizing the health of the baby, a traditional Chinese practice is to use a pregnancy calendar to predict the likelihood of a boy or girl being born in a particular month. Children are also planned for auspicious years.(2)

10 Moons of Pregnancy

Traditionally, Chinese women counted 10 moons and 10 days from conception to birth. As soon as the two Jings interact, a new Shen (consciousness) begins to form. On the third day after conception, the Po – the corporeal, Yin aspect of the soul – enters the fetus. The Po guides the Jing in the creation of the physical body.(3)

During pregnancy, both mother and fetus are influenced by each other. The mother will crave different foods and her body will adjust to the energy of the growing child. Likewise, every emotion, thought, word, touch, and nutrient ingested, as well as the energetic environment of the mother, is directly experienced by the fetus. The mother greatly affects the constitution of her baby by her moods, thoughts, and actions.

> **Note:** there are many practitioners who prefer not to treat pregnant women due to liability issues. I felt it was important to include traditional and contemporary formulas and points. This is valuable information that must be recorded.

1.The health of both parents affects the constitution of the baby. For example, babies born to older fathers have increasingly higher rates of autism and schizophrenia. Ewen Callaway, "Fathers Bequeath More Mutations as They Age," Nature 488 (23 August 2012): 439, doi: 10.1038/488439.a

2.Certain years are traditionally considered lucky, such as the Dragon year for boys and Rabbit year for girls. Also, the luck a child brings his/her parents is revealed in relation to the parents' birth chart.

3. Giovanni Maciocia. *The Psyche in Chinese Medicine; Treatment of Emotional and Mental Disharmonies with Acupuncture and Chinese Herbs.* (Nanjing: Churchill Livingstone, 2009), 48.

This is the foundation for the ancient Chinese practice of "Fetal Education" or *taijiao*. This tradition was heavily influenced by Confucianist thought. Each month carries specific instructions in terms of diet, lifestyle, acupuncture, and herbs in order to heighten development of certain aspects the fetus. There are numerous programs, giving different orders of development of the 5 Spirits and Elements.(4) The programs have modernized. The following are some of the ancient monthly recommendations:(5)

1-3 Moons

It is commonly advised in fetal education to avoid intercourse for the first three months.(6) Sun Simiao(7) advised against sex specifically during the second month of pregnancy. This is to avoid stirring up desire in the gestating woman and diverting energy away from the fetus.

Sun Simiao also recommended avoiding spicy food and extreme temperatures during the second month as it would disturb the Shao Yang (Gallbladder and San Jiao meridians).(8) During the third month he advocated keeping warm and covered at night.

King Wen(9) recommended that during the first three months, the expectant mother wear jade, read poetry, sing songs, perfume the body, and avoid looking at violence.

4-6 Moons

During the second trimester, mothers can begin more intensive fetal education, including singing, reading, talking, and listening to music. During the fourth month, the fetus receives the Jing of Water and uses it to form blood circulation. The fetus can now open the ears and eyes. Sun Simiao recommended eating carp soup (a Blood and Yin tonic) or wild goose broth during this month.

According to Sun Simiao, during the fifth month the Spleen meridian develops. The mother should arise later in the morning than is normal for that season. She should then put on clean clothes and stay in a small room. The mother should eat grains with a rich soup of beef or lamb. The mother should make sure to eat the 5 Tastes (sweet, sour, pungent, salty, and bitter) that are developing the fetus (Chinese nutrition recommends eating the 5 flavors at every meal). The fetus' four limbs are strong now.

During the sixth month, the fetus receives the Jing of Metal and forms the tendons and muscles. Sun

4. Traditionally each month of pregnancy corresponded to a particular Element organ system, and its corresponding Spirit.

5. Fetal education can be found in: Sun Simiao, *Bei Ji Qian Jin Yao Fang Prescriptions worth a Thousand in Gold for Every Emergency Vol. II-IV*, trans. Sabine Wilms (The Chinese Medicine Database: United States, 2008).

6. Shaoting Jing. "TCM Gynecology" (lecture, Yo San University, Los Angeles, CA, July 10, 2003).

7. Sun Simiao (581(?)–682) was an esteemed TCM doctor and author of the earliest known TCM manual on clinical practice.

8. Meridians are the channels through which the Qi flows in the body. There are 12 main meridians that correspond to the Yin and Yang organ systems of each Element.

9. King Wen (1152–1056 BC) was the founder of the Zhou Dynasty. He recorded a detailed program for fetal education.

Simiao's special recommendation is for the mother to go out and watch horses and dogs running. The mother should also stay in dry places to help the Lungs.

7-9 Moons

During the seventh month the fetus receives the Jing of Wood for the bones. Sun Simiao instructs the mother to stay in dry places to help the Lungs. He also advises avoiding excessive crying and talking.

During the eighth month, the fetus receives the Jing of Earth forming the skin. All nine orifices are formed and the fetus can survive on his/her own. The nine orifices are the tai gua: ears, eyes, nostrils, Du 26 (philtrum, under the nose), mouth, urethra, and anus. The Large Intestine is the meridian of the eighth month and the mother is advised not to delay bowel movements.

Sun Simiao states in the ninth month of pregnancy that all the joints and the 6 Fu (Large Intestine, Small Intestine, Stomach, Gallbladder, Urinary Bladder, and San Jiao) are formed. The mother should drink good quality wine and eat good food.(10) The mother should not stay in damp places.

10. Modern medicine does not recommend the use of alcohol during pregnancy.

Birth Through Age 6

Early Development

The Hun – the ethereal, Yang aspect of the soul – enters the body on the third day after birth.[11] This represents the time we become fully embodied; wholly human. The Hun is connected directly to the Collective Conscious (which unifies all living things) and to our concept of God. The Hun exists without the body, while the Po co-exists with the body. Human life cannot exist without the two aspects of the soul. Death occurs when the Hun and Po separate. The Hun leaves, returning to Heaven (the unmanifest realm) while the Po stays with the body and returns to the Earth.

As explained in the Traditional Chinese Medicine Introduction, the 5 Elements are used to describe the major stages of human life. From birth until puberty (the age of 14 for girls and 16 for boys), children are in the Wood Phase of their lives. Their meridians are not completely formed during this Phase. Their Chong[12] meridian is not connected. Early childhood until 7 years old is considered a Yang cycle, with Kidney Yang driving development.

Within the larger cycle of the Wood Phase, early childhood is broken down further into the 5 Phases.[13] The baby begins in the Metal Phase. It is "all about me" at this stage, which is why babies need constant, focused attention to stay calm and happy. All stimuli come through the skin and babies need to be touched. Sometime prior to 1 year of age, the Water Phase begins. Fear arises when they start to see the world as it is. Nightmares can occur when Water is deficient.

At 1-5 years old, children move into Wood. This is the little-tyrant stage. Toddlers begin to exert their will on the world around them and test their boundaries. Children's minds (Shen) are not fully developed and do not restrain the Hun from ages 2-7. They get lost in the world of make-believe; they have imaginary friends, and personify inanimate objects. After age 7 the Shen matures and restrains the Hun. This is a protective measure that allows children to function in the adult world.[14]

At 5 years old, the child moves into Fire. The ability to discern appropriateness in behavior has its first spark. Children start developing the ability to connect and play cooperatively. Prior to the Fire stage, children are not ready for group activities.

At 7-8 years old, children move into Earth. They become more responsible, organized, and stable.

Parental attitudes greatly affect the child's development. Too much discipline creates Liver Fire

---

11. Giovanni Maciocia. *The Psyche in Chinese Medicine; Treatment of Emotional and Mental Disharmonies with Acupuncture and Chinese Herbs*. (Nanjing: Churchill Livingstone, 2009), 25.

12. The Chong meridian is also known as the "Sea of Blood" or "Pemetrating Vessel." It is strongly associated with menstruation.

13. Alex Tiberi, "TCM Pediatrics" (lecture, Pacific College of Oriental Medicine, San Diego, CA, February 28, 2008).

14. Giovanni Maciocia. *The Psyche in Chinese Medicine; Treatment of Emotional and Mental Disharmonies with Acupuncture and Chinese Herbs*. (Nanjing: Churchill Livingstone, 2009), 36-38.

in children. No discipline creates low level stagnation of the Liver leading to no sense of self and insecurity. Excessive nurturing and smothering creates Spleen Damp. Lack of nurturing creates Spleen Qi deficiency.

Typing Children

As children's imbalances are all constitution, rather than condition, it is helpful to understand a child's constitution in order to avoid future problems before they develop. As adults, there are five ways to judge someone's constitution: childhood illness, body shape, shape of hand, personality (likes and dislikes), and health conditions they start having as adults.

Metal Types

Metal-predominant children are very vulnerable to exterior pathogens. They tend to have lung problems, lingering pathogens, latent heat, and Shao Yang level[15] issues. Their skin often looks transparent and weak. The skin may be dry and scaly. Excessive hair on skin is a sign of weak lungs. Metal children will have more trouble letting go of grief and unjust situations. They also tend to be obsessive-compulsive and have a fondness for ritual. They find it difficult to function in disorder.

Water Types

For Water predominant children, development issues are a big factor. They tend towards recurrent ear infections. They suffer from late night bed wetting. They often struggle more with phobias and nightmares. They need to feel safe. When Kidney deficiency is severe, children will be slow to mature physically and struggle to keep up with their peers in cognitive or behavioral development.

Wood Types

Wood-predominant children tend to have strong constitutions, though they may test this to the limit, through a higher incidence of falls, scrapes, bruises, and breaks. Common conditions include hives or hot skin conditions, early night bedwetting, and nail biting. They tend towards anger and control issues. They need freedom to roam and expand.

Fire Types

Fire-predominant children are susceptible to high fevers and hot skin conditions. They tend towards chronic sleep issues. They are overly emotional and cry easily. They need to know they are loved

15. Refers to a stage of pathogenic invasion where the pathogen begins to lodge itself deeper in the body. From the medical text, *Shang Han Lun's 6 Levels of Pathogenic Invasion* written by Zhongjing Zhang around 220 A.D.

on a more consistent and demonstrative level than other types require. Fire very early on requires attention.

Earth Types

Earth-predominant types are often plagued with digestive problems and parasites. They are often preoccupied with food and may hoard snacks. These children often will not wake up after bedwetting. They need to nurture and be nurtured.

Pediatric Tui Na (Massage)

Massage performed by the parents and family members is considered a key tool in optimizing the health and development of the baby in many traditional cultures. In a healthy child, massage assists in developing neuroconnections, improves circulation, and creates bonding between parent and child. In the case of ailments, special massage techniques can be enough to treat the condition of the infant. Whereas the same condition in an adult would require greater intervention and time to see results.

Daily Massage

For the first year of life massage your baby daily. It is best to find five minutes a day to do this rather than do it for a longer period of time once a week. This section contains specific massage techniques you can use. If this is overwhelming, try this routine: gently grasp and knead the infant's arms, legs, and up both sides of the spine. Perform passive joint mobility on each joint. That means very gently take each joint through its full range of motion.

Massage both sides for general health. Traditionally, boys are treated on the left side of the body, girls on the right.

Hands

The micro system of the hand is very important in pediatric massage. (Figure P.1) The Thumb relates to the Earth element, the index finger to the Wood element, the middle finger to the Fire element, the ring finger to the Metal element, and the little finger to the Water element. The Yin organs (Heart, Spleen, Lungs, Kidney, and Liver) are located at the tips of the fingers. In order to tonify (strengthen)

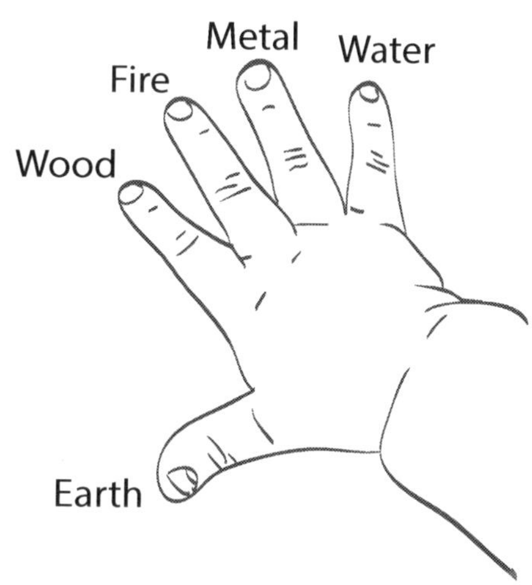

Figure P.1

an organ, rub the tip of the finger. Then use a circular motion to massage the finger, moving toward the hand. This brings Qi in. In order to clear excess from an organ, rub in a straight line moving from the base to the tip of the finger. This draws the unwanted Qi out.

Next is the palm. The back of the hand relates to the Yang side of the body. The palm correlates to the interior of the body in general and the belly in particular. Rub the palm in clockwise direction.

Massage Oils and Remedies for the Medicine Cabinet:

Cooling Tincture:[(1)]

In heat conditions use rubbing alcohol to massage. As you massage it will evaporate and move Heat out. To intensify this further, fill a container 1/3 full with fresh ginger and onion. Fill the rest of the way with alcohol. Let sit 1 week. Strain and use.

Heating Ginger Oil:

Mix sesame oil and dry powdered ginger until the oil turns gritty. This oil is moving and warming. It is particularly good to rub on the spine of babies and small children daily. It is indicated to combat scoliosis and to develop muscle tone. Note: sesame oil is tonifying. Avoid in excess cases (infection or inflammation).

Colloidal Silver:

Purchase concentrated colloidal silver. Dilute and soak with gauze as a compress for any skin irritation or inflammation. Use the compress 10 min., two times a day.

Zi Cao Oil:[(2)]

Powder the herbs to a fine powder: Zi Cao (lithospermum) 30g, Di Yu (sanguisorba) 20g. Melt together over low heat with 500g sesame oil and 160g beeswax. Pour into containers to cool and store. This formula is a favorite with many acupuncturists. It can be used for any Heat condition including eczema, herpetic lesions, burns, and acne. Zi Cao, and its oil, should be a distinct red-purple color.

Huang Lian Gao:

Decoct Dang Gui (Chinese angelica) 15g, Huang Bai (phellodendron) 9g, Sheng Di Huang (raw rehmannia) 30g, Jiang Huang (turmeric) 9g in 360g of sesame oil over low heat until herbs turn brown. Strain out the herbs. Melt 100g beeswax in the oil. Add Huang Lian (coptis) 9g finely powdered once the mixture has cooled a bit but is still liquid. Used to treat infections, acne, and inflammations.

Yunnan Paiyao:

The number one first aid treatment. Use the powder externally on open wounds to prevent infection, minimize scarring, and speed healing. Use internally to move Blood and stop bleeding after traumatic injury.

1. Alex Tiberi, "TCM Pediatrics" (lecture, Pacific College of Oriental Medicine, San Diego, CA, April 12, 2008).
2. Yueying Li, "TCM Dermatology" (lecture, San Diego, CA, September 18, 2011).

Use a pressing and kneading motion on the thenar eminence (the thumb pad). A dark color on the thenar eminence indicates stagnation in the intestines or lymph nodes. Massage the heel of the hand to soothe the emotions.

Massage the wrist crease with both thumbs. Use an opening motion to Clear Heat, especially emotional Heat. Use a closing motion to Move Qi. (Figure P.2)

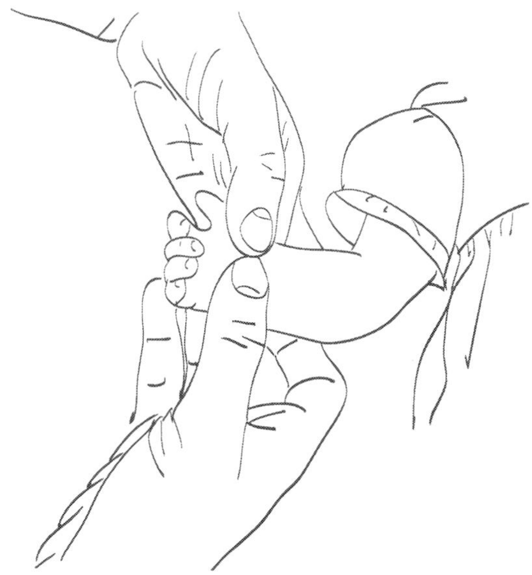

Figure P.2

Arms

When massaging the arms, go against the meridian flow to clear Heat.[16] Move with the meridian to strengthen the organ system. Clear the Lung meridian when there is fever due to pathogens. Clear the Pericardium meridian in cases of internal Heat. Clear the Large Intestine meridian when there is digestive Heat.[17]

Back

Rub your hand back and forth on the back (also called chafing) to create heat and warm up the muscles. (Figure P.3) The most important maneuver for deficiency is pinching and rolling the skin up the sides of the spine. This tonifies the Yang of the body, opens the Du channel, and helps strengthen all the organ systems.[18]

At the sacrum,[19] stroke down to help waste elimination. Stroke upwards for bedwetting. For bedwetting in toddlers, it is also helpful to moxa the sacrum.[20]

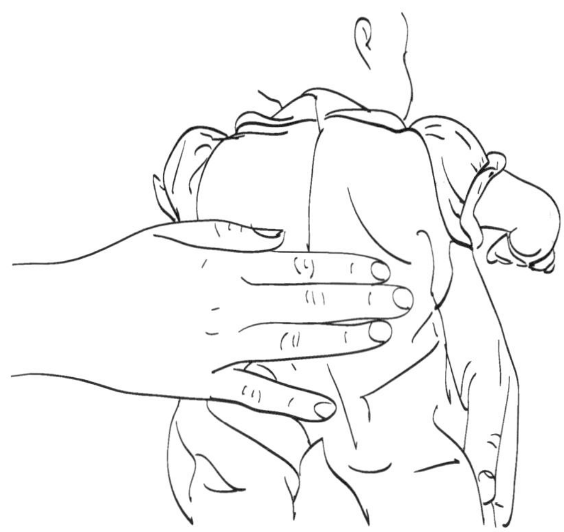

Figure P.3

16. The meridians flow in specific directions. Movement in the direction of the channel's flow tonifies and strengthens the channel. Movement against the channel's flow disperses excess or pathological energy from the channel.
17. Alex Tiberi, "TCM Pediatrics" (lecture, Pacific College of Oriental Medicine, San Diego, CA, April 12, 2008).
18. The Du meridian (sea of Yang, Governing Vessel, 督脈, dū mài) is one of the Eight Extra Merdians that run deeper inside the body than the 12 Meridians. The Du meridian begins in the lower abdomen, runs up the spine, over the top of the head and down to the philtrum under the nose.
19. The sacrum is the large, triangular bone at the base of the spine.
20. Moxa or moxibustion refers to burning Ai Ye (mugwort) on or close to the skin. Light a stick moxa and swirl close to the skin. Keep your hand on the child to mak sure it doesn't get too warm.

Head

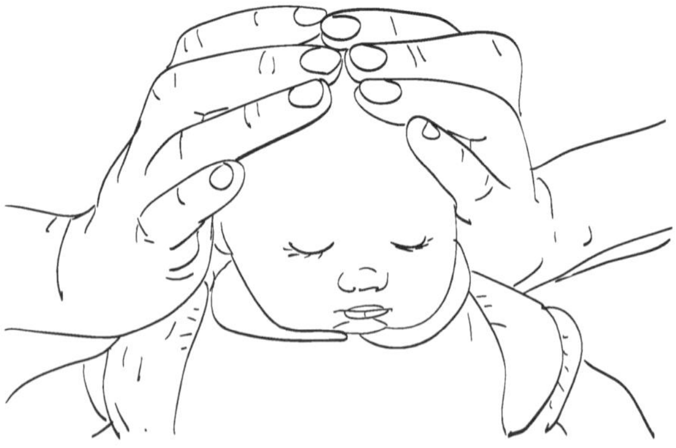

Figure P.4

To stimulate brain function, begin with the middle finger at Du 24, located at the hairline in line on the center line with the nose. (Figure P.4) Using a squeezing and grasping motion, using the whole hand to work down the centerline of the scalp (Du channel). Then use your index and middle fingers to make small circles working until the entire scalp is covered, including where the ears attach. Be very careful to avoid the fontanel (the soft spot on the baby's head where the bony plates have not fused together). Never apply pressure to this area.

Next stroke the face upwards to open the face to release Heat. Use the thumb and index fingers to gently pinch and massage the ears in a circular motion.

Chest & Abdomen

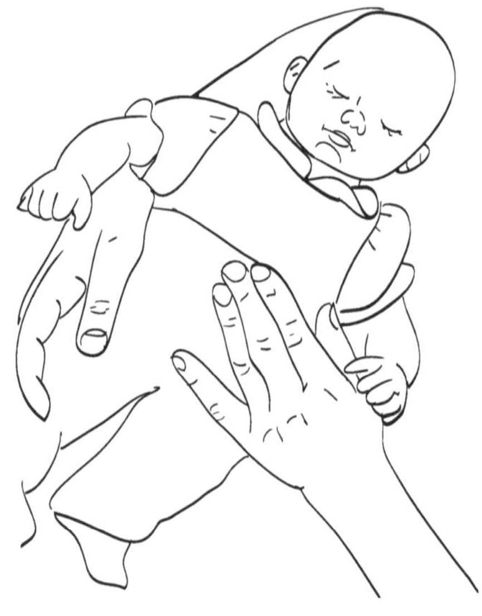

Figure P.5

Do gentle pressure point stimulation with the thumb working down from Ren 15 to Ren 8.[21] (Figure P.5) For stagnation in the Intestines, place the middle finger on the belly button. Circle the finger in a clockwise motion. This also helps food to descend.

The Lower Dan Tian is particularly important. It is located just under the umbilicus and is a major energy center of the body. Gently rub with your palm. For a weak constitution, a vibrating motion is very strengthening.

Legs

The Spleen meridian is used to control bladder function. Stroke downwards to promote urination and treat bladder infection. Stroke upwards to stop frequent urination. Do pressure point massage on Spleen 6 and Stomach 36. Press Kidney 1 when there is wind rising (tremors, headaches, or convulsions) and to stop convulsions. (Figures P.6 a & b).

---

21. The Ren meridian (sea of Yin, Conception Vessel,任脈, rèn mài) is one of the Eight Extra Merdians that run deeper inside the body than the 12 Meridians. The Ren meridian begins under the lower lip, runs downs the front centerline of the body, and ends inside the lower abdomen.

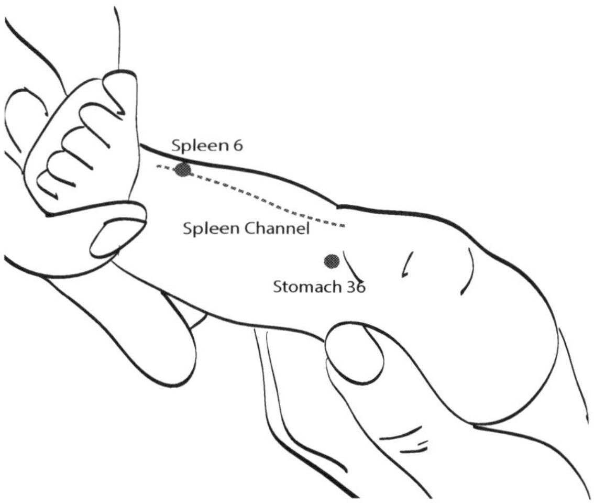

Figure P.6a

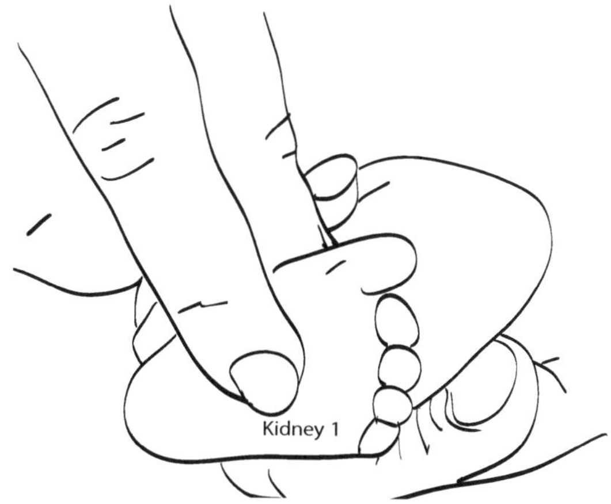

Figure P.6b

PRACTITIONER SECTION: TREATING CHILDREN

Children are not just small adults. They have special aspects to consider during treatment.

Table P.1. Pediatric Diagnosis: Based on Slow Development, and Excessive Softness or Hardness.

5 Slows	5 Softs	5 Hards
Caused by deficiencies in following organ systems:	Spleen Deficiency, Central (Zhong) Qi Deficiency	Liver Stagnation or penetration of Cold in the body.
Slow to: Stand – Kidney & Liver Walk – Liver & Stomach Grow Hair – Kidney Sprout Teeth – Kidney Speak – Heart	Soft: Head Neck Hands and Feet Flesh (hernia, prolapse) Mouth (sit with the mouth open)	Neck (spasms) Mouth (tight jaw, grinding teeth) Hair (thick and course) Feet Muscle Tension

Younger children can be treated with electro-stimulation, magnets, and ear magnets alone. Children can be needled as soon as they are compliant. Glycerin-based tinctures tend to be the best way to administer herbs to children, unless they can be hidden in food.

The Short List of Common Childhood Complaints

Cold Sores (herpes simplex) – Long Dan Cao (gentiana) is an effective herb to denature the herpes virus. Powder and apply topically (use Vaseline or egg white as a medium) and take internally (Long Dan Xie Gan Tang). Chi Shao (red peony) and Pu Gong Yin (dandelion) are also helpful. Stimulate ST 45 (needle, magnet, or electro-stimulation) to drain heat from the Stomach channel.

Diaper Rash – Use Huang Lian Gao, powdered Huang Lian (coptis) with egg white, or colloidal silver saturated in gauze topically. Huang Lian kills candida as well.

Down's Syndrome – This is Kidney deficiency with Dampness. Clear Dampness first. Once the condition begins to shift, begin adding Kidney tonics.

Dyslexia – Stimulate the Yin Qiao (KD6, Lung 7), Yang Qiao (UB 62, SI 3), REN 24, DU 23, 20, 16.(1)

Recurrent Ear Infections – This is due to underlying Spleen Qi deficiency with Phlegm-Damp obstruction. These children often do not hear well and have learning problems. Long-term, tonify the Spleen and resolve Phlegm with Xiang Sha Liu Jun Zi Tang. Acute attacks are often Damp-Heat. Use Long Dan Xie Gan Tang until the acute infection resolves.

Eye Problems – Many eye disorders can be cured if treated prior to the 2nd Cycle (14 in girls, 16 in boys). Use electro-stimulation around the eyes along with magnets or needles to treat the constitution. The eyes at any age benefit from local stimuli. Lazy eye can be treated in children under 7 years old. Use magnets or needles to stimulate LV 3 and GB 37.

Flat Feet - In children this is an indicator of Liver Qi deficiency. Moxa LV 1.

Growing Pains – Nourish Liver Blood to help the tendons keep up with bone growth with a Si Wu Tang-based formula. Needle and massage the tendons in the areas that are painful.

Psoriasis and Eczema – Dilute colloidal silver and make a compress with gauze. Apply for 10 min, twice a day. Next, if there is scaling, mix a liniment with oil and gently rub scales off. Powder Ku Shen (sophora root) and Huang Lian (coptis) and mix in equal parts with egg whites to form a thick paste. Apply to the area twice daily.

Recurrent Sinus and Throat Infections – This is a result of Spleen and Lung deficiency. Give the child Yu Ping Feng San daily to build immunity for 6 months or longer. In case of acute infection, gargle and flush sinuses with diluted colloidal silver. Give the child the appropriate Wind-resolving formula such as Bi Ming Gan for sinus congestion or a Ban Lan Gen-based formula for the throat.

Sleep Disorders – At night, moxa Du 20 to build up the sea of marrow. Waking up at night is related to sugar levels; switch to protein as last food of the day to keep blood sugar stable (this is true at all ages). Sometimes night terrors result from Stomach Heat going up to disturb the Shen (mind). Waking up with fear is not too alarming if it occurs for less than two weeks.

Spinal Development - Parents can hang their baby upside down for 30 seconds or less to self-adjust. Adjust the time according to the child. It should be a fun experience for him/her.

Swimmer's Ear – Always use alcohol to flush out excess water after swimming. Saturate a cotton ball with alcohol. Have the child tilt her head with the ear up and squeeze into the ear. Place a dry cotton ball in the opening of the ear and have her tilt her head with the ear down so the fluids can drain out. Use ear plugs in cold water to protect the eardrums. These apply to adults as well.

Teeth Development – When teeth do not form properly it is Kidney Yin deficiency. When teeth are formed but are not able to push out, it is Kidney Yang Deficiency. The Spleen Qi is responsible for holding the gums against the teeth (use Bu Zhong Yi Qi Tang).

Thrush – This is a form of candida overgrowth and is more common in Earth Element children. Apply Long Dan Cao (gentiana) powder with a cotton swab. This herb is extremely bitter, but very effective.

---

1. My practice of pediatrics was greatly influenced by Dr. Alex Tiberi of Pacific College of Oriental Medicine.

Uniqueness of Children

Children under the age of 7 are different from adults in several ways. First and foremost, they do not have the years of accumulated conditions and complexities that adults have, so their conditions are straightforward. Children are born with constitutional issues, which are strongly impacted by the early environment. By treating childhood conditions, one is treating the constitution directly, preventing future diseases.

All children under the age of 7 have Spleen weakness, which translates into weak digestion and low immunity. This is evident in that most childhood illnesses are the result of digestive disturbance and pathogenic invasion (viral, bacterial, and fungal infections).

All children under 7 also have excess Wood and Fire and a deficiency in Earth, Metal, and Water. This is why they overheat easily. It is also why after having a fever, they easily get Yin fluid injury, causing symptoms such as dry mouth, constipation, insomnia, and anxiety. Children get sick easily and recover quickly compared to adults.

Spleen Weakness

Children's Spleens do not become fully developed until age 7. This is key to understanding childhood diseases and to fortifying their health from a young age. An underdeveloped Spleen means the ability to digest foods, to assimilate experiences, and to ward off pathogenic invasion are not fully developed at this time. It also means there is a propensity towards Food stagnation (upset stomach, poor absorption) and Phlegm formation (runny nose). This has several implications in regards to having a proper diet, building immunity, treating pathogens, and making decisions on immunizations.

Proper Diet

All children have Spleen Qi deficiency with Food stagnation until the age of 7. Without proper diet, digestive weakness will continue into maturity. In these cases children's Spleens will not develop properly and they will carry a Spleen Qi deficient constitution into adulthood, predisposing them to Type II Diabetes, obesity, poor immunity, and many other conditions.

Proper diet is the most important factor in strengthening the Spleen and there is no substitution for it. The diet should consist of fresh, whole foods which are easy to digest and as free of environmental toxins as possible. Many childhood imbalances can be resolved with food, lifestyle, massage, and minor herbal intervention.

Genetically Modified Organisms (GMOs)[22] are the product of genes from plants, animals, viruses, or bacteria that are artificially combined with the DNA of plants and animals to produce "food." The purported benefit is economical; the crops and livestock are more disease resistant and otherwise cheaper to grow and ship. This comes with adverse effects to the health of the environment and humans.

When there is impaired digestion, as there always is in children, these genetically altered compounds further weaken digestion causing allergic reactions and other digestive disturbances. Chemical preservatives, hormones, and pesticides in foods are also hardest on those with weak digestive systems. They destabilize hormonal development and introduce Heat Toxins into the system that may not surface for many years. These should be avoided as much as possible. Limit your child's intake of soda, processed foods, and candy, indulging in them only occasionally. Instead, develop children's palates to enjoy the real taste of natural foods.

Diet for Spleen Qi Deficiency with Food Stagnation (Children's Diet)

Diet Plan

Eat a higher percentage of carbohydrates to strengthen the Qi; 40-60%. The rest of the diet should include 10-20% protein and 30-40% vegetables. Eat mostly cooked foods with a little bit of raw fruits and vegetables. Keep meals simple. Eat congee (rice soup) regularly (Recipes page 325). Follow the directives on Diet page 70.

Foods

Spleen tonics: Yams, winter squash, potatoes, peas, carrots, green beans, oats, rice, beef, chicken. Small amounts of high quality sweets such as dates, honey, fruit juice, dried fruit.

Food Stagnation-resolving: cooked sprouted grains, cooking spices (cardamom, fennel, etc.). Take homemade probiotics with meals (Recipes page 331).

Aggravating Factors

Weaning too early. Not breastfeeding. Excess sweets,[23] poor quality dairy,[24] and processed foods. Cold temperature foods. Raw foods. GMOs, preservatives, chemical additives, hormones, and pesticides in foods. Complex flavors and complicated meals.

---

22. For peer-reviewed research on GMOs see "GMO Myths and Truths," accessed November 5, 2012, http://earthopensource.org/index.php/executive-summary.

23. Generate Dampness and weaken the Spleen.

24. Good quality dairy provides vital nutrients but should not be taken in excess as they promote Phlegm formation.

Formulas

These are available in glycerin-based tinctures. They can be taken three times a day with major meals.

Spleen Tonics:
Xiang Sha Liu Jun Zi Tang, Jian Pi Wan

Food Stagnation Resolving:
Bao He Wan

Include Spleen tonic herbs in cooking:
Huang Qi (astragalus), Tai Zi Shen (pseudostellaria), Shan Yao (Chinese yam), and Fu Ling (poria).

Immunity

Immunity in Traditional Chinese Medicine is tied to the health of Spleen Qi and Blood production. Because immunity in children is not fully developed, it is important to take extra precautions.[25] Furthermore, Wind conditions, such as a cough or runny nose, that are not fully treated can penetrate into the body and become latent Heat Toxins. Latent Heat Toxins are implicated in many modern diseases such as cancer, autoimmune diseases, and many chronic diseases.

1. **Avoid Wind Exposure:** Do not let children go to bed, or go outside in windy or cold weather with their hair wet.[26] Do not leave children in wet clothes. Keep them away from drafts and cold air. Particularly protect the neck and head from drafts and cold air.
2. **Get Ample Sleep:** Overexertion and becoming overtired before bedtime can weaken the Kidneys, Spleen, and Lungs. This applies to adults as well as to children, but is particularly injurious to children because their Spleens and Kidneys are not fully mature. This will also help with bedwetting issues.
3. **Protect the Spleen:** Have your child follow the diet plan for tonifying Spleen Qi and reducing Food stagnation as given above, as well as the dietary guidelines on page 70. Always give your child a Spleen Tonic, like Jian Pi Pian, with meals when taking antibiotics. This protects the Spleen from the harsh cold nature of antibiotics, prevents digestive issues, and prevents chronic respiratory diseases.
4. **Take Immunity-Building Formulas:** To build the immunity give your child Yu Ping Feng San (Jade Screen Formula) first thing in the morning for at least 3-6 months. This is particularly important in cases of recurrent colds, allergies, and exposure to pathogens (such as being in hospitals, schools, or during flu season). It can be taken in powdered, as a patent pill, or in a glycerin-based tincture form. With the first signs of a cold take Gan Mao Ling or one of the home remedies (Recipes page 338). Never ignore a cold in children

25. These guidelines are also true of adults when feeling run down.

26. There is an old Chinese saying that bad spirits can enter the body if you go to bed with wet hair. In modern terms, this describes the propensity to catching cold.

as it can easily and quickly progress into something more serious. If preventive and home remedies do not work, immediately see an acupuncturist or pediatrician for stronger treatment.

Recipe P.1. Caramel Lime & Ginger Tea

This is my mom's family recipe. The caramelized sugar warms the body and creates a high compliance rate. Caramelize ½ cup of sugar. Add 1 cup of milk (or water). Add 1 lime (or lemon) sliced and 1 tsp. minced fresh ginger. Stir over medium heat until the caramel has dissolved. Remove from heat and serve. Give to your child at the first signs of a cold. Put your child to bed and cover him/her up with warm blankets to sweat out the pathogen.

Immunizations

I want to preface this section by clarifying that I am not an expert on pediatric immunizations. I am giving my personal opinion based on observations, what I have learned from parents of autistic children, and what I consider logical conclusions. In 1986 National Childhood Vaccine Injury Act was passed that protected vaccine manufacturers against lawsuits.[27] After this the number of required immunizations in the U.S. increased exponentially. Though these vaccines are "recommended," many parents feel pressured by pediatricians and school mandates to get their children the full list of scheduled vaccines. I would recommend studying the benefits and risks

PRACTITIONER SECTION: TREATING IMMUNIZATIONS

Immunizations introduce Heat Toxins into the body. If the immune system is not strong enough, these will linger in the system and become latent Heat Toxins. Latent Heat Toxins are implicated in many modern diseases such as autoimmune diseases and cancer. A key sign that a child has developed latent Heat Toxin is the development of a red tongue after being immunized.[1]

I recommend administering an anti-toxin formula to children after immunizations as a preventive.[2] Use the anti-toxin formula below or a patent formula such as Huang Lian Jie Du Tang. Children should begin taking the formula soon after the inoculation and continue for 2-3 days. Having children on Yu Ping Feng San long-term to build their immunity is even more effective.

Anti-Toxin Formula: Di Gu Pi (wolfberry root), Lian Qiao (forsythia fruit), Tao Ren (peach kernel), Huang Lian (coptis), Zhi Zi (cape jasmine fruit), Ban Lan Gen (isatis root), Bo He (mint), Xuan Shen (scrophula), Sheng Ma (black cohosh), Jiang Can (silkworm), Gan Cao (licorice), rice.

1. Giovanni Maciocia, "TCM Pediatrics" (lecture, Maciocia Online, November 8, 2012).
2. The same strategy is effective with pets.

27. www.smartvax.com/index.php?option=com_content&view=article&id=66

of individual vaccines as well as the immunization schedules of other developed countries. The decision on immunizations is an individual choice. Do this research prior to bringing children to the pediatrician's office so as to make informed decisions.

It requires reflection that a child is expected to receive 36 immunizations[28] by the time he/she is two years old. Particularly since a child's immune system is not fully developed until the age of 6 or 7. The apparent approach from a public health (and profit) perspective, is that every child should be inoculated for every communicable disease imaginable as soon as possible. From this vantage point, a certain percentage of casualties is acceptable. However, from the individual perspective it can be quite the opposite. It is in the best interest of the individual child to wait as long as possible for their immune system to develop before receiving vaccinations, and then keeping the number of immunizations to a minimum.

When you choose to have your child immunized, here are some basic guidelines you can follow:

1. Never immunize your child if he/she has any signs of a cold (runny nose, slight cough, slight fever, etc) or is going through a stressful time.
2. Only have your child immunized for one pathogen at a time. It is too risky to expose a child with an undeveloped immune system to multiple pathogens.
3. Wait as long as possible to immunize so that your child's immune system will be stronger.
4. Research and make an informed decision on which immunizations are necessary for your child.
5. Take into account the strength of your child. The weaker the Spleen and Jing, the more susceptible the child is to adverse reactions. Build up your child's immunity prior to immunizations with formulas such as Yu Ping Feng San.

Autism

Autism is potentially caused by a variety of factors, such as Jing deficiency (constitutional predisposition), older parents, environmental toxins, and injury by immunizations. The main disease patterns for autism are latent Heat Toxin and Insubstantial Phlegm (Dry-Phlegm) obstructing the mind. Insubstantial Phlegm is Phlegm that is not visible (like a runny nose) but which produces mental and emotional impairment.

Poor digestion is the root source of Phlegm production. Thus, diet is crucial in the treatment of autism symptoms. Experimentation is necessary to find the optimum diet for the individual child. The major culprits are sugary foods, dairy, and cold-natured and cold temperature foods, all of which increase Phlegm in the body. In addition to acupuncture, herbs, and nutrition, many therapies are often necessary in the care of autism.

---

28. www.smartvax.com/images/PDF/gr-autism_and_vaccines_world_special_report1.pdf

PRACTITIONER SECTION: TREATING MENTAL & EMOTIONAL ISSUES

To treat autism focus on clearing Phlegm and latent Heat Toxin and strengthening the Spleen.

Autism Formula:
Dang Shen (codonopsis root), Yuan Zhi (senega root), Shi Chang Pu (sweetflag rhizome), Huo Xiang (agastache), Tian Zhu Huang (bamboo secretions), Chi Shao (red peony), Hu Po (amber), Ban Xia (pinellia rhizome), Fu Ling (poria), Yu Jin (aromatic tumeric), Gan Cao (licorice root), Sheng Jiang (fresh ginger), Da Zao (black date).

Herbs are an effective way to calm children's emotions and help them focus. They can be used to calm ADD and ADHD symptoms. In children with aggression, high anxiety, or Liver Yang Rising symptoms use Chai Hu Jia Long Gu Mu Li Tang. If the child is also very emotional add Tian Wan Bu Xin Dan. Gui Pi Tang is an excellent tonic for the mind that can be used on its own for deficiency-type children. In cases of more neurotic (hypervigilance, irrational fears) behavior, use the following formula:

Yi Gan San:
Dang Gui (Chinese angelica), Fu Ling (poria), Bai Zhu (atractylodes), Gou Teng (gambir vine), Chuan Xiong (ligusticum), Chai Hu (bupleurum), Gan Cao (licorice root).

Parasites

My grandfather was trained as an OB-GYN, but his early practice in a rural region taught him a great deal about herbal medicine, which he used to supplement his medical practice. One day a neighborhood child was brought to him with the bloated belly and skinny limbs of a malnourished child, though she was well fed. The child had a propensity for raw meat, which she would sneak when the cook was not looking. My grandfather diagnosed her with tapeworm and prescribed the following treatment:

The day before treatment, the child was given light food until noon. After noon she had only broth. The next morning my grandfather prepared fresh coconut milk with ground pumpkin seeds and gave it to her first thing in the morning. This was followed by a laxative (he did not use Da Cheng Qi Tang but this would be a good choice). She promptly passed a monster of a tape worm. Note: the head must come out or it can regrow.

Parasites, like parasitic people, take up residence where they sense weakness. This is why children, the elderly, and the chronically ill are most susceptible. The first priority is to strengthen and protect the body. Most treatments in the West focus on annihilating the pathogen, even if it means taking part of the host with it. These parasite cleanses typically drag on for months. This only leads to a chronic condition. TCM prefers quick treatments, as my grandfather used. This protects the digestion.

Parasites are attracted to Spleen deficient individuals, with Dampness or Damp-Heat. Have your child take a Spleen tonic such as Xiang Sha Liu Jun Zi Tang for 3-6 months. This can be administered in a glycerin-based tincture. Older children and adults may prefer pill form. To address the Dampness and Damp-Heat, follow the dietary directives on Clearing Damp-Phlegm page 260 and Damp-Heat page 265. Make sure food preparation is sanitary, foods are fresh, and meals are simple. Avoid rich or greasy foods. Follow the guidelines on Diet p.74 and include fermented foods in the diet to rebuild the digestive flora.

While rebuilding the internal environment and making it inhospitable to intruders, we must also use herbs to clear out the existing parasites. Choose from one of the options in Table P.3.

Table P.3. Parasite Treatments

Parasite	Remedy
Tapeworm	Coconut milk and pumpkin seeds (as directed above)
General Western Herbal Formula	Ding Xiang (clove) - freshly ground cloves to kill eggs Green walnut husk – you can get in tincture form Take for 3 months.
General TCM Formula	Powder the following herbs: Shi Jun Zi (quisqualis, shell removed) 15g, Bing Lang (betel nut) 15g, Dang Shen (codonopsis) 15g, He Shi (carpesium fruit) 15g, Mu Xiang (aucklandia) 3g, Fei Zi (torreya seed, remove shell) 15g For constipation add: Da Huang (rhubarb, powder), add in increments of 1g directly to the rice soup until the desired effect is achieved. For more severe cases add: Ku Lian Pi (melia bark) 15g to the base formula. Add 7-8g of powder to a small bowl of lukewarm, watery rice soup. Take first thing in the morning for 2-4 days on an empty stomach. This is an adult dosage. Adjust dosage according to size of the child. Ku Lian Pi and Bing Lang are slightly toxic and should be used with greater caution.

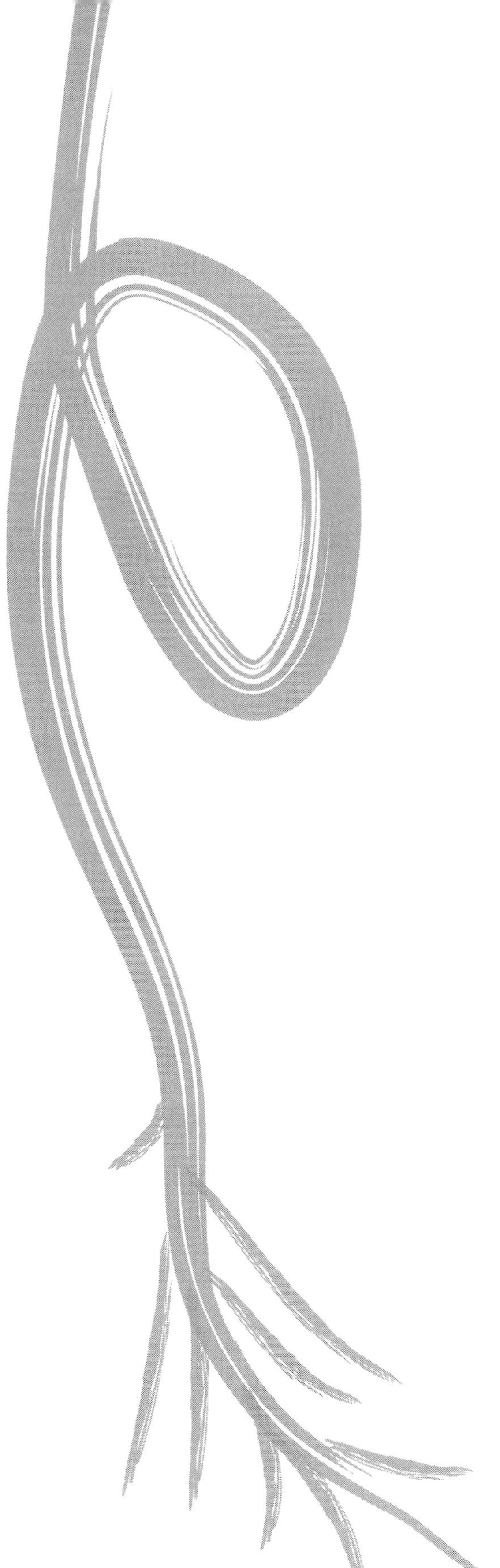

Chapter 1

Age 7

A girl age 7. The Kidney energy becomes abundant, her baby teeth are replaced by permanent ones and the hair grows.
女子七岁。 肾气盛，齿更发长；（7岁）

The 1st Cycle

One x 7 years begins the 1st Cycle in a girl's life. From age 7 to 13 she will continue in the Wood Phase. The Wood Phase is characterized by rapid growth. Children will often plump up in preparation for the big growth spurt. The first stirrings of the Jing begin, manifesting as hints of womanly characteristics.(1) In Western terms, this corresponds to the activation of the pituitary gland signaling puberty. During this seven-year period body hair appears and the breasts develop. There are often emotional swings and vaginal discharge. Any hormonal imbalances at this stage have their root in the Kidneys, as they rule development.

"Don't scare little girls"(2)

The Spleen should be fully developed by the start of the first cycle. This means digestive function and immunity are mature. This also means girls are now better able to digest life experiences. Girl's Kidneys, however, do not become fully developed until the start of the second cycle, at 14 years of age. The relative weakness of the Kidneys accounts for bedwetting and fear of sleeping alone common in small children. It also means girls are more easily frightened, and easily wounded by fright, than adults. Kidney Yang in particular relates to Power, and the ability to protect boundaries. Underdeveloped Kidneys mean that children are more vulnerable to negative energies.

1. Increasingly in recent years these changes are happening at an accelerated rate, and girls as young as 9 are menstruating.
2. Shaoting Jing, "TCM Gynecology" (lecture, Yo San University, Los Angeles, CA, May 22, 2003).

Evil Qi and Negative Energy

Our ancestors interacted with both the physical and energetic realms on a daily basis. They developed tools to deal with energy, tools that children can use to deal with unbalanced energy. They can also be used to help adults with negative life patterns. (For more please see "Transmuting Shadow" on page 162).

It is commonly believed that acupuncture originated from shamanic tradition in ancient China. In the shamanic tradition, evil spirits were considered the cause of disease. These spirits were said to hide in holes or caves and shamans removed them with spears and arrows. In acupuncture, the concept of evil spirits evolved into Evil Qi, xie qi, a term used today to describe pathogenic energy, though it no longer has a paranormal association. Acupuncture points are called xue, which means "cave" or "hole", and acupuncture needles are somewhat reminiscent of spears and arrows.

By the time of the Yellow Emperor's Inner Canon (circa 500-200 B.C.) the focus of ancient Chinese medicine had transitioned from seeing evil spirits as the cause of disease to focusing on healthy lifestyle as a means to immortality.(3) The idea of evil spirits became integrated into this new paradigm; one that focused on balancing the internal environment. Internal imbalance now became what made an individual susceptible to certain pathogens from the exterior. For example, if there was internal Yin deficiency there would be susceptibility to Wind Heat invasion. Certain deficiencies, particularly weakness of the Shen, or Mind, would thus make an individual vulnerable to evil spirits.(4)

These ancient shamanic roots are often seen as shameful or humorous to a medicine that is now finding scientific approval. However, these traditions link us to a part of our humanity that is still relevant. So-called primitive people see the world in archetypes. They experience their Hun, or Ethereal soul, on a conscious level, as do children. This means that they can experience physical reality and non-physical reality at the same time. This ability allows them to communicate directly with nature spirits, ancestors, and universal Source energy. The Hun, being the non-materialized aspect of ourselves, is impersonal and directly connected with everything in the universe.

Artists and energy-sensitive people retain this ability to consciously access their Hun into adulthood; whereas the majority of adults have lost this awareness. Non-physical reality continues to exert its influence on adults; they simply are not conscious of it. What the Hun experiences as negative entities, the conditioned mind experiences as germs, negative life patterns, acts of violence, and shadow aspects of the psyche. Thus, using rituals and symbolic language, as our ancestors did, is the best way to access the Hun and address energetic disturbances.

There are certain conditions that predispose individuals to experience energy consciously. Water is a medium for Qi in the outside world, just as Blood is in the body. Being near water or increased

---

3. The concept of negative entities persisted, however, particularly with Daoist and Buddhist practitioners who incorporated incantations and exorcism in their treatments.

4. Giovanni Maciocia. *The Psyche in Chinese Medicine; Treatment of Emotional and Mental Disharmonies with Acupuncture and Chinese Herbs*. (Nanjing: Churchill Livingstone, 2009), 71-85.

humidity in the air facilitates connection with non-visible reality. This is why there tends to be more spiritual activity in humid climates or by bodies of water. A humidifier will also increase this action in a dry climate.

Adopting a world view that devalues the spirit and natural world in favor of physical reality is the predominant way to lose touch with the unmanifest realm. Individuals who have not undergone this conditioning, or have somehow eluded it, retain the connection with both worlds. Meditation and qigong are ways adults can re-sensitize themselves to non-materialized Qi. People who are near death also begin to experience spirits and a stronger connection with dreams. Another major reason adults lose awareness of energy is that we are so busy rushing and worrying that we are not present enough to pick up on subtle energy.

These factors relate to Qi awareness; both positive and negative. There are additional factors that make an individual susceptible to negative Qi. An undeveloped Spleen can leave children under the age of 6 or 7 unable to secure their psychic boundaries. It is not until the age of 14, when the Kidneys are fully developed, that girls come into their own power. Additionally, the patterns of Qi and Blood deficiency, Gallbladder deficiency, Insubstantial Phlegm misting the Heart, substance abuse,[5] and Kidney Yang deficiency in adulthood can leave the individual vulnerable to picking up on these energies and being deeply affected by them. These patterns all correlate to weakened psychic boundaries. These patterns will also create issues with holding healthy boundaries in relationship and the inability to exert the Will in the world in a clear way. These patterns can either result from physical deficiency or injury from emotional trauma (particularly childhood abuse).

Children require extra protection from negative energy until they are 14, just as they do from other worldly dangers. Both children and adults can use the treatments in Table 1.1. I find Esoteric Acupuncture very effective, particularly the Crystalline Grid Pattern[6] used in addition to the formulas and points below. In young children, use magnets in place of needles.

Preventing Fear at Night

1. Put your child to bed at a reasonable time, before he/she is excessively tired. When children go to bed exhausted, it weakens their Kidneys and makes them more prone to fear. Sufficient sleep deprivation will create paranoia and fear in anyone.
2. Keep your child's blood sugar stable and avoid hunger. This weakens Qi and Blood and creates a perception of vulnerability. A protein-rich snack before bed helps maintain their blood sugar levels through the night.
3. Avoid too much Phlegm-promoting foods. These include ice cream, sweets, and greasy foods. Phlegm accumulation blurs our perception.

---

5. Addiction itself is an attempt to correct an internal deficiency and creates further opportunities for negative energies to attach.
6. Mikio Sankey. *Sea of Life-Cosmic Fire; Esoteric Acupuncture Volume IV.* (Inglewood: Mountain Castle Publishing; 2006), 257.

Table 1.1. Pattern Differentiation and Treatment of Weakened Boundaries

Patterns	Symptoms	Treatment
Qi and Blood Deficiency	Fatigue. Pallor. Feelings of vulnerability. Weakens ability to hold boundaries against external invasion (from pathogens or negative energy).	Yu Ping Feng San, Gui Pi Tang, Bu Zhong Yi Qi Tang (Huang Qi (astragalus) and all types of ginseng are effective). 4 Doors, St 36, SP 6
Gallbladder Deficiency	Timidity and inability to defend oneself. Feeling anxious and fearful. Fear of the dark. Shyness	Wen Dan Tang + An Mian Pian GB40, HT 7, GB 41, SJ 5
Insubstantial Phlegm Misting the Heart	May or may not be physical Phlegm signs. Will present emotional instability including: mental confusion and muddied discernment. Irrational fears. Mania. Sudden outbursts of anger.	Sheng Tie Luo Yin, Chai Hu Long Gu Mu Li Tang ST 40, Pc 8, KD 1
Kidney (and Liver) Yang Deficiency	Lack of strength to assert the Will in the world and to defend healthy boundaries. Fear of the dark.	You Gui Wan, Hong Shen (steamed ginseng) by itself or in formulas KD 7, ST 36, UB 52

Negative energy can accumulate after an argument or any negative event, from stagnancy, or from the presence of misguided entities. Children, and animals, will often experience trouble with entities when there is emotional turmoil in the home.

When I was a child I used to be able to see spirits and was visited by them in my dreams. I had no filter at that stage in my life so what I saw could be angelic or demonic or anywhere in between. Unable to develop proper discernment, I intentionally shut it down. Empowering children at an early age to deal with the ability to perceive the non-visible world will allow them to be able to integrate these abilities as gifts, rather than something to be frightened of.

There are as many approaches to addressing negative spirits as there are fighting styles and weapons to address physical perpetrators. It is important for children to learn as early as possible that they have a right to healthy boundaries and that no one has a right to cross these. This is strengthening their Yang on a fundamental level, where later they will be able assert themselves in the world in a healthy way. This applies to both boys and girls, however, for girls these skills will continue to be honed into adulthood. As women, our physical, emotional, social, and professional boundaries are challenged more often than men.

Predators, whether energetic or physical, are looking for an opening, a sign of weakness, particularly the vibration of fear. Ironically, the gift predators give us is to highlight our own areas of vulnerability. When we are grounded, aligned in our own truth, and clear on what we want in the world, we deny predators a window of opportunity. This also eliminates the need for war or altercation. Recognizing and steeling oneself to negative Qi is a life-long process of development, but nightmares and ghosts in the closet are an excellent starting point.

Exercise 1.1. Steps for Children to Develop Clear Energetic Boundaries

1. **Discernment:** The first step is for your child to discern energy that makes him/her feel expanded and "good," versus energy that feels prickly, makes him/her feel contracted, and "bad."
2. **Right to Say "No":** Next your child needs to know that if something does not feel right, he/she has the right to keep it out of his/her energy field. Period.[7]
3. **Strength to Defend Boundaries:** Have your child connect to a higher power within him/herself which is more powerful than any external threat. You can introduce the concept of the Higher Self or a spiritual figure, use tools such as a mantra, prayer, or a physical symbol of protection. This focuses the child's attention on empowerment rather than fear.
4. **Allow a Higher Power to do the Work:** Once your child has clarity, rejected the energy, and aligned with a higher power, it is spiritual law that this energy cannot remain. Have your child focus on their higher purpose and ask spirit to bind the energy and remove it from their being. Give your child a visual, such as an angel using a net or whatever symbols your child likes. Sit with this until you and your child feel the energy shift.
5. **Have Faith that it is Done:** The final step is to have faith that it is resolved. Our intention is very powerful. If we focus it on what we fear, we will draw the negative energy back to us.
6. **Get Support:** In less severe cases, it is enough for your child to have your support in forming boundaries. In some cases, whether due to the child's sensitivity or the severity of the situation, children need more support. Acupuncture and herbal treatments can strengthen the body. It is also helpful to have someone who performs energetic clearing come to your home and clear the space for you.

Clearing a Space

All spaces should be cleared from time to time. Consider it maintenance just as we clean our physical space. Space clearing is more important where there have been negative events. The approach I prefer is minimal engagement. This means I neither feel animosity toward any energies nor do I feel sorry for them. I do not try to see what they look like or get drawn into their stories.[8]

7. This step often gets damaged in abuse situations, where people are forced to compromise themselves in order to survive. The act of rejecting will produce feelings of guilt or fear. In these cases a new pattern needs to be relearned, whereby as soon as something does not feel right the immediate response is to say "no".

8. Do not seek out haunted places for a thrill or attempt to contact negative spirits as a game. This is disrespectful to those spirits and can leave you open for negative energies to attach.

Exercise 1.2. Steps to Clearing a Space

1. Set the intention to create harmony and allow it to happen in the most graceful way possible.
2. Take a moment to ground yourself to the center of the Earth. Then connect to Heaven by imagining a white light flowing down to the top of your head. Know you are protected.
3. Invoke a higher power to flood yourself and your surroundings with Light to clear the space. Then imagine a great heavenly vacuum pulling up any debris around you that are not for your highest good. Intend not to see any details, just see gray energy. Keep imagining the vacuum until the gray energy turns into clear white light. Then let it go.[9]
4. During this process, use tools that ground your own sense of sacredness. Be sure to work through the entire space, including corners and closets.

If you need support, seek help from a professional space-clearer (such as Feng Shui practitioners, spiritual and religious teachers, or energy healers). There are cases that require professional assistance, either because the negative energy is too strong or there are personal lessons that need to be addressed.

Using props to create a ritual is not necessary, but it helps to create a feeling of empowerment. The more senses you can engage the better. Use lighting, sound, scents, and symbolism to create a sense of sacredness when performing space clearing. A traditional Feng Shui[10] method is to use a knife to cut a symbolic opening in the air for the negative energy to exit. Use whatever tools attract you.

Exercise 1.3. Space-Clearing Tools

1. **Create Open Space:** Open as many windows and doors as is practical to create airflow.
2. **Lighting:** Turn on all lights and open all the blinds. Keep it this way until the space clearing is complete.
3. **Smudging or Incense**: This engages the help of plant spirits and has a long history cross-culturally. Strong space clearing combinations include: sage bundles, sage with cedar, sandalwood, moxa (mugwort), benzoin with lavender and rosemary, frankincense with myrrh, and coffee grounds with garlic skins and sugar. Some of these can be burned as herb bundles or sticks. Alternately, you can purchase charcoal pellets. Light the charcoal and sprinkle the smudging material on it.
4. **Salt Smudging:** A smokeless and odorless alternative is to take 1 tsp. of Epsom salts and ¼ cup of 90% isopropyl alcohol. Place in a deep mug and light it on fire. Use the same way as smudging.

---

9. Jen Leong (author of *Make it Happen with Feng Shui: Attract What You Want*), in discussion with the author September 2012.

10. Feng Shui is an ancient Chinese system for creating and maintaining harmonious living and working spaces. Daoism divides the world into three levels that influence human life: Heaven, Human, and Earthly. On the Heavenly level, Chinese astrology tells us our destiny; our gifts and challenges. On the Human level, qigong, diet, lifestyle, and other choices allow us to alter our destiny and make our own path. On the Earthly level, Feng Shui allows us to optimize our surroundings and change our "Earth luck."

5. **Essential Oils:** This is a way to invoke the protection of plant spirits without using smoke. Essential oils can be blended or used individually and applied to your skin. Powerful oils include: clove, frankincense, myrrh, benzoin, mugwort, sage, and cinnamon.
6. **Vibration:** Sound a singing bowl, tingsa bells, or chimes and cover the entire space as you would with smudging.
7. **Mantra or Prayer:** This is similar to vibration, only you use your own voice and add words which focus your intention. You can choose a meaningful passage from a sacred book to speak aloud, chant a favorite mantra, or sing a prayer.

Building the Foundation for Health

The *Yellow Emperor's Inner Canon*, the first book on Traditional Chinese Medicine written some 2,500 years ago, defined the focus of medicine on diet, lifestyle, and the maintenance of inner harmony. It changed the focus of medicine from fear of disease to the preservation and expansion of good health. The *Yellow Emperor's Inner Canon* saw flowing with natural cycles as the key to longevity and vitality. Here we will cover seasonal living, Chinese Food Therapy (or medicated diet), lifestyle, meditation, and qigong; the primary tools TCM uses for health.

It is important to instill these habits in your child as he/she matures enough to adopt them. Children are building their health based upon how we nurture them. However, what follows here is intended for all ages. We can adopt these habits at any age to create a foundation for health and vitality.

Daily, Monthly, and Seasonal Cycles

Natural cycles occur on a daily, monthly, and yearly basis. When we live in accordance with these cycles it strengthens our vitality. Every day Yin and Yang go through a cycle. "The yang qi moves like the sun" meaning that as the sun rises, so Yang energy rises in the body.[(11)] Yang peaks at midday then begins to decline as Yin rises. Yin energy peaks at midnight.

The greatest physical activity, biggest meals, and most intense mental focus should be when Yang is strong. To increase our vitality we should rise early, between 6 and 8 a.m. We should eat bigger and more complex meals for breakfast and lunch. We should exercise and do our most intense thinking in the morning and early afternoon.

We should rest and renew ourselves when Yin is strong. This means eating a small simple meal before 7 p.m. (some say before sundown). We should relax after dinner and go to bed by 10 p.m. The most restorative time for sleep is between 10 p.m. and midnight.

Each lunar month the moon undergoes a cycle. When it is full, Yin is at its peak. During the New Moon, when it is barely visible if at all, Yin is at its weakest. Like the moon, women's hormones cycle each month. Adapting one's lifestyle according to the menstrual cycle is one of the most important measures a woman can take to stay young, normalize weight, and improve her health. (The menstrual cycle is covered in Chapter 2). Additionally, women should perform moon meditation to increase the Yin in their bodies (see page 85).

In addition to the daily and monthly natural cycles, there are five seasonal cycles associated with the 5 Elements. Even in areas without distinct seasons, energetic cycling still occurs. An additional consideration is that false climates will create pathology. For example, excessive air conditioning

11. Maoshing Ni, *The Yellow Emperor's Classic of Medicine; a New Translation of the Neijing Suwen with Commentary* (Boston: Shambala, 1995), 10.

mimics sudden winter weather causing Wind Cold. Internal heating in winter creates a hot desert climate and can cause Dry Heat.

Spring - Wood - Detoxification

> *"The three months of the spring season bring about the revitalization of all things in nature. It is the time of birth. This is when heaven and earth are reborn. During this season it is advisable to retire early. Arise early also and go walking in order to absorb the fresh, invigorating energy. Since this is the season in which the universal energy begins anew and rejuvenates, one should attempt to correspond to it directly by being open and unsuppressed, both physically and emotionally.*
>
> *On the physical level it is good to exercise more frequently and wear loose-fitting clothing. This is the time to do stretching exercises to loosen up the tendons and muscles. Emotionally, it is good to develop equanimity. This is because spring is the season of the liver, and indulgence in anger, frustration, depression, sadness, or any excess emotion can injure the liver. Furthermore, violating the natural order of spring will cause cold disease, illness inflicted by atmospheric cold, during summer."*[12]

Spring is a time for expansion, growth, new projects, and cleansing. This is the time to do spring cleaning on a physical and mental level; a process of throwing out what is no longer needed and creating space for new experiences. When the Liver and Gallbladder systems are not healthy, the body and mind will not be able to expand as they naturally should. This can manifest as depression, restlessness, anger, volatility, or tendon stiffness.

Spring is the best time for detoxification, especially of the Liver and Gallbladder. Gallbladder cleansing is recommended yearly during this time as a preventive measure (see Liver and Gallbladder Cleanse page 266). If you have a Gallbladder imbalance such as gallstones, do a series of monthly cleansing during the three months of spring.

During spring, we should eat a higher percentage of raw foods (especially in warmer climates), sprouts, young greens (especially dandelion), mung beans, seaweeds, and a more vegetable-based diet. This is the season to enjoy the lightest meals and simplest cooking of the year. Quickly sauté or steam vegetables so that they are partially raw. Focus on sweet and pungent flavors while limiting salty and heavy foods.[13] Eating this way gently, yet effectively, detoxifies our bodies. Spring is the most appropriate time for fasting as well.

Summer – Fire - Abundance

> *"In the three months of summer there is an abundance of sunshine and rain. The heavenly energy descends, and the earth energy rises. When these energies merge there is intercourse between heaven and earth. As a result plants mature and animals, flowers, and fruit appear abundantly.*

---

12. Ni, *The Yellow Emperor's Classic of Medicine*, 5.

13. Paul Pitchford, *Healing With Whole Foods; Ancient Tradition and Modern Nutrition* (Berkeley: North Atlantic Books, 1993), 276-278.

One may retire somewhat later at this time of year, while still arising early. One should refrain from anger and stay physically active, to prevent the pores from closing and qi from stagnating. One should not overindulge in sex, although one can indulge a bit more than in other seasons. Emotionally, it is important to be happy and easygoing and not hold grudges, so that the energy can flow freely and communicate between external and the internal. In this way illness may be averted in the fall. The season of fire and heart also encompasses late summer, which corresponds to the earth element. Problems in the summer will cause injury to the heart and will manifest in the autumn." [14]

Summer continues spring's expansion into fruitful abundance. This is the season for connection, rapid growth, and creativity. If there is pathology in the Fire (Heart, Pericardium, Small Intestine, and San Jiao) systems the body and mind will not be able to grow and connect, or may do so inappropriately. This can manifest as isolation, mania, promiscuity, over-heating, or anxiety.

In summer, eat bright colors to delight the Heart. Continue eating a more vegetable-based diet, but include more variety to reflect the abundance of summer. As in spring, quickly sauté or steam vegetables, so that they are partially raw. Add spicy and pungent flavors to your diet while limiting salt. Be sure to add fluids to cooking to stay hydrated. Rather than using cold temperature foods (i.e., ice cream) to balance heat, use cold-natured foods such as mung bean soup, raw fruits and vegetables, sprouts, cucumber, bitter melon, lotus leaf tea, watermelon, and citrus. Also, use a little spice, such as pepper and fresh ginger, to open the pores and disperse heat.[15] Thai cuisine is the ideal summer food.

Late Summer – Earth - Harmonization

Late summer, Indian Summer, and the transition between each season correspond to the Earth Element. Late summer is a time when Yang transitions into Yin. It is characterized by ease, harmony, tranquility, and moderation. The week before and after each equinox and solstice also belong to the Earth Element.[16] Pathologies of the Spleen and Stomach surface at this time in the form of digestive issues, lethargy, and unwillingness to make necessary changes.

During the Earth Phases moderate food intake, meaning avoid the extremes of fasting or feasting. Meals should be simple and highlight the bland and sweet flavors. Eat Spleen tonifying foods such as yellow foods, yams, greens beans, Yi Yi Ren (Job's tears), and grains.

Autumn – Metal - Introspection

"In the three months of autumn all things in nature reach their full maturity. The grains ripen and harvesting occurs. The heavenly energy cools, as does the weather. The wind begins to stir. This is the changing or pivoting point when the yang, or active, phase turns into its opposite, the yin, or passive,

14. Ni, *The Yellow Emperor's Classic of Medicine*, 5.
15. Pitchford, *Healing With Whole Foods*, 291.
16. Pitchford, *Healing With Whole Foods*, 300.

> *phase. One should retire with the sunset and arise with the dawn. Just as the weather in autumn turns harsh, so does the emotional climate. It is therefore important to remain calm and peaceful, refraining from depression so that one can make the transition to winter smoothly. This is the time to gather one's spirit and energy, be more focused, and not allow desires to run wild. One must keep the lung energy full, clean, and quiet. This means practicing breathing exercises to enhance lung qi. Also, one should refrain from both smoking and grief, the emotion of the lung. This will prevent kidney or digestive problems in the winter. If this natural order is violated, damage will occur to the lungs, resulting in diarrhea with undigested food in winter. This compromises the body's ability to store in winter."*[17]

In autumn, all of nature begins to withdraw and turn inward. This is a time for introspection, to plan, analyze, and focus. It is a time to become clear on what you have and what you want, though not necessarily the time to take action. Metal imbalances tend to show themselves at this time of year in Lung and Large Intestine pathologies: respiratory ailments, dryness, colds, and trouble letting go.

The diet should include heavier foods with higher amounts of protein and carbohydrates. Cook food longer at lower temperatures. Baking and longer sautéing are best for fall. Include root vegetables and concentrated foods (such as broths) daily. Add astringent and sour tasting foods to meals. Include moistening foods to combat dryness.[18] Specific fall foods include pears, pumpkin, winter squash, lemon, and seasonal foods.

Winter – Water - Tonification

> *"During the winter months all things in nature wither, hide, return home, and enter a resting period, just as lakes and rivers freeze and snow falls. This is a time when yin dominates yang. Therefore one should refrain from overusing the yang energy. Retire early and get up with the sunrise, which is later in winter. Desires and mental activities should be kept quiet and subdued. Sexual desires especially should be contained, as if keeping a happy secret. Stay warm, avoid the cold, and keep the pores closed. Avoid sweating. The philosophy of the winter season is one of conservation and storage. Without such practice the result will be injury to the kidney energy. This will cause wei jue, consisting of weakness, atrophy of muscles, and coldness in spring, manifesting as paralysis, wei/flaccid syndrome, arthritis, or degeneration of the bones and tendons. This is because the body has lost its ability to open and move in spring."*[19]

In winter all of nature stores its energy. It is a time of receptivity and stillness. Take extra time to rest. Focus on building up reserves in preparation for the spring. When the Kidneys and Urinary Bladder are imbalanced there may be intolerance of cold, fatigue, low back or knee soreness, or fear of the future.

The diet should include plenty of hearty soups and stews. Eat heavier, concentrated foods. Include warming spices such as dried ginger, garlic, and cinnamon and Yang tonics such as lamb. Roasting

---

17. Ni, *The Yellow Emperor's Classic of Medicine*, 6.
18. Pitchford, *Healing With Whole Foods*, 306-307.
19. Ni, *The Yellow Emperor's Classic of Medicine*, 6.

and baking are favored cooking methods as they pack in warmth. Increase the salty and bitter tastes in the diet.[20]

Diet; Chinese Food Therapy

One half of our Jing is inherited, the other half is created by diet and breath. This makes optimizing digestion a top priority in preserving health. Because the Spleen is weaker in children and the elderly, dietary rules are more important at these times. Following these dietary rules will strengthen the Spleen, which correlates with a stronger metabolism, a healthier immune system, and increased intellectual functioning. We should not wait until we are sick to begin following these guidelines, but rather start them when we are healthy to maintain health.

The Basic Properties of Foods

Traditional Chinese Medicine advocates eating according to lifestyle. For example, if you do heavy physical work you will do better with animal products. However, if you do not do significant physical activity you may be better suited to a vegetarian diet. If you are a vegetarian or want to minimize meat intake, it is important to include Qi- and Blood-building foods and herbs in your diet regularly (page 223).

An easy way to organize the diet is to balance the three major food categories: carbohydrates (grains and starchy vegetables), protein (meat, legumes, eggs), and fruits and vegetables. TCM does not demonize any food group. Rather, when we understand the qualities of foods and our own constitution, we can choose appropriately. Carbohydrates boost Qi in the body and create Phlegm-Damp when eaten in excess. Protein builds Blood and Yin, and causes Phlegm/Damp-Heat when eaten excessively. Vegetables (particularly raw) are clearing and dispersing, and weaken Qi and Yang in excess. Fruits are also clearing, however they are more cooling and their higher sugar content can destabilize blood sugar, making them less suitable for Qi deficiency and Phlegm-Damp constitutions.

Table 1.2 on the next page indicates the percentages of each food group used to balance different constitutional patterns. For example, someone who

Rules of Eating:

1. Chew your food thoroughly.
2. Eat in a peaceful setting; sitting down.
3. Eat food you enjoy. This strengthens the Spleen and digestion. Eating food you dislike weakens your Spleen. Avoid rigidity.
4. Eat in moderation. Avoid over- or undereating.
5. Eat regular meals, at the same time every day. Eat the biggest meal in the morning and the smallest meal for dinner.
6. Eat dinner by 7 p.m.

20. Pitchford, *Healing With Whole Foods*, 314-315.

is Qi deficient requires a higher percentage of grains in order to tonify Qi. Whereas someone with a Phlegm condition should eat more vegetables.[21]

A simple and safe way to cleanse is to eat a higher proportion of vegetables and to eat less "building" foods (carbohydrates and protein) (see Chapter 6 for a full discussion). Women who are anemic, bleed excessively, are pregnant, or are breastfeeding are not the best candidates to be vegan, which is a cooling, clearing diet. It is important to look at individual deficiencies and excesses and choose a diet that balances the condition.

Table 1.2. Diet Plan According to Constitution

Food Category/ Constitution	Qi or Yang Deficiency	Blood or Yin Deficiency	Liver Qi Stagnation or Excess Heat	Phlegm Damp
Carbohydrates	40-60%	30-40%	30%	30-40%
Protein	10-20%	20-30%	10%	10%
Vegetables & Fruits	30-40%	40-50%	40-60%	40-50%

Thermal Qualities of Food

Foods are categorized as either cold, cool, neutral, warm, or hot. Raw foods, juices, and sprouts are cold. Steaming or slight cooking tends to neutralize foods. Roasting, frying, or cooking in soups makes food more warming. Warmer foods are indicated for cold weather or cold disease patterns. Cooler foods are appropriate to balance hot weather or hot disease patterns. Examples of cooling foods include cucumber, watermelon, mung bean, lettuce, seaweeds, and citrus. Examples of heating foods include lamb, garlic, black pepper, mustard greens, peanuts, oats, and wine. Examples of neutral foods include steamed vegetables, pork, and rye.

The 5 Flavors

The 5 Flavors include: pungent, salty, sweet (and bland), sour, and bitter. TCM advocates eating the 5 Flavors daily to stay healthy. However, certain flavors should be emphasized or avoided to treat imbalances.

Sour foods relate to the Wood element. They are astringing and tightening in action. Sour foods balance dryness by astringing the fluids. They also arrest pathological discharges in the body: diarrhea, leukorrhea (vaginal discharge), spermatorrhea (uncontrolled ejaculation), and excessive sweating. Too much sour foods will keep necessary wastes from being excreted and will injure the tendons. Examples of sour foods include citrus, yogurt, royal jelly, pineapple, and vinegar.

21. Will MacClean, *Clinical Handbook of Internal Medicine: The Treatment of Disease with Traditional Chinese Medicine: Vol 2: Spleen and Stomach*. (Sydney: University of Western Sydney, 2002), 870-887.

The **bitter** taste relates to the Fire element. Bitter foods are drying and cooling and balance excess cases, particularly Phlegm-Damp and Heat. The bitter taste curbs the appetite making it a necessary part of a weightloss program, particularly at the end of meals. Bitter foods also promote elimination through urination and bowel movements. Too much bitter can dry out the body and weaken Qi and Blood. In bone disease avoid the bitter taste. Examples of bitter foods include bitter greens (dandelion, watercress), liver, asparagus, coffee, and bitter melon.

The **sweet** taste relates to Earth. It is tonifying, lubricating, and relaxes muscle spasms. Sweet foods harmonize the other flavors and neutralize toxins. Sweet foods tonify Qi and Blood to build healthy muscle tissue, boost energy, and soothe the emotions. Excess amounts lead to Phlegm-Damp accumulation (weight gain, arterial plaque, and tumors). Examples of sweet foods include sweet potato, carrots, peas, rice, wheat, beef, honey, and peaches.

Bland is an additional flavor associated with the Earth element. It drains Dampness and nourishes the Spleen. Examples include Yi Yi Ren (Job's tears), winter melon, and cucumber.

The **pungent** taste is associated with the Metal element. It has a rising and dispersing action on the body. In small amounts the pungent tastes will balance the cloying effects of other foods, disperse Phlegm, and move Qi and Blood. Pungent foods treat poor circulation and sinus conditions. In excess, pungent foods weaken the Qi and dry out the Yin. Examples of pungent foods are most cooking spices, wasabi, horseradish, cabbage, radish, ginger, wine, and mint.

Salty foods relate to the Water element. They have a consolidating and downward action. They also soften hardness. The salty taste lubricates the intestines to promote bowel movements. Too much leads to Dampness and injures the Blood and bones. Examples of salty foods include seaweeds, millet, miso, and table salt.

Organizing Meals

Meals should follow a 3:2:1 ratio. This means eating the biggest meal in the morning, a medium meal at lunch, and the smallest meal at night. Breakfast should also be the most complex meal, meaning you can eat a combination of carbohydrates, vegetables, and proteins.

In Chinese culture breakfast begins with congee, a watery rice soup. This opens the digestion and tonifies Qi and Blood. Congee is the ideal food for anyone who is deficient, sick, or recovering from illness. Congee can be made out of any grain or combination of grains. Simply add 1 handful of grain to 5-6 times the amount of water and cook 8 hours or overnight. This is ideally done the night before in a slow cooker or rice cooker. (See Congee Recipes page 325). If you have a hard time eating breakfast in the morning it is a sign of excess Phlegm. Eat a small bowl of simple congee with Yi Yi Ren (Job's tears), ginger, and tangerine peel first thing in the morning for a few months.

Lunch should be a slightly smaller meal and be based on vegetables and proteins. Dinner should consist of simple, easy to digest foods. A vegetable-based meal of soup with a salad is ideal.

This describes the ideal meals for most people. For those who are deficient or overweight, small meals every three hours are the best choice. Smaller meals are easier to digest. The frequency of the meals maintains blood sugar levels and boosts the metabolism. Some people may also need a different percentage of foods. For example, Spleen deficient individuals might do best with three grain-based meals.

It is very important to eat organic, fresh food. When foods are genetically modified or grown with pesticides they generate toxins in the body. Processed foods contain too many hidden chemicals, sugars, and poor quality salts which generate Dampness as well as toxify the body. Make an effort to cook as many home-cooked meals as possible. The diet should also be regularly supplemented with fermented foods such as kefir, yogurt, and sauerkraut. If there is any digestive weakness, take fermented foods with every meal (recipes page 331). Always keep bone broth or stock in the freezer to use as the base for soups or congee. This will help strengthen your Kidneys and joints and beautify the skin.

Drinking with Meals

The drinking habits of most Americans during meals break major TCM Food Therapy rules. Avoid drinking water within 30 minutes of a meal as it will dilute digestive enzymes and cool the digestive fire. Iced tea and other cold drinks put out the digestive fire, interrupting digestion. Cold milk has both a cooling nature and temperature making it doubly disruptive to digestion. There is probably no good time to drink soft drinks. There are, however, some drinks that improve the digestive process and should be taken with meals.

A quarter cup of probiotic drink, such as coconut water kefir or beet kavaas, will help digestion. A small amount of alcohol, such as a glass of wine, is fine as well, particularly if you have a cold constitution. Clearing drinks such as tea and coffee should only be taken with meals, where they help keep excess fats from being absorbed. Taken on an empty stomach, however, tea and coffee will weaken Spleen Qi.

Tea and coffee assist with the digestion of food. They contain compounds that help break down fats and stimulate digestion. Taken on an empty stomach, however, they can be too harsh and will damage the Spleen. All coffee and tea can be kept in a plastic zipper bag in the freezer to preserve freshness.

Coffee

Think of coffee as a hotter version of tea. Like tea, it contains alkaloids to help cleanse fats from a greasy meal. However, coffee is much more stimulating and warming. It contains higher amounts of caffeine, giving more energy and stronger effect for migraine headaches. It is a Heart Yang tonic and helps stimulate muscle contractions in the body, including peristalsis. It can be too heating and drying for Yin deficient individuals and those with excess Heat. It is not suitable for those who already have too much muscle tension. It is appropriate for those with Cold or Yang deficiency. Yang deficient individuals can use coffee to settle down at night.

Tea

Tea, from the *Camellia chinensis* plant, has alkaloids that cleanse the digestive tract of Dampness and fats from meals. There is a soapy quality to tea you can test by placing it in a greasy bowl in the sink. Tea is more cleansing and cooling than coffee, the degree to which depends on the type of tea. There are five general categories of tea: black, oolong, puerrh, green, yellow/white, and matcha, as well as various flower versions such as jasmine or osmanthus.

Black tea and **Oolong tea** are oxidized. That is, naturally occurring bacteria on the tea leaves are allowed to ferment. Black tea is completely oxidized. Oolong is oxidized to varying degrees. Like all fermentation, this process mellows out the original substance and makes it more digestible. Black tea and Oolong tea are more appropriate for Spleen deficient people than green tea. They have a more warming and tonifying nature.

Puerrh tea is also fermented. Here, specific microorganisms are added to tea leaves and allowed to ferment. Called "black tea" in Chinese, puerrh has a distinct, earthy flavor and is darker than other teas. Puerrh is the most digestive of the teas. It invigorates the transforming and transporting function of the Spleen, inhibits Dampness, while reducing Heat and descending the Qi of the Stomach. Puerrh also counteracts the effects of excess drinking.

Puerrh is divided into two categories: raw (sheng) and ripe (shu). Raw puerrh is aged using traditional methods underground in bricks, cakes, mushroom shapes, and in bamboo. Aged raw puerrh can be very expensive and some purchase it as an investment, like wine. Young raw puerrh has a unique green, astringent, fermented taste that mellows over time to incredible complexity. Ripe puerrh is processed to ripen quickly making it cheaper and rendering aging unnecessary. Ripe puerrh has a rich, less complex flavor and darker leaves than raw puerrh.

Green tea is unprocessed, unoxidized, and unfermented. It has a limited shelf-life and is best when recently harvested. **White tea** refers to the youngest leaves that do not have as much chlorophyll. Green and white teas, like all "raw" substances, are more cooling and clearing in action. They are also the highest in anti-oxidants. Green and white teas are ideal for those who are Hot-natured. Green tea is often paired with flowers such as jasmine. **Matcha** is powdered green tea tips, making it much more concentrated. Matcha takes practice to prepare correctly as a tea but lends itself to adding to smoothies, desserts, or baked goods.

Maté is not of the tea family. I mention it here because it is another good option to drink with meals. It is used as the vegetable to accompany meat meals by gaúchos (South American cowboys). Maté comes in both raw green and roasted. It boosts Qi, contains high levels of chlorophyll, and has a cleansing action.

Table 1.3. Properties of Tea, Coffee, and Maté

Hot Drink	Properties
Coffee	Heart Yang tonic. Resolves Dampness and can deplete Yin. Can aggravate Heat and tension in the body.
Black Tea	Called "red tea" in Chinese. Fully oxidized (fermented) tea. Warming, ascending, diaphoretic qualities.
Oolong Tea	Partially oxidized tea. Beautiful, perfume-like fragrances. Warming, ascending, diaphoretic qualities. Taken with chrysanthemum for high cholesterol and slow metabolism.
Puerrh Tea	Fermented and aged tea. Called "black tea" in Chinese. Earthy, rich flavor. Most digestive. Taken with chrysanthemum to lower cholesterol and increase fat metabolism.
Maté (green and roasted)	Different family. Boosts energy. Allays hunger. Good quality is bright green and fresh tasting.
Matcha Green Tea	Powdered, concentrated green tea.
Green/White Teas	Least processed and lowest in caffeine. Often combined with flowers such as jasmine.

Chinese Tea Culture

As cultures industrialize and become separated from whole foods, liquids become a vehicle for sugar and chemicals to enter the body. The bitter taste then disappears entirely from the palate, and the population becomes obese. There are other factors such as sedentary lifestyle, genetic modification of foods, pesticides, and sick and hormone enhanced animal products, that have injured our society's general health. However, an aversion to drinking pure water and drinks without artificial flavorings is a sign of imbalance. Chinese tea culture stands in opposition to this. Aside from the numerous health benefits, drinking tea the traditional way brings the mind to the present moment and resets the palate. It re-sensitizes the tongue to subtle flavors that have been bombarded with the taste of garish chemicals.

I missed out on well-brewed tea for years because I was turned off by the perceived snobbery and complication of tea ceremony. Chinese tea culture is more about enjoyment of tea than the ceremony. You can learn intricate steps later if you wish, but here I will tell you how to simply enjoy the benefits of tea. A little ceremony is good for centering, and some cute utensils make it fun. Drinking tea the traditional way will transform the experience.

Recipe 1.1. Simple Steps to Good Tea

1. Buy good quality loose leaf tea. Get a tea pot that holds 4-8 ounces of water with a strainer that sits inside.
2. Bring water to a boil.

3. Fill teapot with hot water, then pour the water into the drinking cup. Discard the water. This warms the teapot and the cup.
4. Put about 1 tbsp. of tea into the teapot.
5. Fill the teapot again with hot water. Discard immediately. This washes the tea and is most important in puerrh tea.
6. Fill the teapot a third time with hot water. Allow to steep for about 30 sec.
7. Pour into your cup. Make sure you smell the fragrance of your tea and enjoy the experience of it.
8. A good tea can be steeped 3-5 more times. Add an additional 30 sec of brewing time to each subsequent brewing. This will be 1 min of brewing the second time, etc.

Cooking Medicinal Decoctions

Always rinse the herbs in a colander, just like you wash your drinking tea. Cover with water (usually 4-5 cups) and soak the herbs for 30 min. Simmer the herbs for 45 min. to extract the Yang. Strain. Add more water. Simmer for 45 min. to extract the Yin. Strain and combine with first decoction. If a third cooking is desired, add more water. Simmer for 45 min. to extract the Jing. Strain and combine with the other two decoctions.

Self-Cultivation Exercises

I had incredible spiritual experiences as a child wandering in nature or daydreaming; without any knowledge of spiritual practices. To be with the spirit realm felt to me as if I were spending time with friends. I had no agenda beyond the desire to be in the presence of the Divine and I felt no sense of time. I remember the feelings of awe, innocence, and knowing my place in the universe.

In my teens and 20s, I studied various forms of meditation and spiritual practice. Its supportive structure would invariably grow oppressive to me, however. I would hear, "Oh, I'm not good at yoga (or meditation, etc.)" and feel that self-cultivation was something I could fail at. There were gurus and authorities I was supposed to listen to above my own authority. These disciplines were useful, as long as I did not place spiritual power outside of myself; to a particular practice, movement, or teacher. The moment I handed my power over, I would cease to reach the states I had felt effortlessly as a child.

The purpose of self-cultivation is to make our true selves fully present. The process of self-cultivation requires us to train our intention. It requires that we find a balance between structure and formlessness; between the child and the wise crone within. We must do our work. Then we must develop the patience to wait for Grace to bestow its gifts, on its own time. There is no failing, no competition, and no rush.

As children we naturally get lost in the world of the Hun, the realm of undivided consciousness, if given the time and freedom to do so. Children need to learn to still their bodies and their minds in such a way that trains their intention without harming their natural intuitive gifts. They also need time to explore and be without a purpose. Further, children need to create their play, without too many props, toys, or organized games. As parents, it is our job to create opportunities for children to develop and retain their natural gifts while learning necessary respect and discipline. Women tend to have more intuitive gifts, but self-cultivation is crucial for both males and females of all ages.

This section provides easy exercises that children can use. They are fundamental practices that can be followed for a lifetime, at every age. If you are new to qigong and self-cultivation, this is the place to begin.

Intention

"Intention is everything," is a common saying in Traditional Chinese Medicine and qigong. Our intention refers to what we align our spirit, emotions, thoughts, and body to. We use self-cultivation exercises to train this alignment of intention. Certain exercises focus on developing attributes in the body, others on mental functioning, the emotions, or the spirit. Over time, it all becomes one training.

As we practice self-cultivation, we get to know ourselves. We discover parts of ourselves we like and parts of ourselves we want to change. Internal Alchemy exercises, covered in Chapter 3, are a type of self-cultivation that transform the unbalanced or self-sabotaging aspects of ourselves. For now, use spiritual practice as a time to focus on your soul's purpose or a virtue you hold dear such as peace, abundance, or love. What you focus on in practice will increase in your daily life.

Practicing self-cultivation over time purifies the intention, so that we are naturally virtuous and every part of ourselves is in alignment with these virtues. The competition of our Wood element turns into kindness. The overstimulation of our Fire element turns into peaceful bliss. The worry of our Earth element turns into faith in the Divine acting within ourselves. The grief of our Metal element turns into integrity. The fear of our Water turns into wisdom.

Calming the Mind

Modern society and technology conditions us to be in a state of constant seeking. Quieting the mind is challenging in an over-stimulated world out of touch with natural cycles. Additional tools are sometimes necessary in order to be able to sit in meditation, or relax into a qigong or yoga class. Rigorous physical exercise prior to meditation can be helpful when the Liver is in excess or the body has too much pent up energy. Sometimes it takes the help of another person to quiet us. Acupuncture, massage, and energy work such as Reiki are very effective to bring us back into our bodies and the present moment. These modalities are especially helpful when we are new to meditation so we know the feeling we want to achieve. Herbs and diet can also help us focus. See Table 1.4.

It is important to change our attitude towards self-cultivation. Mystics from different religious traditions often speak of the Divine as a lover. There is no struggle to quiet the mind or stay in the present moment when we are with a lover. This may not be an appropriate metaphor for children, but we need to make self-cultivation time something we look forward to and enjoy. Having this attitude also means that your time consciously connecting with spirit is not limited to spiritual practice, but rather allows it to spill over into every moment of your life.

Table 1.4. Pattern Differentiation and Treatment to Settle the Mind

Symptoms	Diet	Formula
When you try to still your mind, confrontations and resentments come up. You find yourself battling to make it to yoga class and fighting for mat space when you get there. In more extreme cases, you feel drawn to yelling, hitting things, and intensity. Fighting energizes you. Maybe you see yourself as part of the spiritual elite. You find yourself judging others often and have no trouble voicing it.	Follow a Heat- clearing diet: increase percentage of vegetables and raw foods. Decrease meat, alcohol, caffeine, sugars, spices, and garlic.	Shu Gan Wan Long Dan Xie Gan Tang

Symptoms	Diet	Formula
When you try to still your mind it simply will not shut off. Confrontations, deadlines, and resentments come up, but you feel drained rather than energized by them. You feel stressed out and frustrated. Perhaps you feel stuck, depressed, and even worthless.	Eat regular meals and whole foods. Balance fruits and vegetables with healthy protein and carbohydrates. Be present when you eat.	Jia Wei Xiao Yao San
As soon as you try to still yourself you are overcome with anxiety. You are unsettled and you can't ground yourself. Stress has turned to panic.	Eat regular meals and whole foods. Balance fruits and vegetables with healthy protein and carbohydrates. Be present when you eat.	Chai Hu Long Gu Mu Li Tang
When you still yourself you start to cry. You feel vulnerable, unloved, and unable to cope. Maybe it is your hormones or maybe life is just too much. You cannot remember having a decent night's sleep.	Eat Blood and Yin nourishing foods: increase intake of protein and leafy greens. It can also be due to low blood sugar.	Gan Mai Da Zao Tang + Long Gu (fossilized bone), Mu Li (oyster shell)
The flashes of heat disrupt your concentration. You feel irritable and impatient. You find yourself engaging in battles over the thermostat.	Increase percentage of vegetables. No alcohol, caffeine, sugars, spices, or garlic. Take Jing tonics (page 285)	Zhi Bai Di Huang Wan + Jia Wei Xiao Yao San

Rituals and props are helpful to associate with meditation practice so that the mind will more quickly go into a meditative state. They engage the senses. When the senses are stilled, the Po (corporeal soul) is still, which in turn calms the Shen (conscious mind). The Hun (ethereal soul) is then free to connect with Source.[22]

For example, have a favorite blend of calming essential oils or incense burning to engage your sense of smell. Use a singing bowl, tingsa bells, or a gong to engage your hearing. Chanting mantras aloud also engages your ears, as well as creating strong, unifying vibration in the body. Use beads to engage your sense of touch.

Exercises to Still the Mind

Exercise 1.4. Yoni Mudra[23] (Figure 1.1)

"Yoni" is the Sanskrit word for uterus. The Yoni mudra places us in a fetus-like state; internally focused with our external senses closed off.

1. Spread out the fingers of each hand and use them to close your ears, eyes, nostrils, and

22. Giovanni Maciocia. *The Psyche in Chinese Medicine; Treatment of Emotional and Mental Disharmonies with Acupuncture and Chinese Herbs*. (Nanjing: Churchill Livingstone, 2009), 36-39.

23. This mudra comes from kriya yoga (a type of yoga). Mudras are symbolic hand gestures that are combined with special breathing in yogic practice.

mouth as shown in the picture: Close your ears with your thumbs. Cover your eyes with your index fingers. Gently touch your nostrils with your middle fingers so that you can still breathe. Place your ring fingers on the upper lip and the pinkies under the mouth, closing the mouth together.
2. Inhale deeply.
3. Press the nostrils closed and hold your breath for a moment.
4. Release your nostrils. Hum on the exhale so that it sounds like bees buzzing in your head.
5. Repeat.

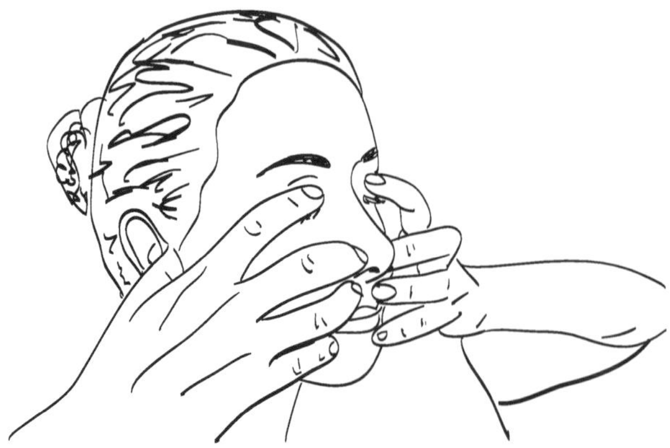

Figure 1.1. Yoni Mudra

Exercise 1. 5. Inner Sight Meditation (Figure 1.2)

This meditation stills the mind and helps develop your inner sight.

1. Take a deep breath in.
2. Swallow and touch your tongue to the roof of your mouth.
3. As you hold your breath, imagine you are looking at your third eye area (the region between your eyebrows) from the back of your skull.
4. Slowly exhale, releasing your tongue. But keep your focus on looking at your third eye from the inside.
5. Breathe in again. Swallow and touch your tongue to the roof of your mouth.
6. Hold your breath and focus.
7. Exhale, relax. Continue as long as you like.

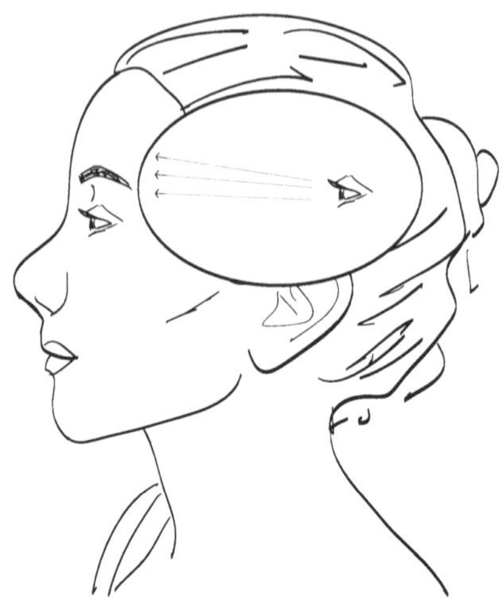

Figure 1.2. Inner Sight Meditation

Exercise 1. 6. Grace Prayer

This is my modification of Thich Nhat Hanh's Meditation Poem.(24) Use it throughout the day to stay connected or in seated meditation. Speak the words to yourself in your mind, not out loud.

1. "In" (inhale)
2. "Out" (exhale)
3. "Deep" (inhale)
4. "Slow" (exhale)
5. "Kindness" (inhale)
6. "Grace" (exhale)
7. "Beautiful Moment" (inhale)
8. "Present Moment" (exhale)

Training Your Right Brain(25)

We live within boundaries of perception that limit our full creative potential. Society promotes the overdevelopment of the left brain (logic, language, rules) while discrediting the use of the right brain (intuition, symbols, creativity). By learning to view the world with our right brain we connect consciously with our Hun, and see the world through the eyes of an artist. An optimal mind is able to utilize creativity and logic equally. The right side of our brains sees the world as an interaction of lines, colors, and textures. To see this you will need to change the focus of your sight.

1. Look at a group of objects.
2. Now look at the negative space around the objects and forget the objects. Notice the shape and color between the objects. Allow this space to become pregnant and alive.
3. Spend an entire day looking at negative space. Forget the names, purpose, or story of the objects around you. Notice how the world immediately opens up and you become present.

Proper use of negative space is what makes a work of art. This same technique can be applied to other art forms. The next time you hear a song, listen for the space between the drum beats. This simple practice brings tremendous insights.

Learning How to Breathe

Breathing and diet are the two ways we take in Qi from our environment. Breathing properly is thus a major component to good health. The breath is also one of the most powerful tools to control the mind. Conscious manipulation of the breath connects us with our Po (corporeal soul). It allows us to affect the unconscious functioning of our body and mind.

24. Thich Nhat Hanh, *The Heart of the Buddha's Teaching; Transforming Suffering into Peace, Joy, and Liberation*. (Berkeley: Parallax Press,1998).
25. Miya Hannan "Using Negative Space" (lecture, Cinnabar Clinic, San Diego, CA, April 15, 2012).

Exercise 1.7. Breath of Fire

The breath of fire is a classic yoga breathing technique. Alvaro Romano, creator of Ginastica Natural, uses this adapted fire breathing exercise to recover quickly during physical exercise. Building lung capacity and breath control in this way increases our power during physical exertion.

1. Begin fire breathing, inhale and exhale quickly and forcefully creating a bellows with your abdomen. To start, place your hand on your belly button. Feel the belly button draw in sharply on the exhale. Feel the belly button distend completely on the inhale. Begin slowly exaggerating the movement, then speed up until you are going as fast as you can. Continue for 1 min.
2. Then inhale quickly and forcefully.
3. Very, very slowly exhale. Alvaro Romano takes a full minute to exhale. At first you may only be able to last a few seconds.

Exercise 1.8. Square Breath[26] (Figure 1.3)

The breath has four distinct phases: inhalation, hold, exhalation, hold. The amount of time spent on each section can be used to affect your energy. Inhaling elevates your energy. Holding on the inhale keeps your energy up. Exhaling grounds your energy. Holding on the exhale keeps your energy grounded. If you spend equal time on each part this is balanced breathing. If you spend extra counts on exhale, for example, you will feel more grounded. If you spend extra counts on the inhale you will feel more elevated.

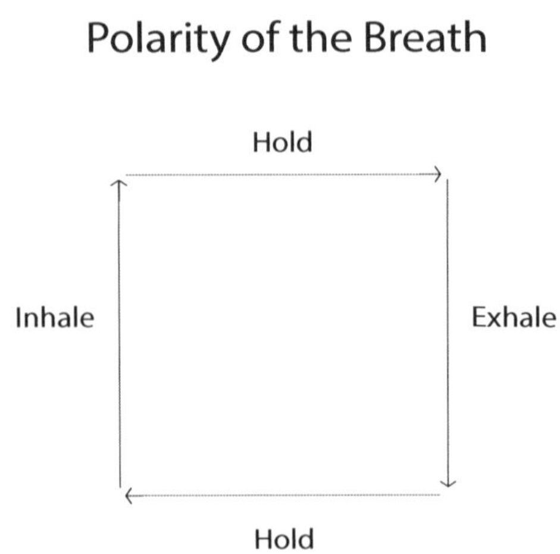

Figure 1.3. Square Breath

Qigong

Infinite styles of qigong were developed over the centuries and continue to evolve. They range from simple exercises to complicated routines, from ancient lineage-based practices to modern forms founded on scientific trials. I find the exercises that work best for me are the simple, repetitive ones. These allow me to observe my breath, my energy, and my thoughts rather than getting flustered on the routine. Others respond better to a complicated pattern. You want something you will perform on a regular basis. There are also impromptu opportunities. A meditation in nature, standing under the stars, walking with your dogs; these can be simple forms of qigong that are readily available. The following are a few fundamental exercises.

26. For more please see: Hidayat Inayat Khan. *Sufi Teachings; Lectures from Lake O'Hara.* (Victoria: Ekstasis Editions, 1994), 106-118.

Exercise 1.9. Shaking

The more tense you are, the less you can feel and the less present you are. It will speed up your practice if you spend a few minutes relaxing. I like to do this whenever I feel myself getting tense. Children take to this one quickly.

1. Stand with your feet hip width apart, knees slightly bent. Now begin to shake. Move from the knees only.
2. After 1-3 min, begin to rotate your torso side to side as you shake.
3. Then begin to bend side to side as you shake.
4. Stop when you are ready.

Shake for at least 3 min. If you continue for 20 min. you will reduce your tension dramatically.

Exercise 1.10. Standing Meditation

This is a foundational exercise used in many qigong traditions. It is incredibly grounding and empowering. Standing meditation takes us in the opposite direction of our overstimulated society. Be prepared for feelings of boredom, anxiety, agitation, and worry to surface. This exercise is particularly effective to control ADD or ADHD, anxiety, and to balance spiritual practice.

1. Begin with your feet hip width apart. Bend your knees slightly. Tuck your pelvis under so that you feel your quadriceps (front thighs) light up and your gluteal muscles (buttocks) relax. Make small adjustments until you find a position that feels almost effortless.
2. Bring your arms up in front of you as if you were hugging a tree. Relax your arms and let your elbows hang. Feel as if your arms are supported from underneath.
3. Touch your tongue to the roof of your mouth and slightly tense your pubococcygeus muscle (muscle that stretches from the pubic bone to the tail bone) to close your circuit.
4. Stand here for 20 min. (Young children will need to begin with smaller increments.) Use a timer or cell phone app so you do not have to look at the time. In most people this will bring up the desire to flee. Allow things to come up and pass through you. You can work up to an hour using small increments of time.

Exercise 1.11. Tapping (Figure 1.4)

Tapping wakes up the meridians,[27] increases circulation, and detoxifies the body. It can be performed prior to qigong practice or as its own exercise. In this exercise we use a loose fist and generally cover the meridians. Some traditions cover each meridian in more detail and use props: rattan sticks (to increase pain tolerance), steel rods (to strengthen the bones and Kidneys), or wooden rods (to increase circulation in the skin).[28]

---

27. Meridians are the channels or circuits through which Qi (energy) flows in the body.

28. These can be found in various qigong websites. For example, Mantak Chia retails metal and bamboo hitters on his website www.Healing-Tao.com and explains their use in his book *Bone Marrow Nei Kung*.

1. Make loose fists and tap the body, following the lines in Figure 1.4. Work down the inside of your legs, up the outsides, ending at the Kidneys. Tap the Kidneys (back of the lower ribs) for a moment.
2. Tap around the chest, clockwise and counterclockwise.
3. Tap under the armpit, down the inside of the arm, up the outside, ending at the top of the shoulder.

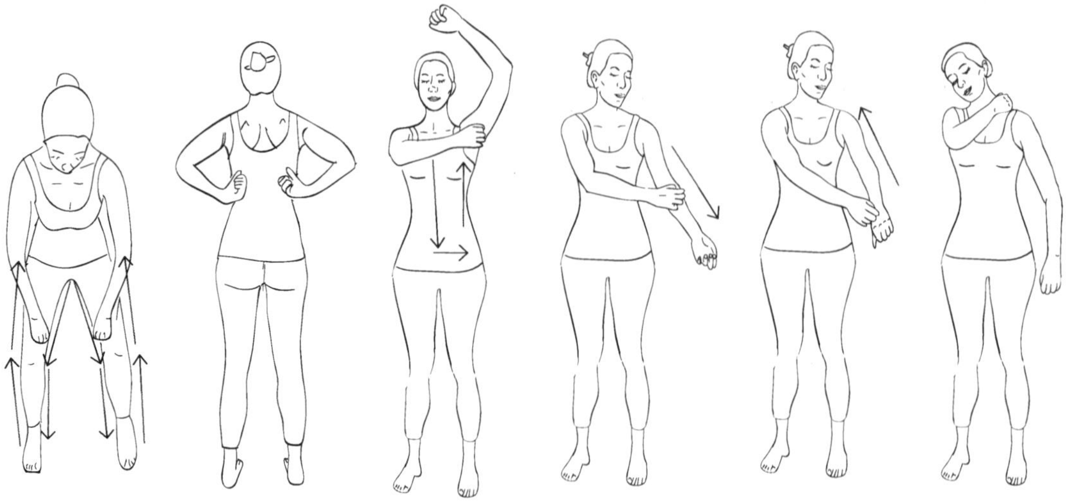

Figure 1.4. Tapping

Exercise 1.12. Connecting with Heaven and Earth

As humans, we stand between Heaven and Earth. When we honor our place in the universe we attain harmony and freedom. The freedom is from our false isolation, arrogance, and over- complication. This simple exercise can be done at any time we need centering.

1. Close your eyes and place your hands over your heart. Bring your attention into your heart space. Imagine this is where you see the world from.
2. Imagine a distant star, the sun, or the moon. Feel that star connect down through the top of your head all the way to your heart. Feel this connection as a loving maternal or paternal energy that loves and guides you in your life. Feel love and gratitude in return.
3. Now imagine the center of the Earth. Imagine it as bright as the star. Feel the Earth's center connect up through the bottoms of your feet, up your lower torso, up to your heart. Feel this connection as a nurturing maternal or paternal energy that supports and provides for you in your life. Feel love and gratitude in return.
4. Rest your attention in your heart. Feel how Heaven and Earth are anchored here. Let this place be your source.

This meditation is especially useful before making a decision or dealing with conflict.

Exercise 1.13. Moon Meditation (Figure 1.5)

Moon meditation is a key exercise for both men and women to connect with monthly cycles. It is particularly important for women to develop a deep connection with the Moon. The Moon is gentle, luminous, and controls the earthly cycles, including our menstruation. This is true Yin Power. Connecting with the Moon increases our Yin energy. Moon meditation is traditionally performed a few days prior to, until a few days after the full Moon, when the Moon is at least half full. You may sit or stand. You have two choices:

Moon Meditation #1

1. Take a moment to connect to your heart.
2. Inhale. Look up to and connect with the Moon.
3. Exhale. Close your eyes and connect down to the center of the Earth. See the center of the Earth as another Moon.
4. Repeat for several minutes or as long as you like. Remember that the purpose is to build a relationship.

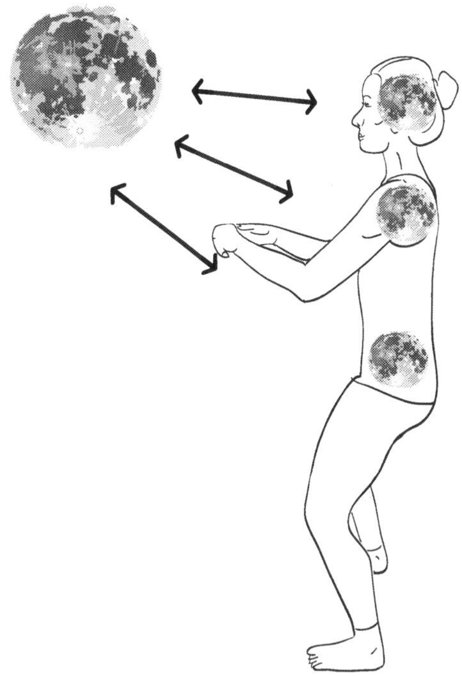

Figure 1.5. Moon Meditation #2

Moon Meditation #2

In Daoist practice there are 3 major energy centers, or Dan Tians. The lower Dan Tian is located in the lower abdomen. The middle Dan Tian is located in the heart area. The upper Dan Tian is located behind the Third Eye area. See Figure 1.5.

1. Close your eyes. Imagine a ball of pearly white light in your upper Dan Tian, behind your third eye. Open your eyes to look at the Moon. Inhale, receive the Moon's loving energy into your upper Dan Tian. Exhale, send loving energy from your upper Dan Tian to the Moon. Repeat until you feel your upper Dan Tian glow.
2. Close your eyes. Imagine a ball of pearly white light in your middle Dan Tian, in your heart space. Open your eyes to look at the Moon. Inhale, receive the Moon's loving energy into your middle Dan Tian. Exhale, send loving energy from your middle Dan Tian to the Moon. Repeat until you feel your middle Dan Tian glow.
3. Close your eyes. Imagine a ball of pearly white light in your lower Dan Tian, below your navel in the area of your womb. Open your eyes to look at the Moon. Inhale, receive the

Moon's loving energy into your lower Dan Tian. Exhale, send loving energy from your lower Dan Tian to the Moon. Repeat until you feel your lower Dan Tian glow.

4. Imagine a rod or cone of pearly white light running down the centerline of your body merging the three balls of light. Take a few breaths to integrate.

As you practice moon meditation you will begin sensing the fullness of the Moon through her cycle.

Exercise 1.14. Sun Meditation

You can perform the same exercises with the Sun and with the stars. Star gazing is particularly healing for Liver Yang Rising conditions. The Sun meditation can be performed daily to increase Yang energy in the body. The Sun nurtures us and our planet in a distinct way to the Moon. The Sun is consistent, bold, and intense.

When connecting with the Sun there are two modifications to the above exercise. First, imagine warm, golden light. Second, do not stare at the Sun directly. Either connect with your eyes closed or gaze at filtered sunlight.

Exercise 1.15. Pouring Your Heart to the Earth

This is my mom's exercise to let go of painful emotions.

1. Lie face down with your heart to the ground; your legs and arms outstretched and your head turned to the side. Relax everything.
2. Connect to your heart. Breathe into it.
3. Feel the connection between your heart and the center of the Earth.
4. Feel into your feelings, letting them run through your heart to Mother Earth. There is no judgment on what you should or should not feel. Feel each feeling fully and embrace it with compassion. Then let it run through you. There is usually another feeling underneath. It may take a while, but you will get to a core feeling. Once you feel it fully and release it, there will be a huge sense of relief. The proper action to take, or not take, will come clearly at this point.

This is the end of preparing the foundation. In the next chapter we dive headlong into puberty and the menstrual cycle of a young girl. It includes directives for all menstruating women, not just girls between 14 and 20.

Chapter 2

Age 14

2 x 7, The dew of Heaven arrives (menstruation), the REN channel begins to flow, the Chong channel is flourishing, the periods come regularly and she can conceive.

二七，而天癸至，任脉通，太冲脉盛，月事以时下，故有子；（14岁）

The 2nd Cycle

Two x 7 begins the 2nd Cycle in a young woman's life. At the age of 14 she will enter the Fire Phase, where she will stay until she is 21 years old. The Fire Phase is characterized by emotionality, new connections, experimentation, and the search for excitement. The Chong Mai, or "Sea of Blood," connects at puberty. Prior to the first menstruation, the Tian Kui, the intricate network of the endocrine system, is activated. The menstruation is referred to as the "Red Dragon" in Daoism, and like the mythical dragon, its first stirring leaves turmoil in its wake. Leading up to and after menarche (the first period) there are often mood swings, changes in physical features, and crisis of identity. Young girls may experience leukorrhea (vaginal discharge) and yeast infections. (The transition of menopause can cause similar disruption).

Menstruation, particularly the early years after menarche, is the first of the three "Golden Opportunities" to greatly influence a woman's constitution. This means the potential exists to either exponentially increase vitality or devastate the constitution. The other opportunities will be postpartum and menopause; two other times of great transition. When hormonal issues are present in girls under the age of 21, treatment should focus on the Kidneys. This is because the Kidneys, and particularly the Kidney Yang, drive development. This chapter covers Traditional Chinese Medical views on the menstrual cycle, the Menstrual Renewal Program, and common imbalances.

The Red Dragon Descends

I first got my period in the midst of family tragedy. My beloved grandfather had just passed away and my mom was in Brazil organizing the funeral. My father had to work so he left my younger brother and I with my paternal grandparents. I had no connection with them so when my period came I did not tell a soul. I figured it would be one more inconvenience for my grandparents. I had also assumed the role as my brother's guardian and felt I had to take care of us. I knew what it was and luckily I bled so little that I was able to use toilet paper. I believe that the circumstances surrounding my first period set the stage for my later hormonal problems.

My mom, in contrast, had had a model experience. When her first period came my grandfather immediately threw her a party to commemorate her transition into womanhood.[1] That my mom was supported by her community, and particularly by her male role model, was such a gift. It sent a clear message that having a period and being a woman is special. My mom never suffered from menstrual problems and she missed her menstruation when she went through menopause.

The first period should be treated as the rite of passage that it is. This is a great gift to a girl as it instills a sense of reverence for the power of her own body. How a woman regards her menstruation directly correlates to how she regards herself as a woman. Menstruation is often referred to as "the curse" or "being on the rag" and other disrespectful names, or it is not spoken of at all as if it were some great secret. This attitude creates disharmony in the body and is a poor example to young girls who are developing their feminine identity. Many women are beginning to refer to their period as "being on their moon," a much more poetic and apt phrase.

Menarche is worthy of a special gift, celebration, or trip. For women who never received this, it is important to treat menstruation as a special time of the month. This chapter covers proper care during the four phases of the monthly cycle. This cycle connects women tangibly to the cycles of the moon and earth. Living in tune with this cycle will regulate weight, increase attractiveness, improve athletic and mental performance, increase emotional awareness, and strengthen health exponentially.

---

1. My grandfather was born into a macho rural Brazilian culture, which was balanced by the strong women who raised him. He showed uncharacteristic reverence for women.

The Menstrual Cycle

The menstrual cycle walks through the circle of Yin and Yang; the cycle of birth, growth, and death; the extremes of feminine and masculine, and balance. This cycle puts women intimately in touch with universal cycles, such as daily solar transitions, monthly lunar cycles, and the seasons. The menstrual cycle also functions as a precise diagnostic tool. Disturbances within the cycle offer immediate, direct information about imbalances in the body.

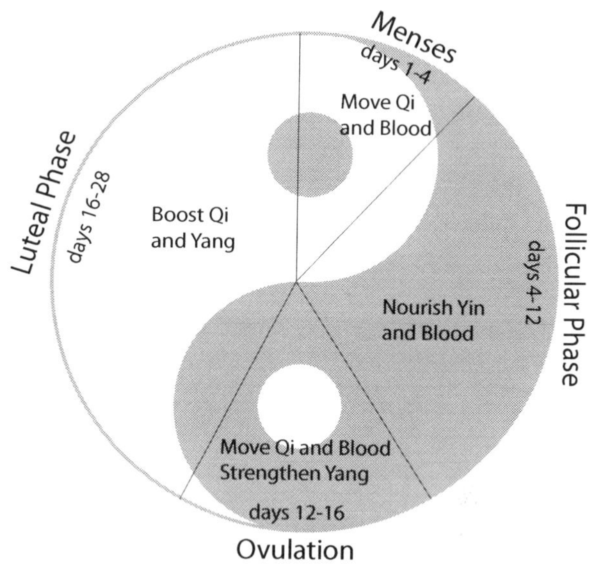

Figure 2.1. Menstrual Cycle

Cycle Overview

First let us define what constitutes a healthy menstruation, as there is a great deal of confusion on this topic. The length of the cycle, the quality and duration of bleeding, and any attendant symptoms are all factors. The length of a normal cycle is 28-30 days. A cycle that is five days longer or shorter is considered abnormal. Additionally, cycle intervals should be regular. A cycle that fluctuates is considered irregular even if each cycle is within normal range; in other words, if one cycle is 25 days long and the next is 35 days long, it is considered irregular.

The normal color of menstrual blood is red, without clots. The normal volume is between 50-80 ml.[(2)] The normal duration of menstruation is 3-5 days. Bleeding less or longer is considered abnormal. Spotting before, after, or between periods is considered abnormal. Also, menstruation closer to the full moon indicates a more excess constitution. Bleeding closer to the new moon indicates a more deficient condition.

After menstrual bleeding has ceased, the body works to restore the Yin and Blood that was lost; this corresponds to increasing estrogen levels. Mid-cycle, ovulation is triggered by a quick surge in Kidney Yang; corresponding to a rise in Luteinizing Hormone which stimulates ovulation. Yang energy stays high until the next menses, corresponding to rising progesterone levels. There is another spike in Yang, in the form of Liver Yang Rising right before the period. Once the Yang reaches its peak, extreme Yang collapses into extreme Yin, and the menses begins, corresponding to a sharp drop in estrogen and progesterone. The menses is a time of rest and heightened sensitivity. It is a little death of the life that could have been.

2. This is considered less useful as a diagnostic. It is tricky to measure unless you use an insert like a Diva Cup. Otherwise it becomes a relative comparison to what is normal for you, or if you are using far more or less sanitary items than other women.

Mapping the Cycle

Using a Basal Body Temperature (BBT) chart to track the cycle offers valuable information about hormonal functioning and the fluctuations of Yin and Yang in the body. It requires taking the temperature consistently each day at the same time, preferably before getting out of bed in the morning, then charting it on a BBT chart. Figure 2.2 below shows an ideal BBT chart. There are lower consistent temperatures during and just after menses (menstruation and follicular phases). Mid-cycle, the temperature spikes sharply within a 24-hour period, corresponding to ovulation. After this spike there are consistently raised temperatures until the next menses (luteal phase), when the temperature drops again. Temperatures that are too high during menses and the follicular phase (from the onset of menstruation to ovulation) indicate Blood and/or Yin deficiency. If there is no mid-cycle spike, this shows there was no ovulation. If the chart fails to show consistently high temperatures after ovulation, there is a deficiency in Qi and/or Yang. A zigzag pattern often indicates Qi and Blood deficiency. Charting creates a sense of connection with the cycle and is helpful in cases of infertility.

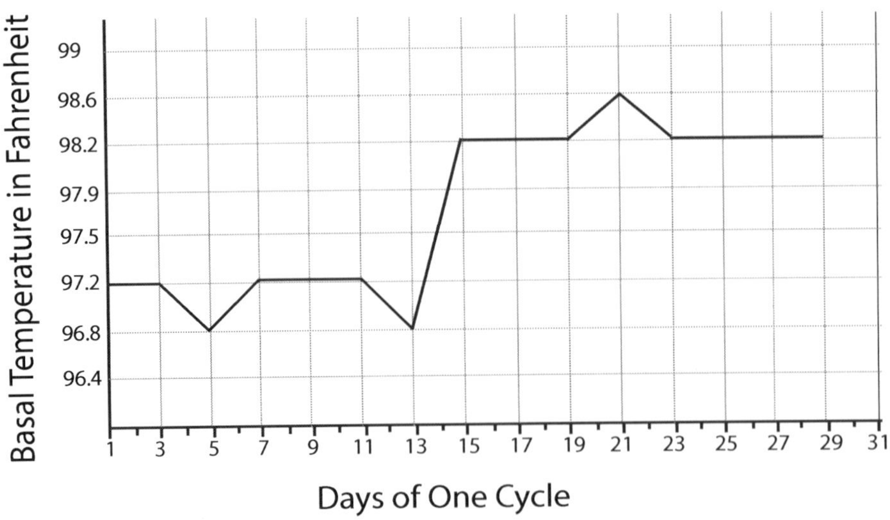

Figure 2.2. Ideal Basal Body Temperature Chart

The Menstrual Renewal Program

Traditional cultures gave women ritualized rest during their menses, often under the guise of "making it safe for the rest of society." This allowed women repose from cooking, cleaning, farming, sex, child care, and the endless other duties expected of them. This monthly period of rest increased vitality and fertility and provided many other benefits.

The Menstrual Renewal Program is a shorter, simpler version of the Postpartum Recovery Program detailed in Chapter 4, and contains the same treatment principles. There are many variations of this program that were practiced traditionally throughout mainland China and Taiwan. The version below is based on the teachings of Dr. Shuqi Zhuang,[3] my teachers, as well as my clinical and personal experience. I include traditional Chinese wisdom which I have adapted to modern life.

Benefits of the Menstrual Recovery Program

Following the lifestyle and dietary guidelines presented in this chapter helps women recover their energy, stay young, balance hormones, maintain their weight, and prevent disease. The Jing (Essence) is tied to the energy used to create new life and is focused in the Kidneys, eggs, and sperm. Women lose Jing through childbearing and menstruation. Men lose Jing through ejaculation. For women to optimize youth and vitality, we must rejuvenate during menstruation and after giving birth. Beyond the physical health benefits, this conserved Jing can be harnessed for spiritual cultivation.[4]

In men, this is accomplished through ejaculation control, in which men learn to orgasm without ejaculation, thus controlling the frequency of ejaculation. Women deplete Kidney Qi with excessive sexual activity, especially when they start too young, during menses, pregnancy, postpartum, when drinking or doing drugs, or when they are over-worked, however it takes far more effort. In my observations, sex is most injurious to women when they are not honored.[5]

The Menstrual Renewal Program is more important today as women are having fewer or no children. There is a trade-off between the number of pregnancies and the number of menstruations a woman has in her lifetime. Liver Blood is lost every month through menstruation and must be replenished. Pregnancy taxes the Kidneys, but gives the woman's body a rest from monthly bleeding, conserving Liver Blood.[6] Thus, more pregnancies mean more strain on the Kidneys, but spare the Liver Blood. More menstrual cycles tax Liver Blood, but spare the Kidneys. If the only factor is the woman's body, multiple pregnancies spaced a few years apart provides the ideal balance. However, this is not the best option for household economics, it shortchanges the individual child, and adds

3. Dr. Shuqi Zhuang is a well-known Taiwanese TCM doctor and authority on women's health.

4. This chapter covers the diet and lifestyle that constitute the foundation for increased vitality. Chapter 3 covers Inner Alchemy, the qigong exercises to lessen menstrual flow and transmute this energy for spiritual purposes. These exercises build on the lessons of this chapter.

5. Please see p.172.

6. This is why Liver Blood deficient women bloom during pregnancy.

to environmental strains of human overpopulation. Having multiple pregnancies also restricts a woman's ability to contribute to society in other ways and is not the best choice for most women. With fewer or no pregnancies, the importance of proper menstrual care becomes critical.

The Menstrual Renewal Program is divided into three categories: rest, practices/prohibitions, and dietary plan. Following it promotes and maintains a healthy cycle. Women with more severe symptoms will need to augment their care with acupuncture, herbs, massage, etc. In the Menstrual Renewal Program, menstruation is treated as a period of convalescence. The practice will seem excessive to most modern women as we have been indoctrinated to ignore our bodies' signals to make us more productive. The Program and the information that follows is applicable to menstruating women of all ages.

Rest

Rest is the most important component of the Menstrual Renewal Program. It is typical for energy to be lower during the first few days of the period. Our hormones are at their lowest. Blood loss creates Qi and Blood deficiency that, depending on the severity, creates physical and emotional vulnerability. Immunity is lowered at this time and women are more deeply affected by emotional stress.

Normal optimal sleep is eight hours a night between the hours of 10 p.m. and 6 a.m. During menstruation, add an additional hour or two of sleep a night. Women should take the opportunity to turn inward, pamper themselves, and conserve their energy. This honoring of the body's needs is a necessary attitude adjustment in preparation for the self-cultivation practices in the next chapter.

Practices

1. Keep Warm

Keep the legs, lower back, and abdomen warm at all times. Wear socks and closed shoes. (Particularly keep the Kidney, Liver and Spleen channels warm). Hot stone massage during PMS and menses alleviates many symptoms.

A traditional precaution during menstruation is to bind the abdomen to protect the Kidneys, womb, and low back from. A girdle or ace bandage wrapped around the low back will suffice. It should not be tight as the purpose is to increase warmth.

2. Moxibustion

Moxa is an important modality in TCM where Ai Ye (mugwort) is dried, then burned directly or indirectly on points. The plant's oils enter the body through the smoke, warming the channels and moving the blood. This makes moxa an ideal treatment during menstruation. Use a moxa stick on the lower abdomen, low back, and along the Kidney, Spleen, and Liver channels (Figure 2.3). Use a swirling or pecking motion until the area feels warmed. A moxa box with loose moxa on the low abdomen and low back is particularly effective in treating dysmenorrhea (menstrual cramps).

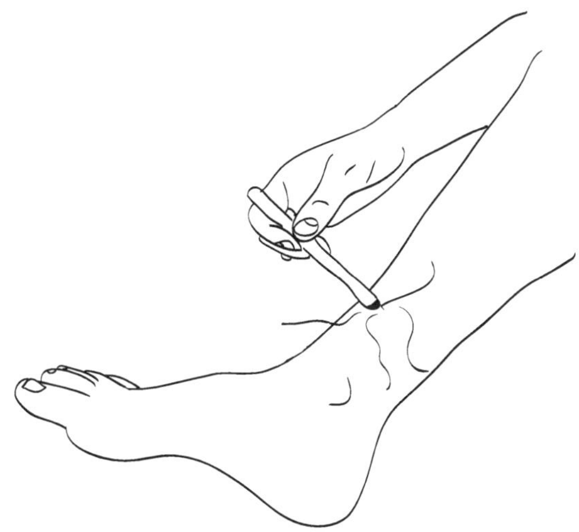

Figure 2.3. Moxibustion of the lower leg

3. Abdominal Massage

Abdominal or hara massage on the days before or on the 28th day will lessen menstrual cramps and promote cycle regularity. Encouraging periods to start on time will eliminate most PMS symptoms, though slight Liver Yang Rising is normal prior to menses. Each day the period is late builds more Liver Qi stagnation, increasing overall tension in the body and exacerbating symptoms.

Prohibitions

1. Do Not Ignore a Cold

The relative Qi and Blood deficiency during menstruation means a weakened immune system. The body is more vulnerable to the external climate and less able to ward off pathogenic factors. Existing pathogens can progress deeper into the body. Upon the first signs of a cold, rest and take the patent formula Gan Mao Ling every three hours, or the immune-boosting recipes on page 338. If the cold progresses see an acupuncturist for cupping and a customized formula. Xiao Chai Hu Tang modifications are typically given for Wind pathogens that invade during the menstruation.

2. Do Not Wash Hair

Do not wash or wet the hair during menses. Either keep the hair braided or clean the scalp with an alcohol solution. To use the Alcohol Wash Method, make a mixture of equal parts 95% isopropyl rubbing alcohol and warm water. Add a few drops of essential oils for fragrance and antibacterial qualities.[7] Use a comb to part the hair and use a cotton ball to apply the alcohol mixture, covering the entire scalp. Comb the hair afterward. Be sure to thoroughly wash the comb with soap and water after each use. Cleanse the scalp with the alcohol mixture daily. Many women will not forgo washing

7. Citrus and rosemary essential oils help to cut oiliness. Clove, cinnamon, and other spice essential oils are antibacterial.

their hair. In these cases, the bathroom should be kept warm and the hair washed and dried quickly. This applies even during summer. Under no circumstances should you walk around with wet hair while you are menstruating.

Reasoning:
The purpose is to avoid Wind Invasion (catching a cold). Dr. Shuqi Zhuang also claims that washing the hair during bleeding will coagulate Blood in the uterus.

3. Avoid Drafts and Exposure to Cold

This includes drafts from air conditioning, swimming, and feeling chilled. Women should pay particular attention to their bodies from the waist down. Keep feet warm, keep legs covered, and protect the Kidneys, low abdomen, and low back.

Reasoning:
Cold entering the channels or the womb will cause constriction and blockage of blood flow. This can lead to menstrual disturbances such as cramps and cycle irregularity. Eventually, it can lead to more serious gynecological issues such as masses, fibroids, or infertility. It is also a precaution to avoid Wind Invasion.

4. Avoid Cold Foods and Drinks

This includes food and drinks that are cold temperature and cold natured. No ice water, ice cream, juices, or raw salads. Eat vegetables and fruits cooked. Warm greens by serving them under cooked food.

Reasoning:
Cold stagnates the Blood. Also, digestion is a hot process. Cold foods consume Qi from the body in order to properly digest (and Qi is weakened at this time).

5. Do Not Lift Weights

Limit physical activity. Avoid lifting weights (above 40 lbs.) or rigorous exercise while bleeding. Wait until the energy recovers to resume normal activity. "Rigorous exercise" means lifting weights at the gym, running, competitive sports, spin class, martial arts, strenuous yoga, etc. In short, anything that causes sweating or fatigue. Following this advice will actually result in an improvement in fitness or physique goals. A rest period is important in any exercise plan and energy levels after the period will increase allowing the woman to return to training with renewed intensity.[8] Additionally, avoid inversions or anything that tilts the uterus above the head. During menses, focus instead on mobility, flexibility, and meditative practices to increase circulation and conserve Qi. Good options

8. Unfortunately, society pushes girls to exert themselves in physical education class and sports without respect for the cycles.

are Dao-Yin qigong,[9] restorative or Yin yoga, and relaxed walking. (These are indicated during any convalescent period.) When training for a particular skill or sport, use this time to greatly decrease the physical output while still going through the motions. This slowing down can offer great insight. Menstruation teaches the value of introspection and the cyclical aspect of life.

Reasoning:
The body is already under strain expelling and replenishing the lining of the uterus. Strenuous exercise forces competing demands on the body for recuperation.

6. Do Not Overwork

During this time, the body naturally wants to sink into a relaxed state. There is heightened sensitivity and receptivity. This is not the time for aggressiveness or high-energy activity. Avoid excessive work. Mental and emotional stress including long hours staring at a computer screen will affect the body much more at this time. Whenever possible, plan for minimizing these activities during the period. This also includes staying out late, excessive drinking, drug use, and other social recreation. Do not push the body on any level and avoid fatigue. If working on a computer, take a break every 40 minutes. This will improve your eyesight and appearance.

Reasoning:
Excess computer work and reading strain Liver Blood. Staying up late cuts into prime recuperation time.

7. Shower, Do Not Take a Bath

Take showers in a warm bathroom.

Reasoning:
The vagina and uterus are more susceptible to bacterial invasion during menses. Soaking in a bath can introduce pathogens into the body.

Menstrual Recovery Dietary Plan

The Menstrual Renewal Dietary Plan is divided into 3 Stages: Stages 1 and 2 are during blood flow, while Stage 3 begins after bleeding has stopped.[10] As long as there is bleeding, the focus is on moving the Blood. As soon as bleeding is over, the focus changes to recuperating Blood and Yin. Day 1 starts the first day of bleeding.

---

9. Dao Yin is an ancient yogaesque style of qigong excellent for rehabilitation and rejuvenation. I learned Dao Yin from Master Huaching Ni and recommend his video. There are other versions available you can try.

10. Shoumei Zhuang. *Your Friend Every Month* (Taiwan: Zhuang Shou Mei Publishing House, 2004). ISBN 957-8807-26-0

During Menstration

Stage 1: Days 1-2

Treatment Principle:
Move Blood stagnation, drain Dampness, while protecting Qi and Blood.

Chinese Herbal Formulas:
Take a Blood moving formula twice a day.

Stage 1 Foods (Recipes page 340)

Organic Liver, 1-2 servings a day:
Liver has an exceptional ability to build the Blood. It also breaks up Blood stagnation, particularly Blood stuck in the uterus.[11] This dual function makes liver the ideal food during menstruation. Invariably when I say this some will say in disgust that liver is a filter and unfit to eat. I believe that organic liver is safe to eat occasionally.

The reason for the concern is that one of the liver's many functions is to clear the blood of poisonous substances which are then excreted in the urine and feces. (Other functions of the liver include production of bile, conversion of glucose into glycogen, storage of iron, and regulating blood clotting.) A 2004 study showed, however, that the liver was no more toxic than lean meat of the same animal.[12] I recommend eating only organic organ meats (and organic meat in general) to minimize exposure to heavy minerals and antibiotics, as well as the inhumanity, present in factory farming methods.[13]

Pork liver is preferred for its neutral thermal property and ability to reduce edema (water retention). Pork is also most similar to our genetic makeup in order to supplement hormones. In terms of taste, I find pork liver is the most challenging to palate. While postpartum women typically will eat anything put in front of them, there is a much lower rate of compliance during menstruation. If you eat pork liver you must soak it in citrus juice (lemon, lime, or orange) or vinegar for 30-60 minutes prior to cooking. Chicken and beef liver are more warming but taste better. For the properties of different types of liver please see p.357).

Rice:
Rice tonifies the Qi and is an ideal food during convalescence. Rice congee, or porridge, is easily digested and assimilated, tonifies Qi and Blood, and harmonizes digestion. It is also an excellent food for sick or recovering patients.

---

11. If you cannot eat liver, eat a rare steak during your period to build your Blood.

12. Irfana Mariam, Shehla Iqbal, and Saeed Ahmad Nagra, "Distribution of Some Trace and Macrominerals in Beef, Mutton, and Poultry," International Journal of Agriculture & Biology (2004), 1560-8530/06-5-816-820, http://www.ijab.org.

13. Many organizations have attacked factory farmng methods on grounds that they are inhumane to the animal, adversely affect the environment, and injure the health of the consumer, compared to traditional farms. Michael Pollan's popular books give accessibe information on the subject.

Red Adzuki Beans, 60g (1/3 cup) daily:
Red adzuki beans eliminate water retention, drain Dampness, and move stagnant Blood. They are diuretic and strengthen the heart.

Yi Yi Ren (Job's Tears), (1/4 cup) daily:
Raw Yi Yi Ren clears Dampness and Heat from the body, and drains edema. Roasted Yi Yi Ren tonifies the Spleen. Add 1/2 raw and 1/2 roasted Yi Yi Ren to cooking grains daily.

Fish:
Fish provides lighter, more digestible protein than meat. Carp is particularly helpful as it reduces edema.

Table 2.1. Stage 1 Sample Meal Plan (Recipes page 340):

30 min Before Breakfast	Blood-moving Formula
Breakfast	1 small bowl of congee, beets and greens, liver or eggs (or vegetarian option)
Lunch	Yi Yi Ren rice, steamed broccoli, liver (or vegetarian option)
30 min Before Dinner	Blood-moving formula
Dinner	Carp soup (or vegetarian soup)
Snacks	Red adzuki bean soup, eggs

Stage 2: Days 3-4 (or until bleeding stops)

Treatment Principle:
Move Qi and Blood. Focus on shrinking uterus and waist.

Chinese Herbal Formulas:
Continue taking a Blood Moving Formula twice a day.

Stage 2 Foods (Recipes page 350)

Organic Kidneys, 2 servings a day:
Eating kidneys tonifies the Kidney energy in our bodies. They also help contract the uterus and waist. Again, pork kidneys are typically used in Chinese tradition as they have a neutral thermal quality. Any organic kidneys may be used.[14] Be sure to cut each kidney in half and remove the white membranes (ureters). Then rinse and soak them in citrus juice (lemon, lime, or orange) or vinegar for 30-60 min. prior to cooking. Different animals have slightly different properties (page 350).

Rice:
Rice tonifies the Qi and is an ideal food during convalescence. Rice congee, or porridge, is easily

14. Pork kidneys and liver are more bitter and stronger tasting than that of beef, chicken, or lamb. If you are new to organ meats, try another one of these options first before trying pork.

digested and assimilated, tonifies Qi and Blood, and harmonizes digestion. It is also an excellent food for sick or recovering patients.

Red Adzuki Beans, 60g (1/3 cup) daily:
Red adzuki beans eliminate water retention, drain Dampness, and move stagnant Blood. They are diuretic and strengthen the heart.

Yi Yi Ren (Job's Tears), (1/4 cup) daily:
Raw Yi Yi Ren clears Dampness and Heat from the body, and drains edema. Roasted Yi Yi Ren tonifies the Spleen. Add 1/2 raw and 1/2 roasted Yi Yi Ren to cooking grains daily.

Fish:
Fish adds lighter, more digestible protein than meat. Carp is particularly helpful as it reduces edema.

Table 2.2. Stage 2 Sample Meal Plan (Recipes page 350):

30 min Before Breakfast	Blood-moving Formula
Breakfast	1 small bowl of congee, steam-fried bok choy, kidney or eggs (or vegetarian option)
Lunch	Stir-fried rice, steam-fried greens, kidney (or vegetarian option)
30 min Before Dinner	Blood-moving formula
Dinner	Fish soup or vegetarian soup
Snacks	Red adzuki bean soup, eggs

PRACTITIONER SECTION: BLOOD MOVING FORMULAS

Formula	Indications
Sheng Hua Tang (page 340)	Gently invigorates Blood and transforms Blood stasis. Specifically moves menstrual blood and contracts the uterus.
Tao Hong Si Wu Tang	Most common formula to invigorate Blood and transform Blood stasis. Specifically moves menstrual blood.
add E Zhu(curcuma zedoaria), San Leng (sparganium), Yan Hu Suo (corydalis), Mo Yao (myrrh), Ru Xiang (frankincense)	In the case of severe Blood stagnation (fibroids, endometriosis, severe cramps).
add Fu Zi (prepared aconite), Gan Jiang (dried ginger)	For Cold in the uterus.

Follicular Phase – Blood and Yin Time

Optimal:
Blood and Yin are depleted after menstruation and are rapidly being replenished during this time. This produces feelings of ease and self-satisfaction. Vaginal moisture increases and changes consistency when approaching ovulation (this is key for fertility). If using a BBT chart, the chart should show a consistently low temperature during this phase. High numbers indicate Excess Heat or Yin Deficiency Heat.

Stage 3: Days 5-7

Treatment Principle:
Tonify Blood and Yin. Only after the bleeding is over and the uterus is clean, can the Blood be directly tonified. Tonifying the body while bleeding can lead to stagnation.

Chinese Herbal Formulas:
Take a Blood and/or Yin Tonifying Formula twice a day.

Stage 3 Foods (Recipes page 353)

The monthly loss of blood makes it more difficult for women to forgo animal products than it is for men. During and just after menstruation, in particular, are the most challenging times to be vegetarian or vegan. If there are no animal products in the diet, it is crucial to take the recommended herbs, Blood-building vegetarian meals, and to supplement with extra protein during this time. I have observed a trend whereby vegan women believe themselves to be healthier because they no longer menstruate or menstruate very little. This is a sign of Blood deficiency, not of superior health.

Organic Chicken, 1-2 servings a day:
Chicken builds Blood and helps recuperate during convalescence. Black bone chicken or Silkie chicken is considered the best to tonify the Blood after menses.

Rice:
Rice tonifies the Qi and is an ideal food during convalescence. Rice congee, or porridge, is easily digested and assimilated, tonifies Qi and Blood, and harmonizes digestion. It is also an excellent food for sick or recovering patients.

Black Beans, 60g (1/3 cup) daily:
Black beans nourish the Kidney.

Fish:
Fish provides lighter, more digestible protein than meat. Carp is particularly helpful as it reduces edema.

Table 2.3. Stage 3 Sample Meal Plan (Recipes page 353):

Before Breakfast	Blood and Yin Nourishing Formula
Breakfast	Millet congee, sautéed vegetables, chicken or eggs (or vegetarian option)
Lunch	Rice, steam-fried vegetables, black chicken soup (or vegetarian option)
Before Dinner	Blood and Yin Nourishing Formula
Dinner	Black bean and fish soup
Snacks	White fungus soup

After day 7, return to the regular diet. Blood and Yin tonics can be continued until ovulation in order to tonify deficiency and regulate the cycle.

Pathology:
When Blood or Yin are deficient, symptoms will be aggravated at this time. For example, fatigue, anemia, feeling wiped out by the period, cramps that begin at the end and just after the period, anxiety, insomnia, feeling vulnerable, depression, etc.

Lifestyle:
Slowly begin resuming physical activity again. If you are generally deficient, avoid excessive exercise, overwork, or fasting throughout the cycle until your body has been built back up. Forcing physical exertion when your body is depleted will only create greater deficiency.

PRACTITIONER SECTION: BLOOD AND YIN TONICS

Formulas	Indications
Si Wu Tang	Classic Liver Blood nourishing formula.
Ba Zhen Tang	Tonifies Qi and Blood.
Gui Pi Tang	Tonifies Spleen Qi and Heart Blood. The Huang Qi/Dang Gui combination generates new blood. Ideal for students, the mentally overworked, and those with emotional issues.
Gui Shao Di Huang Wan (Liu Wei Di Huang Wan + Dang Gui (Chinese angelica), Bai Shao (white peony root))	Nourishes Liver Blood and Kidney Yin. When fertility is desired, use Yin and Blood tonics to increase healthy cervical mucus.[i]

i. Jane Lyttleton. *Treatment of Infertility with Chinese Medicine*. (China: Churchill Livingstone, 2004), 105.

Ovulation – Yang Energy Spikes

Days 11-15

Optimal:
Drastic changes in hormones trigger ovulation, marking the change from extreme Yin to extreme Yang. This correlates with a spike in Qi and Yang energy. Mid-cycle is a key time to regulate if fertility is an issue. Women desiring to increase fertility will want to regulate Qi and Blood at this time and boost the Yang. If using a BBT chart, the chart should spike by 0.4-1°F within a 24-hour period. There is typically a spike in sexual desire and physical stamina at this time. Athletic women often find this is their peak performance time.

Signs of Ovulation and Fertility

1. A spike in Basal Body Temperature.
2. The discharge of cervical mucus of egg white consistency. Lack of cervical mucus indicates Yin deficiency, whereas thick, opaque, or excessive discharge indicates Dampness.
3. The position of the cervix. The acronym S.H.O.W. is used for the ideal state of the fertile cervix: soft, high, open, and wet.
4. Some women will also feel a sensation on the active ovary.

Lifestyle:
Many women find their energy and physical abilities peak at this time.

Pathology:
There are many patterns that can interrupt proper ovulation or cause amenorrhea (the absence of menstruation). Basic patterns with lifestyle and diet advice are given below. The treatment of these conditions is beyond the scope of this book, as whole books can be, and have been, written on the subject. Treatment requires regular acupuncture treatment with customized herbal formulas. Following the diet and lifestyle directives given in this chapter will offer an ideal foundation, to which one should add acupuncture and customized herbal medicine for each stage of the cycle.

Patterns of Ovulation Disorder, Amenorrhea & Infertility

In deficiency conditions and patterns of mixed excess and deficiency, Jing tonics are used, as fertility essentially falls under the function of the Jing. Lifestyle and diet should also reinforce strengthening the Kidneys, independent of the pattern.

Kidney Yang (and Jing) Deficiency

Symptoms:
Long cycle. Fatigue. Feeling cold. Low back and knee soreness or pain. Frequent urination. Pallor.

Diet:
Eat cooked foods. Include: bone broth, yams, sweet potato, rice, oats, lamb, beef, chicken, salmon, kidney, walnut, chestnut, black beans, ginger, onions, garlic, Gou Qi Zi (go ji berries).

Limit salads, dairy, and cold temperature foods.

Lifestyle:
Kidney Yang deficiency is often caused by excessive physical work, too much heavy weightlifting, or excessive sports or dance. Sexual activity before or during puberty damages the Kidneys. It can also be constitutional (Jing-related).

Kidney Yin (and Jing) Defiency

Symptoms:
Short cycles. Scanty menstrual flow. Dryness. Tinnitus. Night sweats and hot flashes. Insomnia. Low back and knee soreness or pain. Thinning skin. Wrinkles. Red cheeks (malar flush) and lips.

Diet:
Eat soups, plenty of vegetables, and drink water. Include: bone broth, seaweed, spirulina, Shan Yao (Chinese yam), millet, oats, wheat, good quality dairy, eggs, black beans, pork, pork kidney, duck, sardine, oyster, seeds and nuts (sesame, chia, hemp, walnuts, almonds, chestnuts, etc.), Gou Qi Zi (go ji berries), mulberries, blueberries, blackberries, Bai Mu Er (white cloud fungus), Hei Mu Er (black wood ear fungus). Be sure to follow the Stage 3 diet plan.

Avoid heating and drying foods like coffee, spices, alcohol, garlic, and citrus.

Lifestyle:
Kidney Yin deficiency is typically caused by chronic stress and overwork for many years, severe febrile disease, or excessive cardio workouts (sweating). Sexual activity before or during puberty also damages the Kidneys. It may also be constitutional (Jing-related). Avoid excessive exercising particularly hot-room yoga, spin, and competitive sports. Include more rest. Avoid overwork. Take special care during menses and post-menses when Yin is depleted.

PRACTITIONER SECTION: PROMOTING OVULATION

The following formula can be taken with modifications to regulate Qi and Blood. Taken at the proper time, it boosts fertility:

Cu Pai Luan Tang (Dang Gui (Chinese angelica) 12g, Chi Shao (red peony root) 12g, Dan Shen (salvia root) 12g, Chuan Xiong (ligusticum) 6g, Hong Hua (safflower) 6g, Ze Lan (lycopus) 9g, Ji Xue Teng (spatholobus) 15g.[1]

1. Jane Lyttleton. *Treatment of Infertility with Chinese Medicine*. (China: Churchill Livingstone, 2004), 397.

Blood (and Jing) Deficiency

Symptoms:
Long cycles. Light-colored and scanty menstrual flow. Fatigue. Emotional sensitivity. Pallor.

Diet:
Eat leafy greens and good quality protein. Include: bone broth, beef, chicken, pork, liver, pork trotters, eggs, black beans, beets, carrots, leafy greens, rice, seaweed, spirulina. Be sure to follow the Stage 3 diet plan, particularly Dang Gui Chicken (page 353).

Avoid excessive salt and sugar, raw foods, and pungent foods.

Lifestyle:
Avoid overwork, particularly excessive computer work. Take special care during menses and post-menses when Blood is depleted.

Liver Qi Stagnation

Symptoms:
Irregular cycle. PMS. Menstrual cramps. Irritability, depression, or anger.

Diet:
Half of the diet should be comprised of vegetables; both cooked and raw. Include: pungent herbs and spices (basil, mint, turmeric, onions, etc.), most vegetables (broccoli, cabbage, turnip, beets, etc.), small amounts of coffee, rye, mung beans, flaxseeds, apples, and bitter melon.

Lifestyle:
Practice relaxation daily such as meditation, tai chi, and soothing styles of qigong or yoga. Exercise is helpful, but avoid competition and extremism.

Blood Stagnation

Symptoms:
Irregular cycle. Menstrual cramps. Dark menstrual flow with clots. Irritability, agitation, depression, or mania.

Diet:
Half of the diet should be comprised of vegetables, mostly cooked. Include: pungent, warming herbs and spices (basil, clove, cinnamon, turmeric, onions, etc.), most vegetables (broccoli, cabbage, turnip, beets, etc.), red adzuki bean, chestnut, eggplant, red wine, seaweed, and Hei Mu Err (black wood ear fungus).

Avoid cold and raw foods.

Lifestyle:
Practice relaxation daily such as meditation, tai chi, and soothing styles of qigong or yoga. Exercise is necessary to improve circulation, but avoid competition and extremism.

Cold in the Uterus

Symptoms:
Long cycle. Menstrual cramps better with heat. Menstrual flow is dark with clots. Feeling chilled during menses.

Diet:
Eat warming, cooked foods. Include: pungent, warming herbs and spices (basil, clove, cinnamon, turmeric, onions, etc.).

Lifestyle:
This is caused by invasion of cold combined with an internal Kidney Yang deficiency. Excessive cold foods and drinks, swimming in cold water during menses, or exposure to cold during menses are common causes.

Phlegm-Damp Obstruction

Symptoms:
Irregular cycle. Excessive vaginal discharge. Sluggishness. May be overweight. Growths, cysts, or Polycystic Ovarian Syndrome (PCOS).

Diet:
Eat a high percentage of cooked vegetables (40-50% of the diet). Include: radish, turnip, lettuce, mustard green, onion, pungent cooking spices and herbs (clove, cinnamon, oregano, thyme, ginger, etc.), horseradish, red adzuki beans, Yi Yi Ren (Job's tears), Bai Bian Dou (hyacinth bean), rye, buckwheat, sourdough, sprouted grain, dry-roasted oats.

Avoid:
Sugar, fruit juice, soda, sweets, bread (sprouted bread is fine), ice cream, alcohol.

Lifestyle:
Diet is both the primary cause and cure for Phlegm-Damp conditions. Follow the dietary directives in section Phlegm-Dampness (page 260).

Luteal Phase – Qi and Yang Time

Days 16-28

Optimal:
The luteal phase is characterized by a predominance of Qi and Yang energy. BBT charting should show sustained high temperatures of at least 98°F. Just prior to menstruation minor PMS is normal: slight breast tenderness, a rise in drive and athleticism, and a mild generalized tension. It should be a slight feeling that signals that the period is imminent, not the incapacitating list of symptoms that have come to be considered normal.

Lifestyle:
Energy for physical exercise and achieving continue to be high. Many women experience a spike in energy, aggression, and physical strength just before the menstruation. This is generally the best time of the cycle for fasting.

Pathology:
Cases of Qi and Yang deficiency will be aggravated at this time. In these cases ovulation may never occur, there may be increased fatigue, digestive weakness, lack of drive, etc. Liver Excess symptoms can also appear as the period draws closer: headaches, moodiness, anger, depression, addictive urges, constipation, and neck and shoulder tension.

Patterns of Luteal Phase Disorder

Qi Deficiency

Symptoms:
Short menstrual cycle. Bloating and fatigue after meals. Muscle weakness. Loose stools. Pallor.

Diet:
Meals should be simple and easy to digest. Eat cooked foods and a higher proportion of grains. Include: white rice, sweet rice, oats, chicken, beef, lamb, sweet potato, yam, winter squash, walnut, pungent cooking spices and herbs (clove, cinnamon, oregano, thyme, ginger, etc.).

Limit:
Salads, raw fruit, seaweed, brown rice, dairy, nuts, and cold temperature foods.

Lifestyle:
Qi deficiency is often caused by poor eating habits, stress, excessive physical work, too much heavy weightlifting, or excessive sports or dance. It can also be constitutional (Jing-related).

Patent Formulas:
Si Jun Zi Tang, Bu Zhong Yi Qi Tang

Yang Deficiency

Symptoms:
Long menstrual cycle. Lack of drive. Fatigue. Poor absorption and loose stools. Feeling cold. Low back and knee soreness or pain. Frequent urination. Pallor.

Diet:
Eat cooked foods. Include: bone broth, yams, sweet potato, rice, oats, lamb, beef, chicken, salmon, kidney, walnut, chestnut, black beans, ginger, onions, garlic, Gou Qi Zi (go ji berries).

Limit:
Salads, dairy, and cold temperature foods.

Lifestyle:
Kidney Yang deficiency is often caused by excessive physical work, too much heavy weightlifting, or excessive sports or dance. Sexual activity before or during puberty damages the Kidneys. It can also be constitutional (Jing-related).

Patent Formulas:
Ba Zhen Tang + Fu Zi (prepared aconite) and Rou Gui (cinnamon bark)

Liver Qi Stagnation

Symptoms:
Intolerance of others. Irregular menstrual cycle. Menstrual cramps. Irritability, depression, or anger. Breast tenderness. Bowel irregularity. Bloating. Headaches. Neck and shoulder tension.

Diet:
Half of the diet should be comprised of vegetables; both cooked and raw. Include: pungent herbs and spices (basil, mint, turmeric, onions, etc.), most vegetables (broccoli, cabbage, turnip, beets, etc.), small amounts of coffee, rye, mung beans, flaxseeds, apples, and bitter melon.

Lifestyle:
Practice relaxation daily such as meditation, tai chi, and soothing styles of qigong or yoga. Exercise is helpful, but avoid competition and extremism.

Patent Formulas:
Xiao Yao San (Spleen Qi and Blood deficiency symptoms: loose stools, foggy-headedness, fatigue, pallor), Jia Wei Xiao Yao San (previous pattern with Heat symptoms: irritability, acne), Shu Gan Wan (pure excess symptoms: anger, rage, acting out)

Liver Yang Rising

Symptoms:
Premenstrual headaches. Tight neck and shoulders. Photophobia (aversion to light). Nausea. Irritability, depression, anger.

Diet:
Eat a higher proportion of vegetables and moistening foods. Include: summer squash, sprouts, seaweed, wheatgrass juice, algae, black sesame seeds, mulberries, Gou Qi Zi (go ji berries), lettuce, cucumber, spinach, eggplant, millet, wheat, white rice, and calcium.

Lifestyle:
Soak feet in hot water at first sign of a headache. Practice relaxation daily such as meditation, tai chi, and soothing styles of qigong or yoga. Exercise is helpful, but avoid competition and extremism.

Patent Formulas:
Tian Ma Gou Teng Yin, Long Dan Xie Gan Tang, (see section "Migraine Headaches" on page 292)

Red Dragon (Menstrual) Disorders

Ancient Chinese culture loved metaphors, and they could not have chosen a more appropriate one for menstruation than calling it a "Red Dragon." A dragon is a powerful, mythical being that is both auspicious and unpredictable. Red is not only the color of blood, it is special in Chinese culture serving as a symbol of happiness and good fortune. When tamed, the Red Dragon would be a blessing. Untamed it could wreak havoc, as anyone with a menstruation knows. In this section we address menstrual symptoms and how to balance the underlying cause. The remainder of this chapter addresses wider issues pertinent to women of all ages, and not necessarily relevant to young girls, though it is important for them to understand why a balanced period will be important for their future.

Our modern lifestyle (poor eating habits, sedentary lifestyle, and stress) is not conducive to hormonal balance. Digestive problems are connected to many gynecological disorders. Eating excess sweets, irregular meals, and stress are great contributors to menstrual issues. It is crucial to keep blood sugar levels stable and avoid excess sugar. Make sure to include the bitter flavor, such as greens and unsweetened tea, in the diet to help counteract excess sweets. This will also help keep tumor formations and acne breakouts at bay.[(15)]

PMS

PMS, or premenstrual symptoms occurring prior to onset of menses, is Liver Qi Stagnation, while menstrual symptoms after menstruation indicate deficiency. Menstrual symptoms during the menses is a combination of excess and deficiency.

Liver Qi Stagnation

Symptoms:
Intolerance of others. Irregular menstrual cycle. Menstrual cramps. Irritability, depression, or anger. Breast tenderness. Bowel irregularity. Bloating. Headaches. Neck and shoulder tension.

Treatment:
Smooth Liver Qi, Regulate Menstruation.

Diet:
Half of the diet should be comprised of vegetables; both cooked and raw. Include: pungent herbs and spices (basil, mint, turmeric, onions, etc.), most vegetables (broccoli, cabbage, turnip, beets, etc.), small amounts of coffee, rye, mung beans, flaxseeds, apples, and bitter melon.

15. Both are due to Damp-Heat or Phlegm-Heat accumulations.

Lifestyle:
Practice relaxation daily such as meditation, tai chi, and soothing styles of qigong or yoga. Exercise is helpful, but avoid competition and extremism.

Patent Formulas:
Xiao Yao San (Spleen Qi and Blood deficiency symptoms: loose stools, foggy-headedness, fatigue, pallor), Jia Wei Xiao Yao San (previous pattern with Heat symptoms: irritability, acne), Shu Gan Wan (pure excess symptoms: anger, rage, acting out). Take as needed to relieve symptoms. These formulas can also be taken throughout the cycle.

Early Periods (23 days or less)

Qi Deficiency

Symptoms:
The menstrual blood is dilute, light-colored, and sometimes pinkish. The flow tends to be heavy. Additional symptoms may include fatigue, shortness of breath, palpitation, dizziness, pallor, dislike of speaking, anxiety, aversion to cold, empty and downbearing sensation in the lower abdomen, and weakness of limbs. The tongue is pale with a thin coating and the pulse is weak.

Treatment:
Tonify Qi and Keep Blood in the Vessels.

Diet:
Meals should be simple and easy to digest. Eat cooked foods and a higher proportion of grains. Include: white rice, sweet rice, oats, chicken, beef, lamb, sweet potato, yam, winter squash, walnut, pungent cooking spices and herbs (clove, cinnamon, oregano, thyme, ginger, etc.).

Limit:
Salads, raw fruit, seaweed, brown rice, dairy, nuts, and cold temperature foods.

Lifestyle:
Qi deficiency is often caused by poor eating habits, stress, excessive physical work, too much heavy weightlifting, or excessive sports or dance. It can also be constitutional (Jing-related). Follow the Menstrual Renewal Program carefully, particularly in regards to rest. Be sure to follow the rules in the Diet section (page 124).

Patent Formula:
Bu Zhong Yi Qi Tang, Gui Pi Tang, Ba Zhen Tang

Heat in the Blood

Symptoms:
The menstrual blood is bright or dark red in color. The flow is thick and sticky with fine clots and tends to be heavy. Additional symptoms may include restlessness, dry mouth, a flushed face, thirst, yellow urine, constipation, and a red tongue with yellow coating. There is a rapid, forceful pulse.

Treatment:
Clear Blood Heat.

Diet:
Half of the diet should be comprised of vegetables; both cooked and raw. Include: broccoli, cabbage, turnip, beets, white rice, mung beans, flaxseeds, apples, and bitter melon.

Avoid heating foods: spices, garlic, and excess meat.

Lifestyle:
Practice relaxation daily such as meditation, tai chi, and soothing styles of qigong or yoga. Exercise is helpful, but avoid competition and extremism.

Patent Formula:
Qin Lian Si Wu Tang

Late Periods (35 days or longer)

Blood Deficiency

Symptoms:
Menstrual blood is pale and scanty. Additional symptoms include: emotional sensitivity, blurred vision, palpitations, pallor, fatigue, and insomnia.

Treatment:
Nourish Blood.

Diet:
Eat leafy greens and good quality protein. Include: bone broth, beef, chicken, pork, liver, pork trotters, eggs, black beans, beets, carrots, leafy greens, rice, seaweed, spirulina. Be sure to follow the Stage 3 diet plan, particularly Dang Gui Chicken (page 353).

Avoid excessive salt and sugar, raw foods, and pungent foods.

Lifestyle:
Avoid overwork, particularly excessive computer work. Take special care during menses and post-menses when Blood is depleted.

Patent Formulas:
Si Wu Tang (classic for any Blood deficiency), Ren Shen Yang Rong Wan (stronger action to regenerate Blood).

Liver Qi Stagnation

Symptoms:
Menstrual blood is normal-colored or dark red with clots. The cycle can be completely unpredictable; at times long and other times short. Additional symptoms may include lower abdominal pain, depression, breast distention, and hypochondriac pain. There will be more severe PMS.

Treatment:
Smooth Liver Qi, Regulate Menstruation.

Diet:
Half of the diet should be comprised of vegetables; both cooked and raw. Include: pungent herbs and spices (basil, mint, turmeric, onions, etc.), most vegetables (broccoli, cabbage, turnip, beets, etc.), small amounts of coffee, rye, mung beans, flaxseeds, apples, and bitter melon.

Lifestyle:
Get abdominal massage and moxa around Day 28 to encourage blood flow. Practice relaxation daily such as meditation, tai chi, and soothing styles of qigong or yoga. Exercise is helpful, but avoid competition and extremism.

Patent Formulas:
Xiao Yao San (Spleen Qi and Blood deficiency symptoms: loose stools, foggy-headedness, fatigue, pallor), Jia Wei Xiao Yao San (previous pattern with Heat symptoms: irritability, acne), Shu Gan Wan (pure excess symptoms: anger, rage, acting out).

Cold in the Uterus

Symptoms:
Menstrual blood is dark red in color and the flow may be light. Additional symptoms include cold sensation and pain in the lower abdomen (which is alleviated by warmth), pale complexion, cold limbs, and aversion to cold. The tongue has a white coating. The pulse is deep and tense or deep and thready.

Treatment:
Warm the channels, Regulate Menstruation.

Diet:
Eat warming, cooked foods. Include: pungent, warming herbs and spices (basil, clove, cinnamon, turmeric, onions, etc.).

Avoid:
Cold foods during menses such as ice cream, cold drinks, salads, and yogurt.

Lifestyle:
This is caused by invasion of cold combined with an internal Kidney Yang deficiency. Excessive cold foods and drinks, swimming in cold water during menses, or exposure to cold during menses are common causes. Get hot stone massage prior or during menses. Moxa the lower abdomen during menses. Avoid exposure to cold, damp weather, and swimming, and cover up during your menses.

Patent Formula:
Wen Jing Tang, Jiang Huang San

Irregular Periods

Liver Qi Stagnation

Symptoms:
Irregularity of any bodily functioning implicates the Liver. Additional symptoms may include lower abdominal pain, depression, breast distention, hypochondriac pain.

Treatment:
Smooth Liver Qi, Regulate Menstruation.

Diet:
Half of the diet should be comprised of vegetables; both cooked and raw. Include: pungent herbs and spices (basil, mint, turmeric, onions, etc.), most vegetables (broccoli, cabbage, turnip, beets, etc.), small amounts of coffee, rye, mung beans, flaxseeds, apples, and bitter melon.

Lifestyle:
Get abdominal massage and moxa around Day 28 to encourage blood flow. Practice relaxation daily such as meditation, tai chi, and soothing styles of qigong or yoga. Exercise is helpful, but avoid competition and extremism.

Patent Formulas:
Xiao Yao San (Spleen Qi and Blood deficiency symptoms: loose stools, foggy-headedness, fatigue, pallor), Jia Wei Xiao Yao San (previous pattern with Heat symptoms: irritability, acne), Shu Gan Wan (pure excess symptoms: anger, rage, acting out).

Painful Periods (Dysmenorrhea)

Be sure to abide by the prohibitions during menstruation as this will alleviate most instances of cramps. Menstrual cramps respond very well to moxibustion (page 94).[16]

Cold in the Uterus

Symptoms:
Menstrual blood is dark red in color and the flow may be light. The cycles tend to be long. Additional symptoms include cold sensation and pain in the lower abdomen (which is alleviated by warmth), pale complexion, cold limbs, and aversion to cold. The tongue has a white coating. The pulse is deep and tense or deep and thready.

Treatment:
Warm the channels, Regulate Menstruation.

Diet:
Eat warming, cooked foods. Include: pungent, warming herbs and spices (basil, clove, cinnamon, turmeric, onions, etc.).

Avoid:
Cold foods during menses such as ice cream, cold drinks, salads, and yogurt.

Lifestyle:
This is caused by invasion of cold combined with an internal Kidney Yang deficiency. Excessive cold foods and drinks, swimming in cold water during menses, or exposure to cold during menses are common causes. Get hot stone massage prior or during menses. Moxa the lower abdomen during menses. Avoid exposure to cold, damp weather, and swimming, and cover up during your menses.

Patent Formula:
Wen Jing Tang, Jiang Huang San

Blood Stagnation

Symptoms:
Heavy dark purple flow with large clots or light flow with lingering spotting. Additional symptoms may include lower abdominal pain (worse with pressure), feeling of suffocation, restlessness. Tongue is purplish or there are engorged sublingual veins. Pulse is thready, hesitant.

Diet:
Half of the diet should be comprised of vegetables, mostly cooked. Include: pungent, warming herbs and spices (basil, clove, cinnamon, turmeric, onions, etc.), most vegetables (broccoli, cabbage, turnip,

16. Practitioners can use strong stimulation of SP 8.

beets, etc.), red adzuki bean, chestnut, eggplant, red wine, seaweed, and Hei Mu Err (black wood ear fungus).

Avoid cold and raw foods.

Lifestyle:
Practice relaxation daily such as meditation, tai chi, and soothing styles of qigong or yoga. Exercise is necessary to improve circulation, but avoid competition and extremism. Get hot stone massage prior or during menses. Moxa the lower abdomen during menses. Avoid exposure to cold, damp weather, and swimming, and cover up during your menses.

Patent Formulas:
Yunnan Paiyao (take 4-6 capsules with a shot of rice wine, sherry, or brandy as needed), Tao Hong Si Wu Tang.

Heavy Flow

If menstrual flow is pale it indicates Qi deficiency. If the flow is red it indicates Heat. If the flow has clots there is Blood Stagnation. A heavy flow can indicate more serious conditions such as endometriosis or fibroids.

Scanty Flow

Most often light flow is a sign of Blood deficiency. It is common in vegans and extreme athletes. It can also indicate a constitutional weakness.

Spotting Between Periods

Do not ignore spotting as it can be a sign of serious disease. Many patterns can cause spotting including Heat, Stagnation, and Deficiency, making it a complicated symptom to differentiate and treat. For any deficiency pattern, E Jiao (gelatin) helps stop the bleeding. For any stagnation, the patent formula Yunnan Paiyao is effective.

Whatever the pattern, it generally requires seeing an acupuncturist and a medical doctor. Red leukorrhea (vaginal discharge) can be mistaken for menstrual bleeding and can indicate serious illness such as cancer. Intrauterine devices (IUDs) can cause irregular or excessive bleeding. There is also a big distinction between minor spotting mid-cycle and heavy bleeding outside of normal menstruation. Mid-cycle spotting is most often a sign of Yin deficiency with Heat. (For more, see "Excessive and Irregular Menstrual Bleeding" on page 303)

Polycystic Ovarian Syndrome (PCOS)

PCOS is a disease in which the ovaries become enlarged with many small follicular cysts. It is characterized by chronic lack of ovulation, obesity, androgen excess, hirsuitism (facial hair), and infertility. Because of better medical diagnostics, more women are being diagnosed with PCOS who are asymptomatic. Women with PCOS have erratic blood sugar levels and insulin resistance and are typically treated in allopathic medicine with Metformin, a diabetic medication. From a TCM point of view, there is either Kidney Yin or Yang deficiency compounded with Phlegm obstruction and Blood stagnation. The Phlegm-Damp component is a key factor of the disorder and must be treated with diet. Eliminate sugars and adopt a Damp-clearing diet ("Phlegm and Dampness" on page 260). The Kidney-nourishing formulas that follow will address the hormonal imbalance and reduce food cravings.

Recipe 2.1. PCOS Formula #1 – Kidney Yin deficiency [17]
Sheng Di Huang (raw rehmania) 20g, Shu Di Huang (prepared rehmania) 20g, Huai Niu Xi (achyranthes root) 30g, Bai Shao (white peony root) 10g, Huang Bai (phellodendron) 10g, San Leng (sparganium) 15g, E Zhu (curcuma zedoaria) 15g, Zao Jiao Ci (gleditsia spine) 15g, Tao Ren (peach kernel) 10g, Zi Cao (lithospermum root) 30g, Zhi Da Huang (prepared rhubarb root) 3-6g, Gan Cao (licorice root) 10g, Sha Ren (amomum) 6g.

Recipe 2.2. PCOS Formula #2 – Kidney Yang deficiency
Sheng Huang Qi (raw astragalus) 30g, Lu Jiao Pian (sliced deer horn) 10g, Ji Nei Jin (chicken gizzard, powdered) 10g, Xiang Fu (cyperus) 10g, Cang Zhu (atractylodes) 10g, Bai Zhu (white atractylodes) 10g, San Leng (sparganium) 10g, E Zhu (curcuma zedoaria) 10g, Zhi Fu Zi (prepared aconite) 3-6g, Rou Gui (cinnamon bark) 3-6g, Gan Cao (licorice root) 6g.

17. Modified from formulas from Dr. Jiling Hu. Jiling Hu. "TCM Endocrinology." (lecture, Yo San University, Los Angeles, November 7, 2003).

Managing Fertility

Fertility has been a source of stress for women throughout history. The excitement and chemistry of a new relationship biologically optimizes fertility, exactly when it is not desired. Then, once a relationship is established and consistent, fertility naturally wanes, exactly when it should be optimal. First, we will address ways of minimizing pregnancy, which becomes relevant in the later teens as girls become sexually active but are not yet ready to start a family.[18] Then we will address how to boost fertility beyond acupuncture and herbal treatment. It is included here as we are addressing the larger topic of menstruation, fertility, and potential disorders. Whether a woman wishes to avoid pregnancy or to have children, she needs to understand her cycle.

Minimizing Pregnancy

The question of birth control is a tricky one, as each method has its side effects. In cases other than a monogamous, long-term relationship, condoms are necessary as they are the only method of birth control to minimize transmission of sexually transmitted diseases during intercourse. When the only concern is unwanted pregnancy, however, there are more options.

The two main forms of birth control, oral contraceptives and the IUD, have negative effects on a woman's health. Oral contraceptives (birth control pills) taken over long periods of time generate Liver Qi stagnation and can create Blood deficiency. Some women do well on them, but for many they cause hormonal imbalances and increase chances of gynecological conditions and blood clots. It is common for the IUD to cause excessive uterine bleeding for the first month or so, after which the woman's body either adapts or the IUD has to be removed.

Natural methods require significant awareness to be effective. Daoist and Tantric ejaculation control practices are not reliable birth control methods. Even if a man is masterful, there may still be mistakes. He may lose control and ejaculate or a small amount of ejaculate may leak out during "reverse ejaculation." If natural birth control is desired, it is best practiced with one of the additional options below.

The Standard Days Method (SD Method) is a modern version of the Rhythm Method created in the 1930s. It is promoted as a birth control alternative for religious

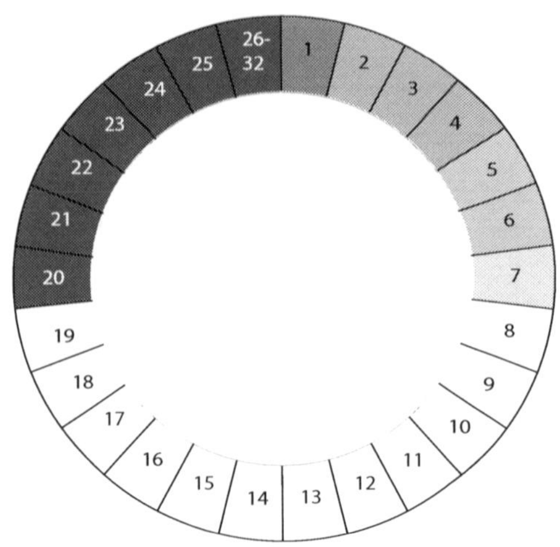

Figure 2.4. SD Method Showing Days of Fertility

18. Though I see adverse affects in using oral contraceptives or injectable birth control methods, they might be the best choice for teenage girls who are not yet responsible enough to use other methods. In these cases, avoiding pregnancy is the bigger concern.

PRACTITIONER SECTION: ENDING UNWANTED PREGNANCY

Note: I do not advocate using acupuncture and herbs to end unwanted pregnancy. The best option is to consult with a physician or clinic where the woman can receive proper counseling and care. If she chooses to abort, she should follow the Postpartum Recovery Program on page 198. Proper recovery care is key. Abortion can present physical and emotional damage because it interrupts the natural cycle. I relay the following as historical information only:

Acupuncturists take extra precautions with herbs and acupuncture during pregnancy in order to optimize the health of the fetus. However, pregnant women are very resilient. Women carry babies to term through famine, war, heavy physical work, and drug use. Using Blood moving herbs and stimulating acupuncture to get rid of unwanted pregnancies is not a reliable birth control method. In some cases, it is effective to use herbs and acupuncture (used with intention) to promote menstruation as soon as the period is late.

Point prescription to encourage menses: Ba Liao points with strong stimulation and electro-stimulation. Sp6, Sp8, 10, LI4, TiTuo, Zi Gong Xue, Kd 14. Electro-stimulation of Sp6 and LI4. Ear Points: Uterus, Abdomen, Point Zero, Shen Men, Sympathetic Autonomic Point.

The following herbs have been used to induce abortion: Fu Zi (aconite) paired with Rou Gui (cinnamon bark), She Xiang (musk), Fei Zi (torreya seeds), Wei Ling Xian (clematis, alcohol extract), Gan Sui (euphorbia), Chuan Xin Lian (andrographis), Tian Hua Fen (tricosanthes root).

Herbs to encourage menses: Tao Hong Si Wu Tang with E Zhu (curcuma zedoaria), San Leng (sparganium), Fu Zi (aconite), Rou Gui (cinnamon bark), Wei Ling Xian (clematis).

reasons, but it applies to those who want another option for health reasons. In the SD Method, couples abstain from unprotected intercourse on days 8-19 of the woman's cycle. When rigidly adhered to, the SD Method has a 5-9 percent failure rate.(19) Such natural forms of birth control are only reliable when the menstrual cycle is very regular and the woman is meticulously charting her days. The SD Method is recommended only for women with a 26-30 day cycle.(20) If choosing this method there is even a smart phone application, iCycleBeads.

The Billings Ovulation Method is similar to the SD Method. However, rather than focusing on the days of the cycle, the Billings Method teaches women to monitor their cervical mucus. It requires more observation, but boasts a lower failure rate of 0-.5 percent.(21) Dryness or static levels of cervical mucus indicate infertility, whereas a rapid change, such as a change in consistency or volume, indicates fertility. Each woman will have her own pattern of cervical mucus she must learn to read.(22) As with the Standard Days Method, unprotected intercourse is avoided during the fertile phase.

---

19. Arevalo M, Jennings V and Sinai I, *Efficacy of a New Method of Family Planning: the Standard Days Method, Contraception*, 2002, 65(5): 333-338.

20. For more details see http://www.natural-family-planning.info/standard-days-method.htm

21. Shao-Zhen Qian, De-Wei Zhang, "Evaluation of the Effectiveness of a Natural Fertility Regulation Program in China." (paper presented at "The Woman of Today and Her Identity: Femininity, Fecundity and Procreation," Centre for Study and Research in the Natural Regulation of Fertility, Universita Cattolica del Sacro Cuore, Rome, Italy, on 8 September, 2000).

22. For more details see http://www.thebillingsovulationmethod.org/

Increasing Fertility

If fertility is desired, the first order of business is to optimize the physical and emotional health of both parents. As discussed in the prologue, a fetus is the product of the Jing of both parents. When parents who are in poor health reproduce it will have adverse effects on both mother and child. Ideally both parents will take 3-6 months to clean up their diet and lifestyle, regulate their weight, as well as treat any imbalances. Eating organic foods is critical as toxins lower fertility.

Some women have erratic periods or none at all and still have healthy pregnancies. This is not the rule, however. Regulating the menstrual cycle balances the body and increases the chances of a healthy pregnancy. When being treated by an acupuncturist for infertility, the first 1-3 months focus on regulating the cycle, during which time the women should not get pregnant. Then, once the mother-to-be is healthy, the next 1-3 months are used to directly boost fertility.

Additionally, prospective parents should consider creating a space in their lives for a new baby. If a couple is already too involved with career and activities, there is no space for a child. Children, particularly babies, require time, presence, and attention. A child will not fit into a tiny space in our lifestyle, rather when a child arrives he/she changes everything.

Fertility is adversely affected by monotony and stress. These take us out of touch with our sensuality and reduce fertility in both men and women. Ideally, a child is conceived out of love between two people; the highest form of chemistry. Couples trying to conceive should increase their loving connection as well as their sexual attraction for one another.

Cultivating Love

To increase love, practice daily kindness, presence, and affection with your partner. This may initially bring up issues with your partner. These will either be healed in the process or possibly highlight an incompatibility. Layers of complexity separate children from adults, but we still respond to the same cues we did when we were infants. Touch and warmth equate to love and connection. Begin with the following steps:

Exercise 2.1. Morning Connection

Connect with your lover first thing in the morning:

1. Begin by placing your hand on your heart. Feel all the love that is there. Feel love for yourself, your lover,[23] and the child who will be born of you both.
2. Now connect with your lover. Be completely present and go with whatever moves you. Gaze into each other's eyes without speaking, kiss, massage each other, or just hold each

23. Think of your partner as a lover rather than a partner.

other. Be sensual, but reserve anything that ends in orgasm for peak fertility days.

3. When you feel fully connected, feel the love between you both creating a warm, safe place for your child to be born into.

Exercise 2.2. Practice Kindness

Take the time to do kind things for each other every day. Make a special dish, perform an unpleasant chore, send a loving message, buy a small gift, compliment each other, etc. Take actions to express what is special in your lover. It is very difficult to hold a grudge when you act kindly on a consistent basis.

Exercise 2.3. Be Affectionate

Kissing, caressing, hugging, and other loving gestures build love between people on an emotional as well as biochemical level. It is natural for connected couples to keep near constant physical connection. For couples who have fallen out of connection it will take conscious effort to reset the pattern. Kiss each other several times a day, one of which lasts at least 10 minutes. Sit next to each other or sit on his lap. Hold hands when you walk together. Cuddle watching television. Take every excuse to touch when you pass each other by.

Generating Attraction

To increase sexual attraction we need to increase polarity and tension. First, reverse the rules for avoiding pregnancy. Namely, abstain from anything that results in orgasm on infertile days and have unprotected intercourse on fertile days. Do not, however, avoid flirting, teasing, or provocative displays of nudity.

Exercise 2.4. Increasing Polarity

1. Physical activity increases our endorphin levels, our feelings of attractiveness, and Yang energy (progesterone and testosterone).[24] For general vitality, both men and women should develop themselves physically. For the sake of increasing polarity, this is more important for men. Specifically, men should train for power (explosive, high intensity movement) and lift heavy weights focused on the lower body (like deadlifts and squats). Be sure to have a snack prior to and a meal after workouts.
2. To increase Yin energy, women should engage their artistic, spiritual, and sensual natures. This can mean taking up artistic projects, getting in tune with Nature, or taking a dance class. Be sure to do the Internal Alchemy exercises (page 135) and Moon Meditation (page 85).
3. When you are not with your lover, you and your lover should spend time with the same

---

24. Excessive exercise and overtraining will deplete these, having the opposite effect.

sex. This will increase the polarity when you are together.

Exercise 2.5. When to Make Love

Our hormones are at their lowest during and just after menstruation. After you have finished bleeding, notice the degree of dryness or wetness of your vagina. This is how you are when you are infertile, and it will vary from woman to woman. As you approach ovulation your body continues to generate Yin, producing a noticeable change in cervical mucus. There will be a distinct slippery quality to your vaginal discharge that signals fertility starting a few days before ovulation. Ovulation is heralded by a sharp spike in Yang energy, and your vaginal discharge will change, becoming less slippery. **The day before your discharge goes from slippery to less slippery marks your most fertile day.** The next 1-3 days will also be peak fertile days. After three days you will no longer be fertile. You can continue to make love freely until you begin your menses. At that point abstain again.

You will also be able to identify ovulation by a spike in your body temperature if you are taking your daily temperature. If you do not observe signs of ovulation, see an acupuncturist. Weekly acupuncture and herbal formulas to regulate the four stages of the cycle are very effective to promote fertility.

Exercise 2.6. Creating Space

During your peak fertility days create a romantic setting. This can be done at home. All it requires is some planning and a little creativity. Be sure to engage all the senses: lighting, color, texture, taste, fragrance, etc. This ensures that you are in the present, enjoying the moment, and not stressing about producing a child.

It is traditionally a man's job to create the set up a romantic setting. This is an extention of his role holding space and creating safety (see page 150). But if it feels right, take on that role yourself. Everyone deserves to experience how special it feels to have your lover put so much energy into creating a beautiful setting for you.

Addressing the Emotions

Not being able to have a child when you feel ready is devastating. It is a hard lesson when we do everything right and do not get what we want. If you are dealing with infertility, you and your partner need to address the range of emotions. Do the Dissolving Energy exercise on page 162 to clear these feelings. Additionally, seek out support groups, energetic healers, and counselors who can help process your feelings. At the end of every challenge there is a gift. There may be deep issues that would never have surfaced otherwise and this is an opportunity to resolve them.

Disorders of the Jade Gate

Many common problems in the vagina and vulva have their foundation in an underlying Qi and Blood deficiency pattern, often due to overwork, excessive drinking, staying out late, not enough rest, excessive caretaking, poor diet, periods of hormonal transition, and stress. Add a new lover, a bubble bath, and hormonal transition and you have the perfect storm for yeast infections, UTIs, and herpes outbreaks

Leukorrhea (Vaginal Discharge)

Occasional white or transparent vaginal discharge with no smell is normal. Stretchy, egg white-like discharge mid-cycle indicates proper ovulation and that the woman is fertile. Other than this, vaginal discharge indicates an imbalance.

Fu Qing Zhu[25] originally categorized leukorrhea into four different types: white, yellow, blue green, and black. Modern TCM has added red and red/white intermingling and omitted the blue green kind. In modern clinical experience, acupuncturists will typically only treat the white and yellow variety, as the others often indicate serious bacterial infections or cancerous conditions.

Table 2.4. Types of Vaginal Discharge

Color	Additional Symptoms	Diagnosis	Treatment
White	Profuse, white/dilute clear that is egg white-like, not due to ovulation. Aversion to cold, fatigue, frequent urination, low backache.	Kidney Yang Deficiency	Jin Suo Gu Jing Wan
	Persistent, excessive, white/slightly yellow, sticky, no smell.	Spleen Qi Deficiency with Dampness	Wan Dai Tang, follow Damp-clearing diet page 260
	With consistency of tofu or cottage cheese, extreme itching and pain. (Yeast infection).	Spleen and Kidney deficiency with Damp Toxin	See Yeast Infection page 126
	Small discharge, may be sticky and thick; Dryness, itching, night sweats, tinnitus.	Kidney Yin Deficiency	Zhi Bai Di Huang Wan + Lian Zi (lotus nut), Chun Gen Pi (ailanthus bark), Huang Bai (phellodendron)
Yellow	Profuse and sticky, fetid smell, lower abdominal pain worse with pressure. May be prolonged menses. Irritability, bitter taste in mouth.	Damp Heat in the Liver Channel	Long Dan Xie Gan Tang

25. Renowned TCM gynecologist, whose writings dating from the early Qing dynasty and form the basis of modern TCM gynecology.

Color	Additional Symptoms	Diagnosis	Treatment
	Profuse with blood and other colors mixed, sticky, odor. Feeling of heat, lower abdominal pain, sticky stool, thirst.	Damp-Toxin	Bi Xie Shen Shi Tang + Pu Gong Yin (dandelion), Bai Jiang Cao (thiaspi), Hong Teng (sargentadoxa vine)

PRACTITIONER SECTION - TREATING CANDIDA

Internal Formula

Patients should be on herbs for 3-6 months. If a patient is open to raw herbs or granules, I like to use the following Shun Gan Yi Qi Tang modification:

Ren Shen (ginseng) 6g, Bai Zhu (white atractylodis) 9g, Bai Shao (white peony root) 9g, Dang Gui (Chinese angelica) 9g, Fu Ling (poria) 12g, Huo Xiang (agastache) 9g, Sheng Jiang (fresh ginger) 3 slices, Ban Xia (pinellia), Sha Ren (amomum) 6g, Chen Pi (tangerine peel) 6g, Zi Su Gen (perilla stalk) (milder for Yin def) or Da Fu Pi (betel nut husk) (more drying) 6g, Yi Yi Ren (Job's tears) 24g.

Modifications:

Qi stagnation - add Chai Hu (bupleurum) 9g

Blood deficiency - add Shu Di Huang (prepared rehmannia) 15g

Kidney Yin deficiency - add Mai Men Dong (ophiopogonis) 9g, Du Zhong (eucommia) 9g, Sang Ji Sheng (mulberry stem) 12g

Damp-Toxin - add Bai Zhi (angelica root) 9g, Ku Shen (sophora root) 9g, Fang Feng (ledebouriella root) 6g

Constipation - add Gua Lou (trichosanthus fruit) 15g

External wash or sitz bath[1]

To relieve symptoms during the acute phase, patients can decoct the following raw herb formula and use it as an external wash or sitz bath, daily for 3-7 days:

Bai Hua She She Cao (hedyotis) 9g, Bing Pian (borneol) 3g, Ku Shen (sophora root) 15g, Huang Bai (phellodendron) 15g, Mu Jin Pi (hibiscus bark) 15g, She Chuang Zi (cnidium seeds) 15g, Hua Jiao (Sichuan pepper) 9g.

Vaginal suppository

This also relieves symptoms during the acute phase. Powder equal amounts of the herbs and put into vegetal capsules. One capsule is inserted into the vagina daily for 7 days.

Peng Sha (borax), Ku Shen (sophora root), She Chuang Zi (cnidium seeds), Da Huang (rhubarb root), Ming Fan (alumen), Huang Lian (coptis), Bing Pian (borneol), Xiong Huang (realgar).

1. Jiling Hu. "Female Genital Disease." (lecture, Yo San University, Los Angeles, November 7, 2003).

Leukorrhea (vaginal discharge) in a Nutshell:

White, sometimes with a cottage-cheese like consistency - indicates yeast infection

Yellow, often with a smell - indicates bacterial infection

Bloody - may indicate cancer

Black - toxic heat, polyps, or tumor

Candida

Candida yeast is a naturally occurring microorganism in the body that grows in excess and mutates when the body's immune system is depressed. First we will cover the systemic candida picture, then we will address yeast infections specifically. Candida is a combination of Spleen Qi deficiency, Dampness or Damp-Heat, with Heat Toxin.[26] This is why treatment can be tricky. Simply draining excess Dampness, as most diets and programs do, can deplete the patient and cause a chronic condition.

Candida most often begins with Liver excess weakening the Spleen. There is an emotional disturbance in the Liver such as stress, anger, or resentment, combined with weakened immunity (overwork, lack of rest) and Dampness (inappropriate diet). There are two classic profiles for chronic candida and yeast infections. The first is a thin, Qi and Blood deficient woman with a driving excess Liver (taking care of too many people and things). The second is an overweight woman who loves her Damp-producing foods (such as ice cream, bread, beer, raw fruits). Chronic candida requires regular acupuncture, herbs, and diet therapy for several months. The only way to treat candida long-term is by strengthening the immune system (Qi and Blood).

The complicating patterns must be addressed concurrently. Soothe the Liver and calm stress. This includes addressing any stuck emotions that have been suppressed. The patient needs to find a healthy way to manage stress. At the same time, tonify Spleen Qi, regulate hormones, and nourish Yin and Blood. Besides their effect on immunity, Spleen Qi and Blood deficiency can create sugar addiction, as the body tries to pull itself out of fatigue, which will fuel candida overgrowth. Make sure to include specific herbs that clear Dampness and help combat candida such as: Bo He (mint), Bai Zhi (angelica), Ku Shen (sophora root), Fang Feng (ledebouriella root), Da Fu Pi (betel nut husk), Zi Su Geng (perilla stem), Huo Xiang (agastache), Sheng Jiang (raw ginger), and Ban Xia (pinellia).[27]

Excess sugar will create Dampness and/or Damp-Heat. Sweet, salty, and sour flavors are all moistening, building flavors. Pungent and bitter foods are clearing. I do not recommend extreme

26. Damp-Heat cases will have additional symptoms of a drawing down sensation in the lower abdomen, burning or hot urination, frequent urination.

27. These are many of the ingredients present in the patent formula Huo Xiang Zheng Qi Tang.

regiments completely eliminating flavor categories long-term, as it can cause more imbalance and failure. Rather, take a few days "fast" from sweets, salt, and sour foods to reset the palate. For most Americans, the bitter flavor, such as greens or unsweetened tea, is sorely lacking. A small amount of bitter is all that is needed and can be added to most meals.

In the case of candida, as with all Damp conditions, diet is critical. Follow the section on Diet (page 124) and clear Dampness (page 260). Take regular probiotics and eat a simple, nourishing diet. Enjoy food and eating. Food addiction often happens because there is a lack of pleasure in life, words that should be spoken are stifled, or there exists a deep unmet need for emotional nourishment. Attacking the only avenue for pleasure—eating—without addressing the underlying issue will only create more unhappiness.

Yeast Infections

Yeast infections are a special class of annoyance. Yeast infections often occur at times of hormonal instability and change such as puberty, pregnancy, and menopause. Stress and any immune suppressant can also bring them on. They can also be caused by local irritation, such as wearing restrictive clothing or sex after a period of abstinence. Certain soaps or bubble baths (containing detergents or irritants) can be enough to cause a yeast infection in some women.

Internal Formulas:

Yu Dai Wan is a common patent for vaginal discharge that tonifies the Blood while clearing Damp-Heat. If there is more Heat present combine with Long Dan Xie Gan Tang. Alternately you can combine Huo Xiang Zheng Qi Tang with the appropriate tonic or harmonizing formula.

External Treatment:

Yin Care is a patent concentrated herbal liquid that can used as a douche or a wash to alleviate local symptoms. A raw herb formula can also be used as a wash, douche, vaginal suppository,[28] or sitz bath. With a sitz bath, or vaginal steam, the woman sits over the steaming decoction allowing the herbal steam to penetrate the tissue.

PRACTITIONER SECTION: UTI FORMULA

This is a Bi Xie Shen Shi Tang modification:

Bi Xie (dioscorea root) 12g, Yi Yi Ren (Job's tears) 12g, Huang Bai (phellodendron) 12g, Mu Dan Pi (tree peony root bark) 10g, Chi Shao (red peony root) 10g, Ze Xie (alisma)10g, Hua Shi (talcum) 15g, Che Qian Zi (plantago) 12g, Jin Qian Cao (lysimachia) 15g, Hai Jin Sha (lygodium spore)15g.

28. A tampon is soaked with an herbal decoction then inserted in the vagina for a short period of time.

Urinary Tract Infection (UTI)

The key symptoms of a UTI are burning urination, dark urine, and heaviness in the lower abdomen. Urinary Tract Infections can be triggered by dehydration, sex, soap, tight clothes, poor hygiene, and hot weather or foods. To avoid introducing bacteria to the vulva or urinary tract, women should always be sure to wipe from the front to the back when using the toilet. Also, be strict that lovers may only touch this area with clean hands or genitals.

Burning urination can be a symptom of a yeast infection and may not be bacterial in nature. If there is cloudy urination with no burning or heat sensation, it is an indication of Dampness. Follow the Damp-clearing diet (page 260).

In case of a UTI, avoid spicy foods, citrus (astringes the pathogen), sugar, and dehydration. Eat cooling, hydrating foods, such as soups and congee. Drink ample water and cranberry juice.[29] At the first inkling of a UTI, take Yu Mi Xu (cornsilk) tea continuously throughout the day. To make it, fill a pot with cornsilk, then cover with water. Simmer for 45 minutes. Strain and drink hot or cold.

Sexually Transmitted Diseases

Sexually transmitted diseases (STDs) that are bacterial and acute in nature are easiest treated with antibiotics. Antibiotics have a bitter cold nature that damage the Spleen. Be sure to support Spleen functioning while taking antibiotics with formulas such as Jian Pi Wan or Xiang Sha Liu Jun Zi Tang taken with meals, along with the steps to promote intestinal health (page 248). Also be sure to take probiotics to rebuild healthy intestinal bacteria.

Herpes

The herpes family of viruses are a particular scourge on humanity. All forms of herpes are associated with nerve pain prior to an outbreak of itchy, fluid-filled vesicles. Here we will focus on the sexually transmitted variety, herpes simplex I and II, which can occur on the mouth or genitals. Shingles (herpes zoster) is covered on page 319. The herpes virus is highly contagious and can be passed to a sexual partner when the first signs of tingling or itching begin (prodome phase), as well as through contact with herpetic lesions. Avoid contact during any time the virus is active. Condoms may not cover the area of a lesion and should not be relied upon to protect against the virus.[30]

Herpes simplex reoccurs in similar circumstances to yeast infections. Herpes is a Heat Toxin that lies dormant, resurfacing when the body is weakened. Qi and Blood Deficiency (from overwork, illness), complicated by Liver Qi Stagnation (stress), Damp-Heat (poor diet and stress), provide the perfect

---

29. Take the pure, unsweetened version from the health food store. Dilute with water and add stevia to sweeten.
30. This is the consensus of the medical establishment for safer sex practices.

PRACTITIONER SECTION: HERPES SIMPLEX

Internal Treatment

Herbs that control active outbreaks of herpes simplex include Long Dan Cao (gentiana), Ban Lan Gen (isatis root), and Chi Shao (red peony root). I give Long Dan Xie Gan Tang in pill form in order to get compliance. Megadoses (14 or so teapills) of Long Dan Xie Gan Tang can be taken for 1-2 weeks, 2-3 times a day. Patients with herpes should have a bottle on hand and begin taking at the slightest sign of an outbreak. For patients who get an outbreak pre-menstrually, have them begin taking the formula at a normal dose one week prior to their menses. Zhi Bai Di Huang Wan is more gentle for use during menstruation and long-term. Give patients formulas such as Jian Pi Pian to take with meals to protect their Spleen.

Once the active lesion has subsided, the focus shifts to treating the underlying condition. There is typically a combination of Liver excess, lower jiao Damp-Heat, combined with a deficiency pattern. Modify harmonizing formulas such as Jia Wei Xiao Yao San and Xiao Chai Hu Tang with Qi, Blood, and Kidney tonics as appropriate. This formula should be taken for 3-6 months to build up the constitution. During the dormant phase continue to calm the Shen during acupuncture treatments. Be sure to educate your patient on diet and lifestyle.

Topical Treatment

Herpetic lesions respond to needling and bleeding methods just as shingles lesions do. Unfortunately, local treatment of herpetic lesions is too painful in the mouth or genital regions for many patients. If a patient is sufficiently uncomfortable to accept such treatment, use the Circle the Dragon technique. Use a thin gauge needle (I use 40 gauge Seirin needles). Circle the lesion with needles. Then needle the center. Alternately, use a lancet to gently open the lesions. These lesions cannot be cupped, but allow them to ooze and bleed on their own after removing the needles into a cotton ball. Note: It is crucial in this process to avoid cross-contamination and pay extra attention to sanitation, including wearing gloves.

Next, apply a compress by saturating a cotton ball in the external wash below and leave it on for 10 minutes. Finally, apply a powder to the lesion while still moist. These last two steps can be used daily by the patient at home.

External Wash - Make a decoction or sitz bath and use for 3-7 days. Alternately, use smaller amounts of herbs in the same proportion to make a smaller batch and use as a compress:

Huang Bai (phellodendron) 40g, Long Dan Cao (gentiana) 40g, Ku Shen (sophora root) 75g, Ban Lan Gen (isatis root) 40g, Ye Ju Hua (wild chrysanthemum flower) 40g.

External Powder - equal parts: Long Dan Cao (gentiana), Huang Lian (coptis), Bing Pian (borneol), Liu Huang (sulphur), zinc oxide.

environment for outbreaks. This makes stress management, long-term tonics, and proper diet key for keeping outbreaks under control. Acupuncture and herbs are most effective if used before the lesion erupts[31] and should be used as preventive care.

31. Prior to a lesion, there is a distinct nervy sensation on the surface of the skin.

Proper lifestyle is critical for those with chronic outbreaks. Manage stress by scheduling relaxation time regularly (yoga, meditation, etc.), avoiding clutter, removing drama and dramatic people from your life, and spending time in nature. Avoid overworking and be sure to sleep eight hours every night. Face emotional issues. Follow a Damp-Heat clearing diet page 265. Jiao Gu Lan (gynostemma) is a particularly effective adaptogenic herb for herpes simplex and zoster, and can be taken daily long-term to keep the immune system strong.

A Word on Safe Sex

Unfortunately, anything that happens below the waist in our culture is often imbued with shame. Any dysfunction involving the genitals or digestion requires a hushed tone and a break in eye contact. It is very important to adjust this attitude whether you are a practitioner or a lay person. Clear communication about sexual health history, including any current and previous infections, modes of protection used, and birth control are necessary conversations prior to engaging sexually with anyone.

The only thing more awkward than frank talk about the logistics of sexuality is sharing true intimacy and discussing needs and boundaries openly. Safe sex conversations should include expectations and needs in sexual relationship. Emotional and spiritual safety is just as important as physical wellbeing. The first step is to assess what your needs are, then craft a concise version to share with potential lovers. This goes beyond adhering to safer sex practices (such as using condoms) or the established norms of a relationship. Personal rules should be based on individual needs, values, and goals. Any ambiguity in establishing boundaries will lead to tension and drama later.

Once the personal rules for sexuality and relationship have been established, honor them at all times. This is a practice of integrity with yourself. The Po, through the physical, gut intuition, will always signal when a situation or lover is not in alignment with our highest good. It is a combination of conditioning and lack of value for the self that keeps us from listening. Bringing true needs and values to conscious awareness will make it easier to sense when you are in danger of compromising yourself.

A good rule, for example, is to have sex only when your body, heart, and mind are in alignment with that decision. This means there is physical chemistry, emotional safety and connection, and spiritual alignment. It takes time to achieve clarity on what we want and need. See your mistakes as lessons on what you do not want.

There is another facet. As women we often do not know the value of what we offer during sexual experience. Physically, we grace our lovers with Yin Qi, which flows effortlessly through us. There is a natural emotional healing that emanates from our hearts. Additionally, there are the gifts earned from our personal cultivation, which may include providing spiritual healing and advancement to our lovers.[32] Knowing that we, as women, possess this innate value makes us more inclined to expect that our needs and values be honored by our mate. Once the rules have been established, always expect a lover to stand by his/her word.

Levels of confidence and self-worth are greatly influenced by the health of the body. This is why building up our physical health is so important. For example, building Qi and Blood makes us less emotionally needy for, or in, a relationship with others, romantically or otherwise.[33] A strong Gall Bladder creates decisiveness and lessens the influence of outside opinions. Healthy Yang Qi provides the power and resolve to protect personal boundaries. Soothing Liver Qi makes us less dominant, controlling, and impatient in relation to others.

Crafting a Quick Safe Sex Speech

Ask yourself, "what do I need to have joyous, fulfilling sexual experiences that enrich my life and relationships?" Now answer the question as honestly as possible. Some common sub-questions might be:

1. What level of openness and transparency do I want from my sexual partners? Do I believe I can never have too much information or, do I like keeping certain things private?
2. Do I need celibacy, monogamy, or polyamory for my highest good right now? Exactly what does this mean to me? What will that look like? (The answer to this question may vary widely based on the time in your life).
3. What level of connection do I need from a particular lover? Do I want daily connection or do I prefer a more casual relationship? The degree of spiritual, emotional, and physical commitment desired needs to be established prior to engaging sexually.

When Should A Girl Become Sexually Active?

The answer to this question varies dependent upon physical and emotional maturity. Sex before a girl completes puberty injures her Jing. This can create issues with fertility, menstrual cycles, and her vitality later in life. During the first years after puberty, a girl's body is still vulnerable to injury from sexual intercourse. For most girls, full maturity does not happen until the late teens, though girls have been undergoing puberty at younger ages compared to statistics in the 1950s and 60s. Once women are physically mature, our bodies can handle a great deal of sexual activity, which, in the right context, strengthens us. Whereas men must learn techniques such as ejaculation control in order to make love often and for extended periods without injuring their Jing, a woman naturally has this ability.

32. Men have similar gifts to offer such as Yang Qi, a safe container, and love. Many men do not value the gifts they have to offer either. Instead, they often erroneously believe their value is based on sexual performance or what they can take from a situation.

33. Observe how, because pregnancy conserves Liver Blood, women become more self-sustained during this time.

Our emotions and spirit, however, can be injured by sex with the wrong partners or when we are not receptive. Girls should abstain from making love until they have learned to adequately discern among potential partners and have the strength to stand by their decisions. Until a girl is able to take responsibility for her physical and emotional health during sex, she is not ready. Women should ideally wait until their early twenties to have children, thus birth control should be taken very seriously at this age.

In this chapter we covered the 2nd Cycle along with the general topics of menstruation, fertility, and gynecological disorders. In the next chapter we will discuss the 3rd Cycle along with the energetics of sexuality, Internal Alchemy, as well as some of life's heavier lessons.

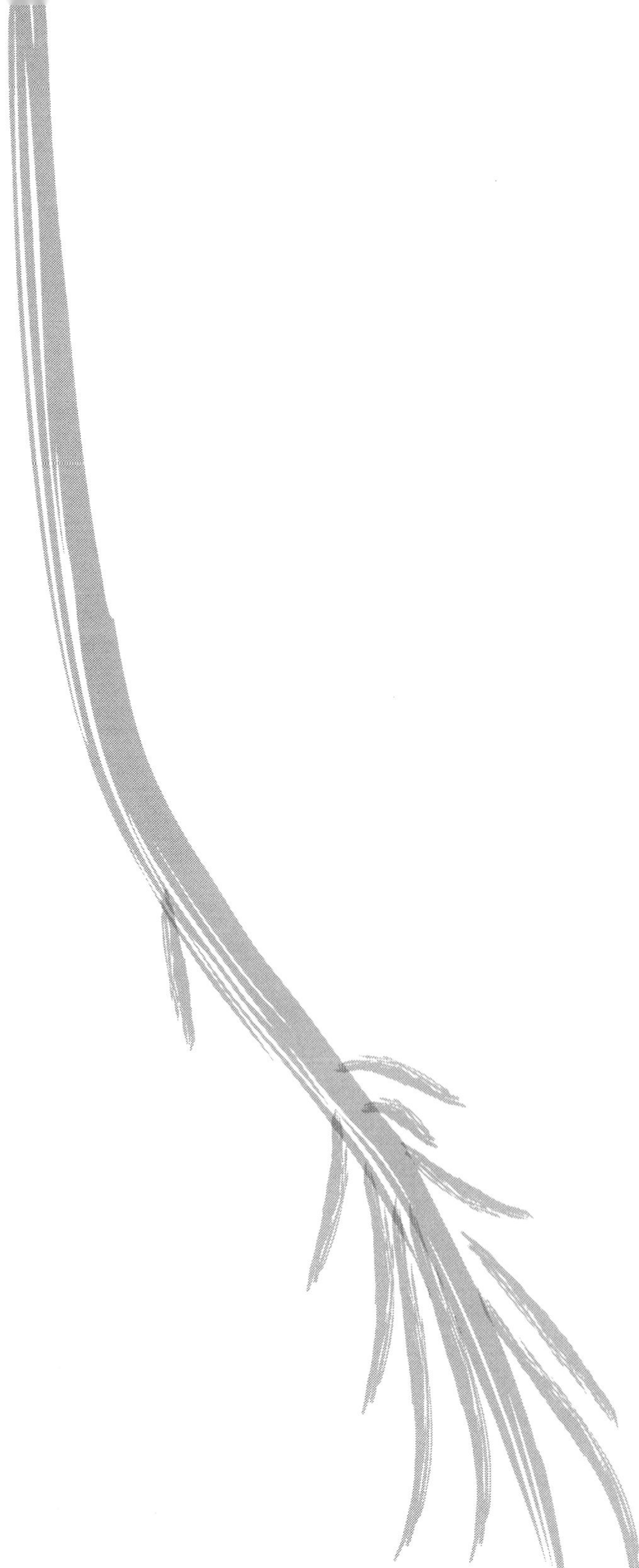

Chapter 3

Age 21

3 x 7, Kidney Essence peaks, the wisdom teeth come out and growth is at its utmost.

三七，肾气平均，故真牙生而长极；（21岁）

The 3rd Cycle

Three x 7 years begins the 3rd Cycle in a woman's life, when she reaches physical maturity. The 3rd Cycle begins at age 21 and extends to the age of 27. This Cycle begins the Earth Phase, representing a peak of physical vitality that continues through age 34. Like Earth, this is a time of building security, attachments, and nurturing relationships. It is also the phase of life that is most material and Earth-bound.

In ancient Chinese culture, the beginning of the 3rd Cycle was considered the most appropriate time for women to become sexually active. In a time without reliable birth control, the ancients believed that women should reach a fuller level of physical and emotional maturity before facing the dangers of childbirth. It also speaks to women reaching a certain sense of self and inner strength prior to engaging with partners. This chapter centers on sexual cultivation, drugs and alcohol, personal empowerment, physical development, and life's heaviest lessons. These are all relevant topics as young women step out into the world.

The Kidneys and personal power should be sufficiently strong. The Liver is the primary focus when treating hormonal imbalances occurring between 21 years of age through menopause. This is due to the deep connection between the Liver and menstruation. The Liver Blood is depleted after monthly bleeding. Also, in adulthood, Liver Qi Stagnation is almost inevitable, as Liver Qi Stagnation is the disease of unfulfilled desires and thwarted growth.

Sex and Self-Cultivation

The Jing is stored in the Kidneys, eggs, and sperm. This reproductive energy is the raw creative power used to manifest in the physical world. It is like a great furnace that is used to power whatever we want. In an unconscious state, humans will allow their vital energy to run out of them, treating every moment as if it were the last opportunity to reproduce offspring. When procreation is not desired this becomes wasted energy. Daoist alchemical practices center on cultivating, or conserving, this energy to create health in the body and for use in spiritual cultivation.

The primary way men lose Jing is through ejaculation, whether through sex with a partner or masturbation. Women lose Jing through loss of their eggs, either during menstruation or pregnancy. Thus men's sexual cultivation practices focus on mastering non-ejaculatory orgasms. Women's cultivation focuses on stopping or lessening menstrual flow, menstrual and postpartum recovery, and spacing out the birth of their children.[(1)]

Dual cultivation, or alchemical practices with a partner, facilitates the harmonization of Yin and Yang energy in the body. Women release Yin Qi and men release Yang Qi during sex and orgasm, which is then absorbed by their partner.[(2)] In a harmonious, loving interaction all parties are rejuvenated. Predatory or manipulative behavior regarding sexuality results from an individual's own dysfunctional Yang Qi or Yin Qi. Whether or not one is on the giving or receiving side of the interaction, both parties are damaged by it.

It takes more for a woman to injure her body through sex. The most common ways are: excessive sex when a woman is depleted, sex before a girl is fully developed, or sex while using drugs or alcohol. These all can cause Kidney deficiency including exhaustion, accelerated aging, and chronic vaginal discharge. A woman is more at risk of emotional injury from sex. Any sexual interaction that is not empowering for a woman is depleting and can damage the Shen (spirit). Women must avoid anything less than a loving, deeply honoring interaction. Sexual injury is often seen, for example, in prostitutes or women who abuse drugs.

A primary component of Daoist self-cultivation is learning how to refine and store sexual energy so that it can be used for spiritual advancement. Modern practice uses Daoist self-cultivation practices as a means of increasing health and youthfulness. These practices are included in the 3rd Cycle as this is when most women have achieved sufficient maturity to begin the practices, though they can be started at any age with significant spiritual, health, and beauty benefits. A woman can use these practices her entire life.

1. Proper menstrual and postpartum practices are covered in Chapters 2 and 4, respectively.

2. This is based on traditional roles. Whether a man or woman gives Yin or Yang, or in the case of same sex couples, I think what is important to note is that where there is sexual chemistry there is polarity. When those opposites come together they offer what is missing in the other and together they form a whole.

Inner Alchemy (Nei Dan)

In the Tang and Song dynasties (circa 618-1279), Daoists shifted from external alchemy to Internal Alchemy. Rather than turning lead (in this case cinnabar)[3] into gold, the focus shifted to transforming oneself into higher material. This section covers the basic components used to transmute energy that sabotages our progress into energy that fulfills our purpose.

The Three Energy Centers

There are three Dan Tians (cinnabar fields) as shown in Figure 3.1 which are the three major energy storage centers of the body.[4] These energy centers connect each individual to the Heavenly, Human, and Earthly realms. The **Lower Dan Tian** is located two finger widths below the navel and one finger width deep inside the body. It can extend to include the Hui Yin (perineum, located between the genitals and anus) and the Ming Men[5] (Life's Gate) in the low back. The Lower Dan Tian relates to the Earthly Realm.

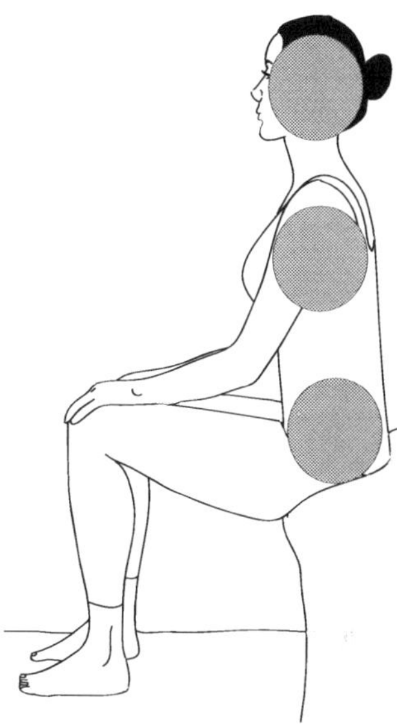

Figure 3.1. Three Dan Tians (Energy Centers)

The **Middle Dan Tian** is located in the chest and includes the Heart. This relates to the Human Realm. It is considered the most important Dan Tian for women's cultivation. The **Upper Dan Tian** is located between the Third Eye and the center of the brain. This is the seat of the Heavenly Realm, intuitive sight, and connection with the Heavens. There is usually too much mental activity which is why practices often focus first on developing the lower and middle centers.

Fire and Water

Besides strengthening the three major energy centers, Internal Alchemy focuses on harmonizing Fire and Water within the self. Several levels of symbolism can be found in the internal harmonization of Fire and Water. Firstly, they represent opposite aspects of human nature, like Yin and Yang.

Fire represents the Heart Shen (spirit) which allows loving connection with the outside world. Water

3. This is why cinnabar (dan) is used extensively in describing inner alchemical practices. External alchemy used the mineral extensively. It holds both Yin and Yang properties. When cool, it is red and hard. When heated, it becomes liquid and silver.

4. These are distinct from the Indian concept of the 7 chakras.

5. Du 4, located in the depression below the spinous process of the 2nd lumbar vertabrae.

represents the Kidney Zhi (willpower); the deep, still, spiritual aspect of self that connects to Divine Love and Purpose. The harmonization of Heart and Kidney creates an ability to experience Divine Love internally and externally.

Fire and Water also come together to make mist in alchemical practice. This mist combines the virtues of Love (Fire) and Truth (Water) and is capable of transforming everything it touches. As nothing can be destroyed, the negative aspects within the self must be transformed. Using mist or cloud visualization to dissolve and transmute unwanted emotions is a primary tool of Inner Alchemy.

Fire and Water represent opposite energetic movement, both of which are necessary for balance. Fire ascends like rising flames up the spine. Water descends like rain down the front centerline of the body.

The two elements further represent the key ingredients necessary for dual cultivation practices. Practitioners cultivate these virtues within the self, in relation to the Divine, and in relationships with others. Fire relates to Love. Water relates to Truth. Truth dispels the illusions of Love, while Love softens Truth. Fire relates to appreciation or adoration. Water relates to safety. Both are necessary for alchemical transformation. The simultaneous intent on Love and Truth keeps the student on a clear path. When the practitioner creates safety for his/her practice and holds a feeling of adoration it exponentially speeds growth. These same principles can then be applied to the external world with loved ones, in dual cultivation practices, and in healing work. These principles apply to men and women. The following practices are specific to women.

Cutting the Red Dragon

It is not until the Qing period (1644-1911) that we find detailed written instructions on women's Inner Alchemy (nu dan). From this time on, the foundational practice for Daoist women was to cut the Red Dragon, or stop menstruation. According to these texts, women must first convert their Blood into Qi. After this, women may proceed as men, transmuting their Qi into Shen, and finally emptiness (xu wu). Different sources offered variations, but the foundational practices were breast and ovarian massage, meditation, breathing techniques, and transmuting negative emotions. Breast massage, in particular, was used to divert the course of their menstruation back up to their Heart.

A subcurrent to these texts implied that these exercises would make a woman more like a man. She would return to her prepubescent state and lose much of her womanly characteristics. There is a sense that a woman's blood was impure and her emotions too erratic for spiritual development.[6] We have to remember that when we look at recorded history we are often looking through the lens of patriarchy. In many Eastern traditions it was (and sometimes still is) thought that enlightenment could only occur in the body of a man. Women today live in a time and place with much greater

6. Elena Valussi, "Female Alchemy and Paratext: How to Read Nüdan in a Historical Context," Asia Major 21, no. 2, (2008): 153.

freedom. We have choices on birth control, are no longer dependent on men for survival, and can express our sexuality with less severe consequences. Additionally, menstruating has become more convenient and sanitary. We must thus select what still works for us and what is no longer useful.

The current practice of women's Inner Alchemy has been adapted to this modern world. Women have created their own systems. Even teachers from patriarchal traditions cater their teachings to an empowered female audience, as in the West the ones who spend money on spirituality are mostly women. Most current systems of Women's Alchemy do not advocate completely halting menstruation, only lessening it. Also, the practices that once were used to create chastity are now used to enhance a woman's sexuality and femininity. They are also used for health purposes, not necessarily linked to any spiritual pursuit.

In practice, completely halting menstruation is an extreme accomplishment. Stopping the menses altogether can be dangerous if not under the direction of an expert teacher. If the uterus does not cleanse itself each month, as is the case in some menstrual disorders, it creates Blood stagnation. This has negative effects on the Shen and leads to masses accumulating, and even cancer. If women stop their menses they need to be adept at qigong exercises that keep the built-up Blood and Qi circulating. It is debatable whether this is worth the effort. There are great spiritual, beauty, and health benefits to practicing Inner Alchemy for the purpose of lessening menstrual flow. It is readily attainable and does not produce any negative side-effects.

What is good in moderation can become negative when taken to the extreme. I have the same concerns with women completely stopping their menses as I do with men stopping ejaculation. Some become too extreme in their sexual cultivation. For instance, a colleague related once how he did not cuddle after sex, lest his partners absorb his Yang Qi. The intent of ejaculation control is to avoid excessive leakage of vital energy and the ideal frequency of ejaculation varies according to the age and vitality of the man along with his lifestyle. In other words, the practice is used to balance the body. Older men might do well to not ejaculate for weeks or even months, whereas younger men can develop severe Shen Disturbance (mental issues) by going the same time period. Men who elect to place severe restrictions on their ejaculation are already predisposed to extremism. Either they have become excessively stingy with their energy or they wish to maintain an unbalanced lifestyle of excessive sex. The purpose of any health practice is balance. If something is creating imbalance, it should be discontinued. The purpose of any spiritual practice is not the practice itself but rather a spiritual state. Exercises are never important in and of themselves; they are simply tools. By aligning the mind with the desired state, the exercises happen of their own accord and eventually can be discarded. Fixating on an exercise or particular skill creates obsession and imbalance, the opposite of what is intended.

The second major shift in Inner Alchemy for women is that it is now used to increase sexuality. Women's Alchemy moves sexual energy. Previously, women were advised to transmute this energy for spiritual purposes. Now many women use this cultivated sexual energy to increase their beauty, youthfulness, and sexual vitality.

The third major shift is that women are using Inner Alchemy solely for health purposes. These exercises balance women's hormones and cycles, reduce cramps, and protect against masses in the breasts.

Intention

Intention is everything when it comes to working with energy. There are many potential benefits to Women's Alchemy practices. Be clear on what you want out of your practice. Do you want to cultivate energy for spiritual goals, such as spiritual advancement or to improve your healing work? Do you want to increase your sexual vitality and youthfulness? Do you want to balance your cycles and increase your general health? Or perhaps you want to ground the Divine Feminine in your body. Once you are clear on your intent, begin the exercises in the sections on Breast Massage, Ovarian Massage, and Jade Egg Practice, by taking a moment to focus on your intention. This focus is more important than the details of the exercise, as, in time, it will manifest the desired energy into reality.

Inner Alchemy unifies all your energy behind your intention. This is accomplished by 1.) transmuting negative energy within that blocks you and 2.) keeping energy from being wasted.

Universal Yin

In addition to magnifying internal virtues, women's Inner Alchemy connects us with and allows us to channel higher Universal energies, including Universal Yin. All living things are channels for energy, and we naturally channel what we focus on. Men can channel Universal Yin as well, and women can channel Universal Yang. Daoist practice advocates such energetic transgenderism as a means of balancing internal energies. For the specific purpose of the exercises for the feminine reproductive organs, Yin energy is the focus. This also creates a polarity for future dual cultivation. I find connection to Universal Yang easiest with physical exercise, as described later on in this chapter.

Universal Yin is akin to the Divine Feminine and is the primordial Yin force of creation. Unfortunately, this energy has either been repressed or strictly contained for many centuries crossculturally. Soft, fluid, mysterious, intuitive energy is destabilizing to hierarchical power structures, so it had to be isolated and rendered vulnerable. Repression of Yin blocks everyone's progress and freedom. A healthy person experiences the constant interplay of Yin and Yang energies which gives rise to new growth. It is important to rediscover the natural eruption of feminine energy within the self.

Exercise 3.1. Connecting with Universal Yin

Experiencing Yin Qi is unforgettable. It is gentle, loving, soft, radiant, healing, and Divinely powerful. Yin Qi follows no schedule and comes of its own accord. Yin Qi elicits absolute surrender, but not by instilling fear or inflicting pain. Rather, anything touched by its gentle grace is overcome with awe and love.

1. It is helpful to find a symbol of Yin energy, such as the Moon, a beautiful natural setting, a flower, or other personal symbol. As you focus your eyes on the object or scene, feel the Divine Feminine energy within it. She is at once beautiful, sensual, powerful, and angelic. Allow yourself to feel adoration and gratitude for this energy that birthed you and everything in existence. Stay here as long as desired.
2. Feel the love and adoration mirrored back to you, as the Divine Feminine outside of you sees and acknowledges the Divine Feminine within you. Imagine this energy pooling in your Third Eye, your heart, and your womb. Stay here as long as desired.

It may take time to connect with Yin Qi or it may come instantly. Over time, the internal connection with Yin Qi will grow and become easier to connect with the Yin Qi in others.

Breast Massage for Lessening Menstrual Flow

Breast massage is the primary exercise of women's Inner Alchemy. Regular practice regulates the hormones and lightens the flow of menstrual bleeding. Each month Blood flows down from the Heart center so that a woman can menstruate each month. Breast massage diverts sexual energy, which is raw creative energy, from leaking out during menses and sends it up to the Middle Dan Tian (heart center). Stimulating the breasts mimics the energetics that occur during and just after pregnancy, when Qi and Blood are diverted up to the breasts and there is a cessation of bleeding. The body puts its best into nourishing the new life with breast milk, prioritizing this over menstruation. Regular breast massage has the added benefits of eliminating breast lumps, firming the breasts, and sometimes increasing their size.

You can start this practice at any age, from puberty to post-menopause. It was considered ideal to stop the menses as young as possible to preserve the vitality. However, even the old texts recommended Inner Alchemy to women who no longer menstruated to rejuvenate them to a premenopausal state.(7)

For most of the benefits, you can begin the breast massage practice at any time during the cycle. If you want to lessen your period, first begin breast massage when you feel premenstrual symptoms:

> *All those who practice refinement for female perfection, must first ... sit until the qi within the body circulates freely. One day before the menstruation, at the hours of zi and wu (midnight and noon), start the practice. At midnight, put a robe on and sit with the legs crossed, with the two hands holding firmly to the sides of the ribs. After (the qi) has ascended and descended within the body a few times, press the left heel against the vagina and the rectum, clench the teeth, close firmly the eyes, shrug the shoulders, and lift up with great strength, thinking of the two red channels of qi that rise from the womb through the weilü* 尾閭 *pass and the three passes [weilü, jiaji* 夾脊, *yuzhen* 玉枕*], ascend to the niwan* 泥丸*, descend to the root of the tongue, and pour into the two breasts. In this manner, practice this continuously until the body is warm and then stop. Then use a white silk kerchief and*

7. Elena Valussi, "Female Alchemy avnd Paratext,"153-193.

insert it into the vagina to compare the quantity (of blood) to last month's and to see if there is any. Again, like before, (use) the circulation (of the qi) to scatter the blood and qi in order to avoid illnesses. In less than a hundred days (the period) will be cut by itself.[8]

Intention is very important here. A desire to avoid inconvenience or dislike of womanhood will not produce positive results; just as fasting for spiritual purposes is vastly different than refusing food out of hatred for the body.

Note: a light menstrual flow does not in itself indicate mastery or the superiority of a particular diet. It can also be a sign of anemia. Consciously lessening menstruation is not the same as causing Blood deficiency, a condition where there are not enough reserves to menstruate, as in the cases of excessive exercise or deficient diet. Chemically halting or lessening menstruation, as with birth control pills, causes Liver Qi stagnation and Blood deficiency, and will not produce the same results.

The following is a simplified routine. Some sources include more exercises, however I find simpler routines allow for more frequent practice.[9] Additionally, complicated routines distract the focus from feeling the energy. Perform breast massage daily except on the days of menstruation. If time is limited, the most important is Exercise 3.2b.

Exercise 3.2a. Opening the Lymph (Figure 3.2)

1. Use the fingers of your right hand to massage from under the clavicle at the center line of the body to the left armpit.
2. Grab the tissue at the juncture of the armpit and chest and pinch.
3. Repeat on the other side.

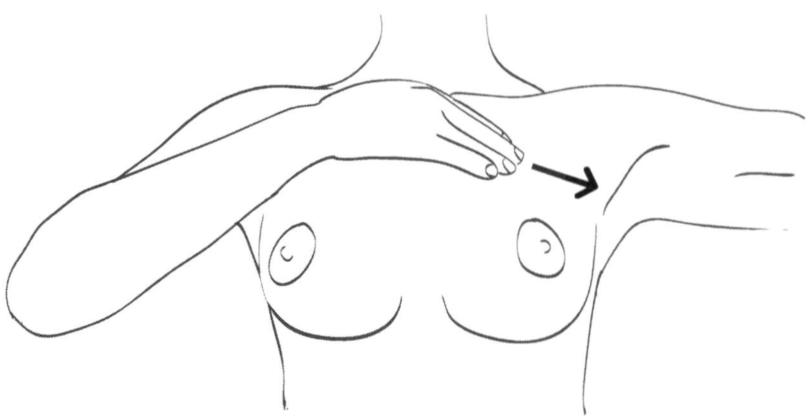

Figure 3.2. Opening the Lymph

8. Duan honglong 斷紅龍, p. 2b, in Shangcheng xiudao mishu si zhong 上乘修道秘書四種, in Daozang jinghua 12.2.
9. See Resources p. 453.

Exercise 3.2b. Performing Static Circles (Figure 3.3)

The greatest experiences in life happen when there is no expectation. Maintain an attitude of openness and curiosity. This puts the body and mind into a relaxed state of awareness. Focus on feeling the energy in the body.

1. Focus on the womb and ovaries. Feel them filled with Golden Qi.
2. Feel the Golden Qi rise up to the Heart. Visualize that this energy, rather than nurturing a baby through breast milk, instead resides in the Heart, where it can be used to love and heal on a universal scale.
3. Rub the hands together until they are warm.
4. Place the palms of the hands on the breasts and press in towards the rib cage, avoiding the nipples. Press firmly as if to touch your ribs. Make slow circles, moving up and inwards. Repeat 36 times, or until the energy shifts. This will build and increase the breasts.
5. Make slow circles, moving up and out. Repeat 36 times, or until the energy shifts. This will disperse breast lumps and stagnation. Normally it is recommended to perform them both ways (clockwise and counterclockwise). If deficient, focus on the inward circles. If excess, focus on the outward circles

Note: Perform the circles using arms and shoulders as one. Feel the scapulas (shoulder blades) move over the rib cage. This exercise opens connections in the entire upper torso.

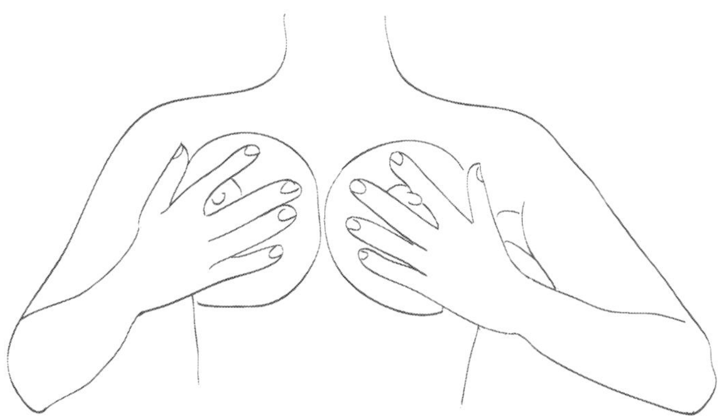

Figure 3.3. Static Circles

Exercise 3.2c. Performing Moving Circles (Figure 3.4)

1. Use the pads of the fingers to massage in small circles. Move up and inward. Repeat 36 times, or until the energy shifts.
2. Perform the same exercise, moving downward and outward. Repeat 36 times, or until the energy shifts.

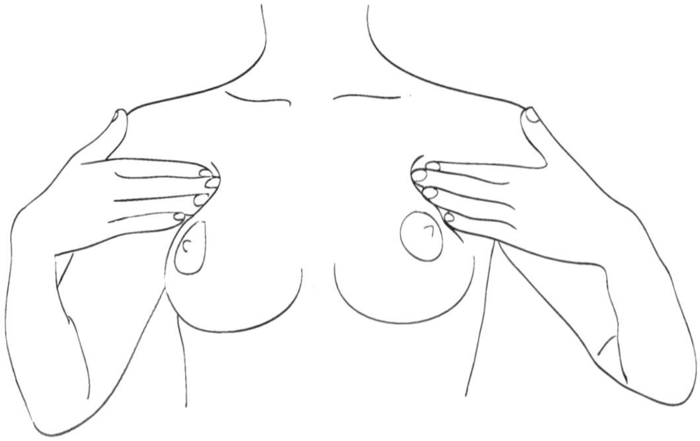

Figure 3.4. Moving Circles

Ovarian Massage to Boost Hormones

The ovaries, in holding our eggs, are the seat of our reproductive power and a primary site for storing our Jing. Inner Alchemy places great importance on maintaining and rejuvenating the ovaries. Daily ovarian massage circulates our sexual energy, moves stagnation, keeps the ovaries young, and stimulates healthy hormone production (increasing fertility if desired). During menopause the ovaries can shrink considerably. Performing daily ovarian massage can minimize this in premenopausal women and turn back this process if you are postmenopausal. Your ovaries are located about four inches below the umbilicus and three inches lateral on both sides.

Exercise 3.3. Ovarian & Uterine Massage

1. Rub your hands together to warm them.
2. Make a triangle with your thumbs and index fingers (see Figure 3.5). Place your thumbs at your umbilicus, forming a straight line from thumb to thumb parallel to the ground. Place the tips of the index fingers together to form a triangle, with your other fingers pointed toward your pubic bone. Where the tips of the pinkies and ring fingers rest are your ovaries. (This is the location of the extra point Zi Gong Xue). Where the tips of your index and middle fingers rest is your uterus.
3. Use your pinkies and ring fingers to massage your ovaries with a circular motion 36 times in each direction.

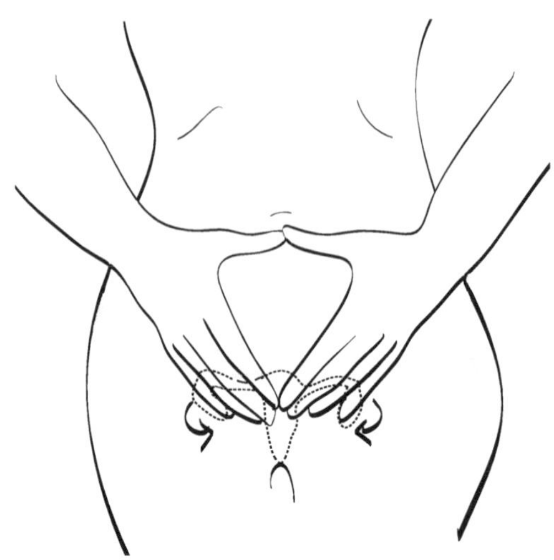

Figure 3.5. Ovarian Massage

4. Use your index and middle fingers to massage your uterus with a circular motion 36 times in each direction.
5. Keep your hands on your lower abdomen. Feel the warmth from your hands penetrating and rejuvenating your reproductive organs. Visualize them filled with a gold light.
6. You can proceed to circulating this energy through the Microcosmic Orbit (page 145).

Jade Egg Exercises to Strengthen Vaginal Muscles

Vaginal strengthening exercises can be started at any age to improve vitality, sexuality, and body awareness. They are necessary before and after childbirth for easing delivery and vaginal rejuvenation, and in older age to avoid atrophy and urinary incontinence. Vaginal exercises increase sexual responsiveness and enhance the ability to build and circulate sexual energy during cultivation exercises.

These exercises focus on developing the perineal muscles, particularly the pubococcygeus muscle (PC muscle). The PC muscle originates in the pubic bone and inserts at the base of the coccyx, forming the pelvic floor. It controls contraction and relaxation of the urethra (urine flow), vagina (during orgasm and childbirth), and anus (helps avoid hemorrhoids). The PC muscle holds the weight of our internal organs.

Jade eggs were a tool used by ancient Daoists to facilitate mastering the vaginal muscles. The exercises in this section may be performed without an egg, though using the jade egg will exponentially increase their efficacy and progress. Using a jade egg provides instant feedback and resistance, just as lifting weights does versus performing bodyweight exercises. It also serves to increase sensitivity and body awareness within the vagina. Jade was chosen for its ability to nourish Yin. Modern women can choose jade eggs, eggs made of other types of stone, and stainless steel versions in various shapes. They are most often marketed to decrease incontinence.

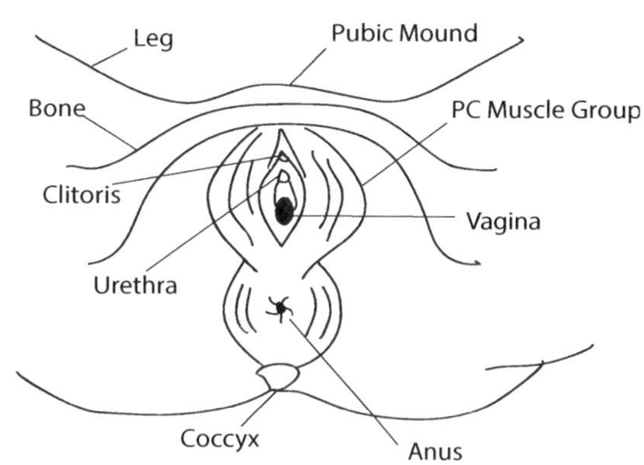

Figure 3.6. Pubococcygeus (PC) Muscle

Choosing Your Egg

Choose your egg carefully. It should be made of a non-porous material such as a hard stone or metal that can be sterilized. It should have a hole drilled through it. Dental floss or a sterile string is threaded through the hole and tied allowing for safe removal (like removing a tampon). As practice progresses, the string can be used to hang weights. Eggs come in three different sizes: small, medium, and large. Most women begin with a medium size and progress to a small one, which is more difficult to control. Women who have experienced vaginal delivery or muscle atrophy may prefer to begin with a large egg.

Always thoroughly disinfect a new egg by boiling it in vinegar and water for 15 minutes. Remove from the pot and cool prior to using. After every use, wash with mild soap and water and store in a clean dry place.

Exercise 3.4. Vaginal Strengthening Exercises

At first you might want to practice lying down until you get used to using your muscles. Otherwise they can be performed standing. Short daily practice is preferred to longer sporadic practice. Choose one or two exercises at a time. Some women go about their day with the jade egg in. More advanced practices involve controlling multiple eggs and adding weights to the string.

Basic Kegels
To find the PC muscles, the next time you urinate, practice stopping and allowing the flow. These are your PC muscles. Once you have found them, squeeze as hard as you can, then relax completely. A fully functioning muscle can perform the full range from tension to relaxation. Perform 100-200 repetitions daily.

Varying Tempo and Tension
Once you have mastered the basic exercise, begin varying tension and tempo. For example, practice slowly squeezing and slowly relaxing the PC muscles. Then do a few quick tenses and relaxations, pumping the muscle. Begin playing with full tension and then only half tension. Relaxing halfway rather than relaxing fully.

Horizontal Isolation Exercises
Next, begin to isolate three zones: the clitoris, the vagina, and the anus. This will seem impossible at first. Focus your attention on each zone and imagine that you are tensing and relaxing only that zone while keeping the others relaxed. Over time imagination will turn into actual muscle control.

Vertical Isolation Exercises
Isolate the muscles up the vaginal canal. First imagine that the entire canal, from entrance to cervix, is divided into 5 rings. Practice tensing and releasing each ring up, then each ring down. Progress by undulating up, then undulating back down. If using an egg, imagine moving the egg up and down the vaginal canal. Then side to side.

Hip Movements
Doing hip isolations rejuvenates the Kidneys, frees sexual energy, and keeps the joints of the lower body supple. When performed with a jade egg it strongly activates the neuroconnections within the vaginal canal. Figure 8s can be performed by the hips in four directions: up, down, forwards, and backwards. Practice moving very slowly. Once you have the movement, initiate the movement from the muscles holding the jade egg. See Hip Figure 8s on page 213 for instructions on hip movements.

Inserting the Jade Egg (Figure 3.7)

Tie a piece of dental floss through the hole drilled in the egg. This allows you to safely remove it.

1. Warm the egg in your hands and place it next to your heart.
2. Charge the egg with Divine Love. Envision it having the power to dissolve any unwanted energy that may be trapped in the genitals.
3. The egg is inserted wide side first. Place at the opening of the vagina. Imagine the vaginal muscles pulling the egg inside the vagina as you gently push it in.
4. Take a moment to feel reverence for your womb and genitals. See the vaginal canal as a conduit between Heaven and Earth energies and connected closely with your heart.

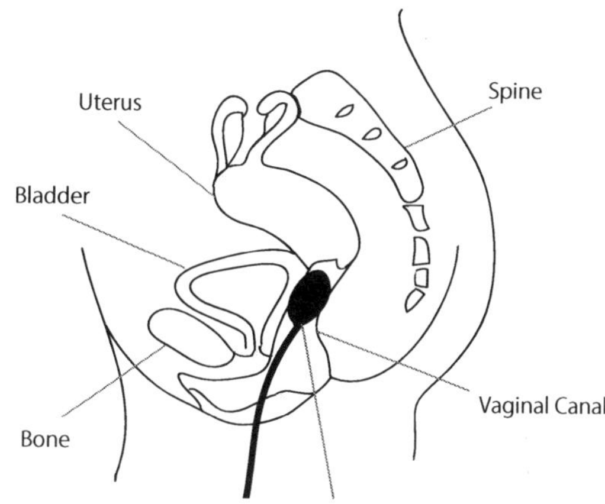

Figure 3.7. Inserting the Jade Egg

The Microcosmic Orbit to Circulate Sexual Energy

The Microcosmic Orbit refers to the connection of the Ren and Du channels as seen in Figure 3.8. Qi naturally flows up the Du channel, up the spine, and down the Ren, the front centerline of the body. Touching the tongue to the upper palate and squeezing the PC muscles[(10)] during qigong practice closes the circuit so that the Qi and Jing are contained within the circuit. Self-cultivation practices in both sexes focuses on opening, circulating, and building energy through these channels.[(11)]

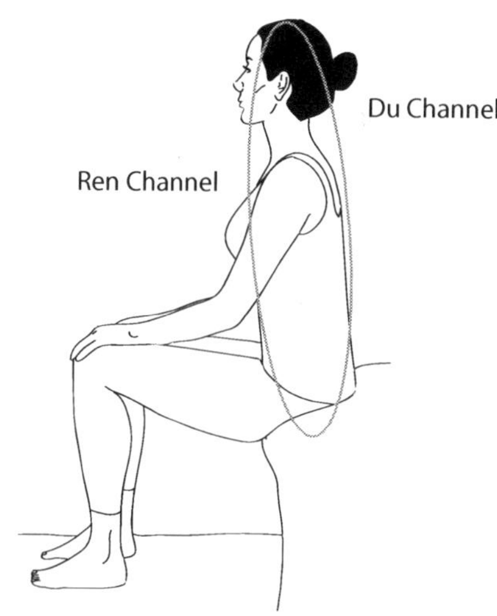

Figure 3.8. The Microcosmic Orbit

10. The pubococcygeus muscle. It originates in the pubic bone and attaches to the coccyx. Made famous by Kegel exercises, you can control them by tensing the muscles you use to stop urinating. Tightening these muscles keeps Qi from leaking out of the body during qigong exercises.

11. The Microcosmic Orbit, largely popularized by Master Mantak Chia in the West, is a staple of Inner Alchemy for men and women.

Exercise 3.5. Pearl Exercise

In this exercise we consciously move energy through the Microcosmic Orbit. This allows us to feel for blockages. Do this exercise after Breast and Ovarian Massage or at the end of other qigong exercises.

1. Slow and deepen the breath.
2. Touch tongue to the upper palate. Tighten PC muscles.
3. Focus on the Lower Dan Tian in the lower abdomen. Imagine the gold light of the Sun and the silver light of the Moon coming together to form a luminous pearl there. Concentrate love and gratitude on this ball of energy for several breaths.
4. Now begin to move the pearl. Exhale, send the pearl down the lower belly, across the perineum, to the tailbone. You can add a slight tuck of the tailbone to help the Qi to the spine, then release.
5. Inhale, move the pearl up the spine to the top of the head.
6. Exhale, bring the pearl back down the front of the body to the Lower Dan Tian.
7. Repeat as many times as feels comfortable. Then bring the pearl back to the lower abdomen. Place the hands on the lower abdomen for a minute.

Exercise 3.6. Primordial Circle Meditation[12]

This is a gentle method that allows the connections to open at their own pace. I like to do this exercise before going sleep at night. It can be done sitting or lying down. See Figure 3.9.

1. Slow and deepen the breath.
2. On the exhale, imagine warm light entering the nose and going down into the Heart. Inhale, relax. On every exhale collect more warmth in the Heart.[13] Do this exercise for 3 days.
3. After 3 days, begin the exercise as before. But now when the Heart gets warm, let the warmth overflow down to the lower Dan Tian.[14]
4. On the inhale, relax. On the exhale, bring the warmth down through the nose, the Heart, down to the Lower Dan Tian. Repeat steps 1-4 for 1 week, collecting warmth in the Lower Dan Tian.
5. After 1 week, begin with steps 1-4. Once the warmth builds up in the lower Dan Tian, expand the heat to the whole lower abdominal region. With practice the perineum will become warm. [15]

---

12. Based on an exercise by the same name brought by Master Hong Liu to the U.S. Merle Morgan-Drennan. "Medical Qigong" (lecture, Yo San University, Los Angeles, August 1, 2001).

13. A sensation of warmth is one of the ways we feel Qi moving in the body.

14. The lower Dan Tian is located 2 finger widths below the belly button and 1 finger width deep.

15. Located between the genitals and the anus.

This is as far as conscious connection of energy goes. The pathways will start to open up on their own allowing the warmth to flow through the entire orbit.

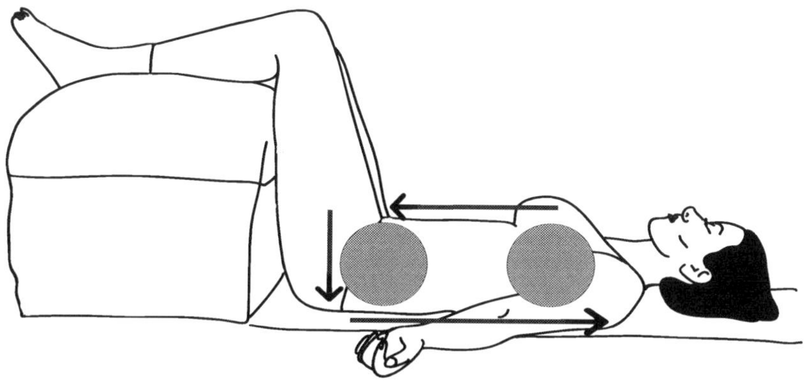

Figure 3.9. Primordial Circle Meditation

Dual Cultivation

"Semen is Latin
for a dormant, fertilized,
plant ovum -
a seed.
Men's ejaculate
is chemically more akin
to plant pollen.
See,
it is really
more accurate
to call it
mammal pollen.

To call it
semen
is to thrust
an insanity
deep inside our culture:
that men plow women
and plant their seed
when, in fact,
what they are doing
is pollinating
flowers.

Now.
Doesn't that change everything between us?"[16]

---

16. Stephen Harrod Buhner, *The Taste of Wild Water: Poems and Stories Found While Walking in Woods. (Raven Press,* 2009), 48, by permission of the author.

Inner alchemical practice is necessary prior to dual cultivation. It allows for better discernment in partner selection (choosing partners who are an energetic match) and better relationships. Once there is personal development, dual cultivation can be added. The term "dual cultivation" encompasses alchemical practices involving a partner. This can include anything from casual practice partners to sacred partnership.[17] When two or more people come together with the intention of giving, it exponentially increases the love and spiritual growth in their lives and those around them. At its best, it brings lovers to their most vulnerable state so that they may be fundamentally transformed. I recommend only practicing in the context of loving, committed relationships. True dual cultivation is not for the faint of heart. It is not a superficial romantic ideal, nor a sexual fantasy. It is one of the most powerful ways to transform ourselves.

There are thousands of particular techniques, which lovers should explore and experiment. What I discuss here are some foundational principles, without which the alchemical process cannot occur, no matter how high we swing from the chandeliers or how masterful we are with our jade eggs.

Attracting a Partner

Dual cultivation requires attracting the right partner. Practicing the Moon Meditation on page 85 increases women's magnetic Yin energy which attracts masculine energy. However, unwanted relationship patterns must be cleared, or else one will simply attract more of the same. Whatever relationship patterns we inherited, we have the power to change them. It requires holding reverence for ourselves, fearlessly rooting out unwanted patterns, dissolving them, and infusing a new energy in its place. In order to create something in our lives, we need to make space for it. Use the dissolving exercise on page 162 whenever unwanted feelings or patterns arise. You can then infuse what you want in their place using the following exercises:

Exercise 3.7. Holding Reverence for Yourself

Every woman is the embodiment of the Divine Feminine. Few women, however, are received into the world this way. Spend extra time during the Moon meditation and jade egg practice feeling reverence for yourself. Practice daily until this reverence is firmly rooted in your body. The rest of the world will respond to the reverence you hold for yourself.

Exercise 3.8. Receiving Love Meditation

Babies are wired to love whatever they receive from their primary caretakers. If the caretakers are abusive or neglectful, a baby will be wired to feel love whenever she encounters that abusive or neglectful pattern. In these cases a new healthy pattern will have to be consciously put in its place.

1. Every night before bed, focus on the energy a loving partner would possess. How would

17. Sacred partnership is used for a commitment where two people walk a spiritual path together.

they greet you, talk to you, interact with you? What would their energy feel like to you? What is it that you most need to feel from a partner?

2. Imagine this person sitting in front of you. Do not focus on their physical appearance, focus on the quality of their energy. Imagine this person loving you the way you want to be loved.
3. Receive this loving energy fully. Resistance m ay come up.[18] If so, it is an opportunity to do the dissolving exercise on page 162.

Adoration and Safety[19]

Once we have practiced seeing the Divine within ourselves through self-cultivation, we are ready to look deeply into our lover and see the Divine in them. When the Divine aspect within us sees the Divine aspect in another, there is an instantaneous sense of adoration that springs forth; a mixture of awe, honor, appreciation, gratitude, and love. Adoration is the manifestation of the highest aspect of Fire.

The second element that is necessary for the alchemical transformation is safety. True vulnerability cannot exist without a container of safety. We must have a desire to protect, to put at ease, and to create a soft resting place for our lover and we must be received in kind. Only in this way can our deepest wounds surface to be healed. (Otherwise our wounds surface to be re-injured).

Within our own selves, healthy Kidney Yang is the power that provides safety for healthy Kidney Yin (Divine Love). This harmonious interaction of Yin and Yang in the Kidneys produces wisdom, stillness, and peace. In relationships it is the role of Yang to provide a container of safety. Though this manifests in both genders, it is more commonly the role of men. Sexually, Yin Qi will not show up in its full expression unless a woman feels safe. Safety, and the peace it creates, is the highest aspect of Water, which balances Fire.

These two ingredients of adoration and safety cannot be bypassed. A woman cannot repress her true nature nor can she compensate for a partner who has not done his/ her work to fulfill this role.

Radical Honesty

Once adoration and safety, the essential ingredients for alchemical transformation are in place, a third ingredient can be added: the deepest honesty. Honesty means being transparent with yourself and your lover about your deepest truth. There is no issue too small and anything that disturbs inner peace must be addressed. It means sharing your fears, wounds, dreams, wants, and needs. It means staying when you feel like running, and being vulnerable when you feel like armoring up. With this

18. The vulnerability of an open heart can be very scary and difficult to sustain at first.

19. For more information see: Tom Kenyon, Judi Sion. *The Magdalen Manuscript: The Alchemies of Horus & the Sex Magic of Isis.* (ORB Communications, 2002).

process, the most hidden aspects of the psyche surface to be transformed. Radical honesty is the hardest, most frightening, and most healing practice we can engage in.

Entering Into Resonance

Ever since I can remember, when I was in deep connection with something, it felt like we resonated within each other. It is how I learned to communicate with animals, plants, spirits, and the natural world around me. It took me many years before I was able to explain the process with my conscious mind.

Resonance is how we can feel into the pain in a patient's body or know intuitively what a lover needs or hear the energetic call for help from a child or pet. Everything in creation has this ability and it is far more accurate than spoken language. Many people have consciously forgotten how or they may not have the words to explain it. Resonance helps us establish a deep rapport with our lovers.

Exercise 3.9. Finding Resonance:[20]

1. Get a singing bowl (or wine glass) and make it sing.
2. Listen for the tone. Where are you listening from? It is not just your ears. I most often listen from my heart, but others may listen with their hands or other centers of their bodies. When you make a bowl sing, you and the vibrating object are entering into resonance.
3. Once you get it, practice with others. Be sure to always ask permission. Close your eyes and feel into that part of you that is listening. Now turn your focus outward.
4. Next time you are watering your plants, feel into that place within you and listen to what they are saying.
5. When your dog or cat is in a relaxed state, feel into that place within you and from there connect with their heart.
6. Lay or sit heart to heart with your lover. Feel into that place within you. Move up to your upper Dan Tian (Third Eye) and from there connect with their upper Dan Tian. When you get it, it feels like you have an open door into their space, as they do into yours. You literally become one vibration. Take your time here. Now move down to your middle Dan Tian (heart) and repeat. Then move down to your lower Dan Tian (lower belly) and repeat.

When you are both done, gently fall out of resonance and come back to yourself. Sometimes plants and animals are easier to start with as they already know this way of communicating, and are eager for you to finally start listening to them.

Resonance requires a state of heightened awareness within and outside ourselves concurrently. When we enter into resonance with someone, our energy naturally flows well with them. When the connection does not serve us, we can simply come out of resonance with each other.

20. Modified from an exercise from Reid Mihalko. "Sexual Energetics." (lecture, August 5, 2012).

Connecting through resonance is a much cleaner form of connection than "cording" or "hooking." Hooking is when someone places an energetic hook into another person. This can happen consciously or unconsciously. The person being hooked will feel unbalanced and controlled by the relationship. Hooking is a common element in addictive relationships. Once you experience a connection that feels good, you will be able to feel immediately connections that are intrusive or unbalancing. You will be able to feel the hook within your own body and simply dissolve it.

Always ask permission, verbally if possible, or mentally before entering another's space. We always have the right to accept or refuse connection. Like the elements of adoration, safety, and honesty, resonance is not limited to dual cultivation or romantic relationships. These are ways we can relate within ourselves and with the outside world.

Sexual Energetics

Sex is based on polarity. When we make love we balance our Qi with the energy of our lover. Daoist teachings often have rigid rules about the role of the woman and of the man. There is similar polarity in same sex couples, or there would not be attraction. Also, the roles of Yin and Yang shift within healthy heterosexual couples. I believe developing this fluidity is important. I say this because I want you to find freedom and creativity in your sexuality, not a litany of rules and restrictions. When you hear masters espousing rules, view them as guidelines. Assimilate the information in a way that makes you and others feel empowered.

There are a number of mechanical differences between men and women. It is said that men are Fire, quick to ignite and burn out, while women are like Water, slow to boil and inexhaustible. Men and women enhance the sexual experience by balancing their own natures and supporting their lover.

Men typically must do more to connect their sexuality with their spiritual and emotional natures. They must learn to slow their desire and avoid distractions. Within the drive for sex is a desire for acceptance that men attain from being received by a lover. When men heal their need for acceptance, they can choose consciously when and with whom to have sex. When men are unconsciously led by their sexuality, they are easily manipulated by any woman who passes by. Many women both lament and enjoy the power this brings. However, when men are empowered and conscious they have much more to offer.

Another step men must take is to control their ejaculation. This means learning to delay ejaculation to keep pace with their lover and to orgasm without ejaculation to conserve their vitality. Controlling ejaculation creates mastery in other ways. Men's orgasm and sexuality is more focused on the genitals, whether through cultural teaching or biology. Women naturally have full body orgasms. Through ejaculation control men learn to experience sexual ecstasy in their whole body. Also, in unconscious ejaculation, men discharge their unprocessed emotions into their lovers, for them to process. When ejaculation becomes conscious, men can ejaculate positive energy into their lovers, for healing, for the attainment of a common goal, or for health.

Additionally, men have the special function of anchoring the Divine Feminine.[21] This is a spiritual function of the Divine Masculine that occurs cross-culturally during spiritual ceremonies. When men create a safe container, practice adoration, and exhibit radical honesty, women can relax into themselves and channel Divine energy into manifestation. When men learn to fulfill this role during lovemaking, it becomes a sacred event with magical effects.

Women's cultivation is different but no less challenging. We must also learn to center ourselves, ignite and circulate our sexual energy, and master our PC muscles. However, the real achievement for a woman is stay in her heart and to be receptive. We must clean out unwanted energy within us and develop the proper filters of discernment. This empowerment allows us to receive our lovers and to allow Divine energy to flow through us at the same time. This level of surrender takes preparation. It takes great courage and power to stay in this state.

If you are in a relationship, make a daily practice of making love. This balances energy, generates intimacy, and helps manifest your dreams. Be sure to use the Dissolving Exercise on page 162 to cleanse your own energy.

The Proper Place of Power

Power is only useful when it is in its proper place; as a servant. Within yourself, keep power as the servant to the innocent, vulnerable, and pure part of yourself. This is the lesson behind chivalric imagery. The knight (power or ego) is in service to God (the Divine within) first and the fair maiden (the vulnerable and pure) second. Within the physical body, power is concentrated in Kidney Yang; the right kidney symbolically. It must be equally balanced by spiritual love and awareness in the left kidney, where Kidney Yin is symbolically stored. When your power is balanced with love, rather than instilled with fear, you empower those around you. When power is too weak, this can lead to victimization. When spiritual love and awareness is too weak, this can lead to predatory or tyrannical behavior. As our knowledge of manipulating energy increases, so does our responsibility to use it properly. Without proper emotional balance, the same power that is used to heal becomes highly destructive.

Part of our purpose is to harmonize polarity. In order to learn balance we must often experience the extremes of imbalance. In the process we face our fears and learn awareness. The next section covers the darker aspects of ourselves and our world. As we develop awareness and discernment we learn to live in peace in a world of shadow and light.

21. I use the terms man and woman to represent the polarity of Yin and Yang. Individuals, regardless of gender can switch roles.

Pimps, Vampires, & Spiritual Gurus

"It is much easier to make good men wise than to make bad men good."

--Henry Fielding, 1749

Since early antiquity, a pimp would size up a potential prostitute. He would observe her and intuit her weaknesses. He would then call her out on these deficiencies of character and convince her she needed him. Over time he would break her down until he convinced her she could not exist without him. The truth to any outside observer is obvious. It is the pimp who cannot survive without the prostitute, whereas the prostitute is infinitely better off without him.

You do not need to study psychology or energy. You need only understand this basic mechanism to avoid the vast majority of predators. Every bully, con artist, sociopath, parasite, false guru, abuser, malevolent ghost, etc. is simply using pimp psychology. The basic mechanism is this: a wounded person feels out of control of his[22] internal environment so he seeks to control people and circumstances outside of himself. He studies weaknesses in others and develops strategies on how to make them dependent of him. He himself is bound by his misuse of power. In order to control someone else, he must believe the source of power is outside of himself as well. He develops no self-reliance and his very survival depends on his victims. Thus he will never connect with the source of his own power, which is within himself. All a pimp needs is to find someone looking outside of him/herself for an answer; someone who does not realize their own power.

Patriarchal Influences

Pimp psychology is born of patriarchal values, which in turn are based on fear, the illusion of separation, and disempowerment. Traditional practices and philosophies largely emerged out of male-dominated cultures that accepted exploiting women, children, and those who were of "lesser value." Our own culture has not emerged out of patriarchy which is why these practices continue, albeit more covertly. I received a thorough education on the misuse of spiritual and sexual power in churches, self-help groups, shamanic circles, Wicca, Daoism, and Tantra. The sad truth is that predators find refuge in spiritual, educational, and religious institutions, where people are at their most vulnerable and trusting.[23]

I had developed a disdain for Daoist and Tantric sexual cultivation. I had observed far too many men reverently quoting ancient texts on uniting Yin and Yang and honoring the Divine Feminine only to find them preying on young women in the most cynical fashion. I had seen women who called themselves goddesses, priestesses, or whatever spiritual name was in vogue, manipulating others to extract Qi and money. I came to realize that I need not avoid these philosophies altogether. Rather

22. I use the masculine pronoun to keep with the pimp metaphor, though it applies equally to women. I use the masculine pronoun to keep with the pimp metaphor, though it applies equally to women.

23. The molestation of children by priests and coaches that has recently been made public is an example of this.

I needed to be in a constant state of self-awareness so that I could discard teachings or teachers misaligned with my ethical beliefs. We now have the liberty to discard these darker practices.

Sexual Vampirism

> *'If you are able to change women with great frequency, the benefits you will gain are numerous. When a person constantly mounts a single woman, [her] yin qi will turn weak and the [health] benefits [for the man] will also be reduced. The way of yang is modeled after fire and the house of yin is modeled after water. Water is able to control fire, and yin likewise disperses yang. If used for a long time without stopping, yin qi will surpass yang and yang will then be diminished instead. What you obtain does not supplement what you lose. Nevertheless, if you are able to mount 12 women and not ejaculate repeatedly, this causes the person to not grow old and to have a beautiful complexion. If a person can mount 93 women and keep himself secured [i.e. without ejaculating], he will live for 10,000 years.' Sun Simiao, the King of Medicine (581?–682)* [(24)]

Sexual vampirism refers to a broad range of practices employing spirituality and sexuality to steal life force energy from unsuspecting victims in order to advance one's own physical vitality and spiritual powers. Various forms of sexual vampirism and black magic surfaced wherever sacred sexuality evolved.[(25)] Such practices are part of the history of Daoism and Tantra. Just as individuals developed methods to grow and evolve, others found ways to misuse them. Practices developed to rob sexual energy (life force energy) from others and to use magic to manipulate them on a physical, emotional, and spiritual level with huge karmic ramifications. Sexual vampirism is an ancient concept that has made its way to the West in Daoist, Tantric, and Tibetan Buddhist circles. There is also a "seduction community" (like pick-up artists and other groups) that uses modern manipulation techniques such as neuro-linguistic programming (NLP) to con women into bed. The seduction community and traditionalists sometimes cross paths, which is why I include them here; one uses black magic, the other nefarious psychology.

Sexual cultivation is meant as a mutual path of advancement. It becomes predatory for the same reason a pimp seeks a prostitute; the illusion of external control. Vampires see everything outside of themselves as a means to gather energy, attain higher states, and achieve immortality. The central fallacy of sexual vampirism is this: he/she can bring him/herself up spiritually by stepping on someone else, that by disempowering others he/she increase his/her own spiritual power. When reduced to its essence it is a comical idea. However, the practice is often carefully hidden in disinformation and theatrics.

Some sexual cultivation practices still largely serve to disempower women. Reverse ejaculation, for example, is a means to make opposite the energetics of sex, whereby a man sends energy to a woman, or rather they share their energy. Instead the man gives nothing and reverse ejaculates his

---

24. "Nurturing Life in Classical Chinese Medicine: Sun Simiao on Healing without Drugs, Transforming Bodies and Cultivating Life," The Journal of Chinese Medicine, accessed November 11, 2012, http://www.jcm.co.uk/product/catalog/product/view/10293/nurturing-life-in-classical-chinese-medicine-sun-simiao-on-healing-without-drugs-transforming-bodies-and-cultivating-life.

25. This is why I tentatively recommend teachers and books.

energy along with the woman's up his spine to his brain. Men in these groups are encouraged to engage in multiple partnerships and avoid loyalty or connection to any one woman. More than sex objects, women are sources of Qi for their own enlightenment. The women believe they are fulfilling a spiritual purpose, when in truth they are being used. Women have their own history of sexual vampirism, with their own techniques and following, which operate on the same central fallacy.

The best defense against hidden predators is self-awareness. Our instincts will alert us when we come in contact with someone who wishes us harm. Many of us ignore these instincts because we do not trust them, because we are conditioned to be nice, or because it is incomprehensible that someone could be so evil. It can be a process to learn to trust your instincts again. Forgive yourself if you falter and see it as valuable knowledge you received. Sexual vampires exhibit similar signs as spiritual abusers, see below.

Spiritual Abuse(26)

The topic of sexual vampirism is linked to the larger issue of spiritual abuse. Spiritual abuse refers to an abuser using their power within a framework of spiritual belief or practice to satisfy their own needs at the expense of others. Spiritual abuse is another form of the basic pimp con using spirituality in order to gain fame, money, power, and sex.

Modern media and information outlets have both unmasked and fostered the growth of new false healers, spiritual leaders, and gurus. Students and patients can seem like easy prey for unscrupulous teachers and healers due to basic human psychology. People often revert to a child-like state in order to learn or to be healed. Spiritual abusers tend to display certain characteristics. The following list is only to help you begin seeing the pattern. However, do not rely solely on this list as con artists are always adopting new tricks.

Common Signs of Spiritual Abusers (Pimps)

1. **Self Aggrandizement** – In traditional religions this would be called apotheosis (being raised to a god-like status). In spiritual circles you will see elaborate self-appointed titles. Whatever the semantics, the spiritual abuser is the one, the only, the best, and necessary for your spiritual advancement. He/she also does not have to play by the rules of mere mortals.
2. **Theatrics** – There is always music, lights, and other smoke and mirrors to keep you distracted from the fact that they are not really saying anything new or important. Some spiritual abusers have honed their theatrics to the point where they literally mesmerize their audience with their presence.
3. **Sexual Inappropriateness** – Spiritual leaders, teachers, and healers have a parent-like

26. Spiritual abuse is a term originally used to describe misuse of power by Christian clergy. It has currently been popularized by authors such as Steven Lambert. The term has grown to encompass religious and spiritual leaders in all faiths who misuse religious power including the growing number of false gurus. I have adapted the signs to what I have witnessed in a wide variety of spiritual, religious, and self-help settings as I believe the foundation is the same.

relationship with their followers, students, and patients. Their role is to create a safe place for learning and healing. Sex or romantic relationships with followers, students, or patients is a sure sign of a spiritual abuser. This may seem obvious, but many sexual predators have found safe haven in spiritual and religious communities.

4. **Angry Exes** – Every movement, teacher, or healer will have people who move on to other things. Spiritual abusers can amass a number of disgruntled ex-followers. This is a sign that people felt deceived.
5. **Cult Following** – The spiritual abuser cultivates a cult following, has an elite inner circle, and handlers to keep everyone in line.
6. **Inability to Take Criticism** – They grow angry or defensive if anyone dares question their behavior or their teachings.
7. **Denial** – They will have irrational reasoning to explain why it was okay for them to sexually abuse someone, steal money, or other outrageous behavior. They passionately repeat it, perhaps until they themselves believe it. Common themes are that their state of enlightenment makes it okay for them; or that their actions are to help their disciples grow. They refuse to take responsibility for their actions.
8. **Disempowering** – The spiritual abuser looks like a big, shiny object, and yet you find yourself feeling bad about yourself in their presence or after they leave.

Black Magicians

Black magicians are pimps who have learned to manipulate energy. They externalize the internal alchemical practices. Rather than mastering their own mind and emotions, they seek to control those of others. This places them at an advantage to manipulate those who are unaware of their energy.

You may not be able to see a black magician, but you can sense him/her by your own gut feeling. Many times the true face of a black magician will appear to you in a dream, even if your conscious mind believes the façade. Those who do harm to others carry the dark, heavy cloud of their karma with them. You do not need to be especially psychic to feel this. Every living thing has this instinct. We need to cultivate this awareness. The instant we are aware we can choose to disengage.

Staying Safe

The lesson of the pimp, whatever his/her form may be, is for you to realize what he/she does not understand; that the Divine within us is the only source of power. Use your qigong, meditation, and Inner Alchemy practices to cultivate self-awareness. This is their fundamental purpose. It will soon become very clear when you are in the presence of someone who is trying to disempower you. A spiritually evolved being will leave you feeling lighter and more empowered, the opposite of a pimp. Trust this unequivocally. All you need to do is see it for what it is, disengage, and let them go. If you become afraid, feel sorry for them, get angry, or offer them energy in any way, you will only give them an opportunity to hook you. Pimps need you to make them relevant. The best you can do is ignore them. (It might also be appropriate to warn others.) As long as there is someone to use they have no hope of rehabilitation.

When we are empowered we do not need anyone outside of us to validate us. Hold no person, place, or thing above the Divine within you and you will be safe. If you are ever tempted to believe yourself inferior to a pimp, remember, they need you, not the other way around. If you find yourself seeking outside of yourself look at it from a 5 Element point of view. The Elements present as follows: Wood seeks the perfect cause and becomes addicted to being aroused. Fire seeks the perfect lover and becomes addicted to love. Earth seeks the perfect family and becomes addicted to being needed. Metal seeks the perfect system and becomes addicted to rigidity. Water seeks the perfect teacher and becomes addicted to either learning or being protected. Whatever the hook is for you will tell you which Element needs balancing. This process will get you to the root of why you are seeking and heal that void.

Practicing Integrity

"Be silly, be honest, be kind" is a famous quote by Ralph Waldo Emerson. It is that simple to create a better world for ourselves and others. If you choose to do the practices in this book or other personal cultivation practices, be aware that they increase sexual attractiveness (energetically), energetic awareness, and spiritual power. Our moral responsibility increases in direct correlation. Understand that others may not be on the same playing field.

Exercise 3.10. Relating with Integrity

1. Be clear on your own boundaries. For many women and those who were brought up to be nice, this is a process. Be gentle with yourself as you learn how to say "no."
2. Always honor the boundaries of others. You do this by asking permission, supporting others in making conscious decisions, and then honoring their decisions (especially if you do not like it). This simple step avoids untold pain and karmic debt.
3. Be clear with yourself on what you want and communicate this to others. For example, in a romantic relationship, ask yourself: What are you real motivations for engaging? Is it pure attraction? Is it an expression of love? Do you want spiritual cultivation? Are you expecting to get something? It is crucial to communicate clearly what your needs and expectations are.
4. Take 100% responsibility for your actions.

These steps for integrity apply to all interactions.

Healing Ourselves

Traditional Chinese practices offer tools to understanding and healing emotional and spiritual wounds. I felt it was important to include the following information in this Chapter which focuses on young women because the earlier we begin the healing practice, the sooner we can become a healing presence in the world.

Understanding Abuse

In order to heal ourselves and others we need to understand how abuse and trauma affects the individual organ systems. People will experience issues with the organ systems that are constitutionally weaker, which explains why the same abuse affects individuals differently. Supporting these organ systems with acupuncture, herbs, and diet therapy will expedite progress in therapy.

Abusers share the following characteristics: they take no personal responsibility for their actions, they lack compassion or true connection with their victims, and they are in denial about their actions. If these did not exist they would cease to be abusers. Victims will either buy into the lie imposed by the abuser or reject it, based on their strength in relation to the severity of abuse. Abuse survivors will recover, or not, based on the strength of their organ systems. This explains why people can remain altered after being victimized and unable to heal while others are able to heal and move on. Weakened systems must be nourished so that survivors have the strength to process their experiences. Stagnations must be moved to facilitate letting go of old thoughts and patterns.

The Earth system, which rules bonding, trust, and sense of community, is often hard hit from abuse. This is particularly so if the offense occurred in early childhood when the Spleen was not fully developed. When the Spleen is not strong enough, the abuse survivor will not be able to properly digest what happened. There will be denial, and they will absorb the shame, guilt, and responsibility that rightfully belong to the abuser. The pattern of victimization is often stored in weak Spleen Qi. There will be irrational feelings of inferiority to the abuser and others, lack of self worth, dirtiness, shame, or guilt.

The potential for Earth injury is greater the more dependent the victims are on their abusers for survival. In the case of abusive parents or hostage situations, victims can develop deep denial and ingratiate themselves to their abusers. They may even develop feelings of love and loyalty towards their abusers that continues long after dependency ceases. This phenomenon is termed Stockholm syndrome, and results from the human psyche being hardwired for survival, at all costs. I have seen instances of child abuse survivors vehemently defending and adoring a horribly abusive parent. Such denial takes patience, time, and energy to unravel. Practitioners must provide consistency to heal the Earth element.

The Wood element governs the establishment of boundaries, decisiveness, courage, and the ability to reject false statements about the self. In order for abuse to occur this natural mechanism must be undermined. When someone is unable to defend him/ herself in the moment it causes Liver Qi stagnation. Abuse survivors often struggle to establish healthy boundaries. Either they become overly guarded and confrontational (Liver excess) or blame themselves for the abuse (Liver overacting on Spleen). For Liver excess, meditation techniques such as the Dissolving Meditation page 162 are helpful to move anger in a gentle manner. Acting out anger in such cases can create a habituation of, and addiction to, anger. These patients need strong Liver clearing formulas such as Long Dan Xie Gan Tang or Shu Gan Wan. In cases of Liver overacting on Spleen, patients need extra support expressing suppressed feelings, particularly rage. In these cases, physically acting out anger, such as hitting a pillow or shouting is therapeutic. Use harmonizing formulas such as Xiao Yao San.

Further injury occurs when victims who have a strong Wood system, speak out, and either are ignored or reprimanded. Many families and institutions would rather quiet the victim than face the change required in confronting the abuser. In cases where victims were silenced, energy gets lodged in the throat. The Esoteric Heart Shao Yin pattern is very effective to recover the voice.[27] Use

PRACTITIONER SECTION: HEALING EMOTIONAL & SPIRITUAL WOUNDS

Esoteric Acupuncture is very effective for emotional and spiritual issues.[1] Dr. Sankey's Cube on Cube and Heart Shao Yin Patterns are particularly helpful in these cases. The following are two traditional point prescriptions that can be used to assist healing of a wide range of emotional and spiritual damage:

Clear Dragon Treatment

This is an old "exorcism" treatment. It is effective in moving chronic depression and stubborn emotional patterns. This is an intensive treatment on both patient and practitioner. Patients may go into a healing crisis or there may be some turmoil around them for 24 hours or so after treatment. Practitioners should spiritually cleanse the room before and after, and do no more than one per day.

Begin by using sage or some other space clearing method that is meaningful to you to clean the space. Intend that the situation be transmuted gently for everyone's highest good.

Needle: Ren 15, ST 9, 25, 38, 40, Pc 6, Si Shen Cong Repeat clearing the space.

Sun Simiao's 13 Ghost Points Treatment[2]

Indicated for severe emotional and spiritual issues. Needle the points in this order and remove in reverse order. Begin on the left for men and the right for women.

Du 26, Lung 11, SP 1, Pc 7, UB 62, Du 16, ST 6, Ren 24, Pc 8, Du 23, Ren 1 (don't needle, apply direct moxa), LI 11, Hai Quan.[3]

---

1. Esoteric acupuncture was developed by Dr. Mikio Sankey. His fourth book has an extensive list of point prescriptions.
2. From the Qian Jin Yao Fang, 652 A.D., as repeated in Maciocia, *The Psyche in Chinese Medicine*, p.85
3. Extra point. According to Deadman, located in the center of the frenulum of the tongue between Jinjin and Yuye (M-HN-20) The tongue should be rolled back to locate and treat this point. If required the practitioner should roll the tongue back using a gauze swab or wooden spatula. If the deeper method is used, the tongue then rests on the needle with the mouth closed. To needle: 0.1 to 0.2 cun or prick to bleed; or 1.5 cun directed towards Yamen Du15.

appropriate formulas to move stagnation such as Yue Ju Wan (general stagnation) or Ban Xia Hou Po Tang (specific for the throat). Such patients must also be supported in appropriately speaking out and feeling heard. Practitioners must provide respect for boundaries to heal the Wood element.

The Fire system, which pertains to the Heart Shen (spirit), can be deeply injured by abuse. In such cases there will be chronic Blood deficiency and anxiety disorders. Humans are social animals and it is heartbreaking to be betrayed and injured by those we are designed to trust and connect with. The emotional blow of cruel words or the rage absorbed by the victim of physical abuse injures the spirit. The Heart Shen is particularly vulnerable when there is a spiritual nature to the abuse, as in the case of religious or spiritual leaders molesting children or assaulting followers in their care. Calming the Shen and Tonifying the Blood will be part of the treatment principle. Gan Mai Da Zao Tang with Long Gu (fossilized bone) and Mu Li (oyster shell) is a good general formula to settle the Shen in deficiency cases.

The chronic fear and moments of shock attendant to many cases of abuse and trauma cause injury to the Water element. Besides Kidney weakness symptoms, there may be generalized fear, irrational phobias, and flight responses. This Kidney weakness is a key component of post-traumatic stress disorder (PTSD). These patients have a deep need to feel safe.

When the Metal system is injured there will be a great deal of grief and inability to let go. Survivors will isolate themselves and feel as if their boundaries are constantly breeched. Yu Ping Feng San and Qi and Blood tonics are very helpful. Coming to terms with a sense of Divine Justice, particularly when earthly justice is not possible, is very important. They will also be concerned with protecting others and changing laws.

Integrating the Shadow

During each lifetime, the dark shadowy aspects of the psyche surface in order to be healed and integrated in a healthy manner.[28] A main focus of self-cultivation is to make this unconscious process conscious, thereby avoiding or mitigating painful life experiences. Conscious healing of shadow energies requires two steps: 1.) unearthing hidden aspects of the self and 2.) transmuting them into positive energy.

Unearthing Shadow

Meditation and dreamtime offer direct conscious access to the Hun (Ethereal Soul). During dreams and meditative visions, the unmanifest aspect of the soul (Hun) is able to communicate directly with the conscious mind (Shen). The Hun carries the unconscious aspects of self, karmic lessons, as well as a direct connection to the Universal Qi that flows through everything in creation.

28. Shadow refers to unconscious aspects of the psyche, which may or may not be negative.

Learning how to consciously utilize meditative visions and dreams allows us to make deep changes: resolve karma without acting it out physically, live life in alignment with our higher purpose, and clear negative patterns on a universal level.

It takes patience and practice to work consciously with the Hun. The Hun does not speak in linear terms. It communicates in the form of symbols, archetypes, and imagery. Do not expect linear, logical explanations.

Exercise 3.11. Developing Consciousness in Dreams and Meditative Visions[29]

1. Intend when you go to bed at night and before meditation that shadow aspects, negative life patterns, and your greatest fears come up in a form that you can understand and remember. If you are struggling with a particular issue, ask specifically that it come up to be resolved.
2. First thing in the morning, or right after meditation, make a habit of journaling dreams and visions. Include every detail possible and date it. This begins the practice of bringing the Hun into conscious connection with the Shen.
3. As you practice this, energy patterns will be cleared during dreams and meditation. You will be given guidance on how to clear residual patterns in waking life.

Transmuting Shadow

Every time a painful feeling surfaces, either due to a dream, during meditation, or in response to a life experience, there is an opportunity to transmute unwanted energy. Transmuting this energy is the basis for alchemical transformation of the self and spiritual evolution. I recommend making a daily practice of this. No upset is too small to be cleared. Life's challenges become opportunities to transform suffering into greater happiness. The bigger the trauma, the bigger the gift that awaits.

Exercise 3.12. Dissolving Unwanted Energy

There are many variations of this simple meditation which form the basis for Daoist alchemical transformation. For a more complex version see the 5 Cloud Meditation on page 311.

1. Any time you are faced with an overwhelming emotion or situation, ignore the impulse to run away mentally, and sit still. Bring up the person or event and imagine it in front of you.
2. Fully feel whatever is present. Feel acceptance and compassion for yourself for having these feelings, as if you were comforting a crying child. Look inside yourself to see where the feelings are located.
3. Take a moment to connect with Heaven and Earth (page 84).
4. Imagine the most loving, compassionate energy. You can use spiritual or religious imagery such as Buddha or Jesus. See this compassionate energy take the form of a Golden mist.

---

29. Carissa Schumacher. "Understanding Our Dreams." (lecture, San Diego, November 16, 2012).

5. Go back to where you felt the unwanted feelings and direct the Golden mist to dissolve it.
6. Stay present until it is dissolved.
7. Focus on the virtues you want to place in the new space that opened up. For example: peace, ease, patience, love, kindness, strength, etc.
8. Trust that it is done.

Exercise 3.13. Changing the Outcome of Dreams

A shift happens when we realize that we are never at the mercy of our dreams. We have complete power to confront and clear any negative occurrence or energy within a dream. A nightmare is often a warning or a shadow issue coming to the surface.

1. The next time a painful event is about to occur in a dream, simply stop and re-script it. For example, if you dream you are being chased by a predator, imagine you grow very big and powerful, turn around and effortlessly stop the predator. Or, imagine that a flock of huge birds comes and carries the predator away forever. Make it as fantastical as you want. Just change the energy.
2. See a Golden mist dissolve any residual unwanted energy.
3. Infuse positive energy in its place: healing, love, abundance, health, peace, etc.
4. Know it is done. Changing energy patterns in our lives can be as simple as deleting a computer file.

Forgiveness

"Resentment is like drinking poison and then hoping it will kill your enemies."

--Nelson Mandela

Forgiveness has been a process for me and for many of my patients. I understood conceptually that resentment and guilt merely keep us locked in old energetic patterns. I knew that resentment blocks our good from entering our lives. I knew that forgiving myself and others was key to spiritual progress, and yet at times it seemed very difficult. It did not help to beat myself up for not being able to just let it go. I finally came to understand three things that make the forgiveness process easier:

First, forgiving does not mean absolution of responsibility. Whatever someone does to another, they have already done to themselves. When a person commits a wrong against another, they set in motion instant energetic ramifications, even if those ramifications do not manifest physically for some time. Divine justice, unlike human justice, is absolute. The Universe takes care of it. Whether I choose to forgive or hold resentment, those feelings only affect me.

Second, forgiveness does not mean accepting bad behavior. Forgiveness is not denial. It is candid acceptance and a choice to let go of unwanted energy. Discernment still applies. If someone is violent, unscrupulous, etc. I avoid having them in my life. Forgiveness also would not keep me from taking appropriate action to protect myself or others.

Third, forgiveness does not leave you vulnerable to attack. In certain environments wearing an armor of anger feels necessary to avoid victimization. However, resentment does not protect me from harm. My discernment, my intuition, and what I have learned from past lessons do. The more present I am in the moment, the easier it is for me to access these gifts. I cannot be present when I feel resentment.

Resentment can also become a habit or an addiction. This requires re-patterning with daily forgiveness. Herbs, acupuncture, and other therapies that move physical stagnation in the body help dislodge trapped resentments and emotional blockages.

I use the following exercises to practice forgiveness as I need to.

Exercise 3.14. Forgiveness Exercise

1. Bring up a person or situation for which you hold resentment. See the person or situation in front of you.
2. Go into the most painful aspect; the part you most want to avoid. See the details of the situation and bring up the pain
3. See the Golden mist dissolving this pain.
4. Bring up any blame you place on yourself, such as "I should have known better", etc. See the Golden mist dissolving these thoughts and feelings.
5. Ask yourself what you believe about yourself to stay locked in this situation. Do you believe this person has power over you? Do you believe this always happens to you? Use the Golden mist to dissolve these beliefs.
6. Ask yourself if there is a secondary gain to holding on to this resentment. Do you get out of facing something? Use the Golden mist to dissolve these beliefs.
7. If resistance to forgiveness comes up, accept it and dissolve it.
8. Feel yourself grow larger than the situation.
9. See the Golden mist dissolving the image of the other actors.
10. Create a new scene and feelings you want to replace the old one.

Exercise 3.15. Practicing Atonement

1. This can be used to process an infraction you committed on a living thing or group. It will both help in their healing and dissolve your own guilt. It is often harder to forgive ourselves.
2. Go into the most painful aspect. See the details of the situation.
3. Feel deeply into what prompted your behavior.
4. Imagine a Golden mist transmuting this aspect of yourself into a virtue. For example, if you acted out of fear, bring in courage in its place.

5. Empathize with the one(s) you hurt. Feel into how they must have felt.
6. Experience the pain you inflicted on them in your own body. Everything you think you did to another, you have done to yourself.
7. Imagine a Golden mist dissolving the pain in your body.
8. Offer a heart-felt apology and a gift of grace. See them made whole again and bright.
9. See the Golden mist dissolving the image of the role you played. See yourself transformed into a higher aspect of yourself. See yourself behaving as you wish you could have, from a place of higher consciousness.
10. See yourself as forgiven.

A New Identity

"Thinking there is a problem to be solved is the problem to be solved."

--Matt Wuchner

Our egos love wounds and traumas. Once these have cleared, there is often a moment of "who is this stranger?" We find ourselves responding differently to life situations. The energy within ourselves feels different. There may be a moment of wanting to revert to old familiar patterns. No matter how painful those patterns were, there is always a perceived gain, so that letting go of the pattern will register as a loss of something. This is the last hurdle. It is common to miss the drama and excitement of negative life patterns. Many people are at first uncomfortable with peace.

The paradox is to both fully acknowledge our deepest wounds and to realize that these wounds are not our identity. Trauma is just the gift wrap covering lessons and gifts. Once a trauma has been addressed, healed, and forgiven, it is to be discarded, and only the gift retained. No one is truly broken or a victim. These are temporary illusions, though they feel very real at the time. The real you is deeper than any life experience can injure.

This is challenging because you will reach the point where the ego is at risk. In dissolving old traumas and thought patterns, our very identity is questioned. We can no longer be the victim or unloveable. The world can no longer be a scary place. All the illusions that we have clung to must fall away, leaving us in unknown territory.

Altered States

Inebriants are used for a variety of reasons: to escape, to relax, as medicine, and as a tool for self-exploration. This section covers inebriants used as medicine, for self-exploration, and addiction.

Inebriants as Medicine

The ancient Chinese viewed herbs with hallucinogenic or mind-altering properties as unbalancing, and therefore largely excluded them from their pharmacopeia. However, they used alcohol extensively as a medium for internal and external application of herbs.

Alcohol

Fermentation has a long history with humanity. It has the ability to extract nutrients and compounds (and some say the very "spirit") that would otherwise be unavailable. Traditionally fermented alcoholic beverages were social and spiritual affairs. They contained plants with nutritive, medicinal, and mind altering abilities. In its proper place, alcohol is warming, promotes Blood circulation, and is used to extract favorable compounds. Minor, occasional inebriation can open stuck states of consciousness. In excess, it generates Damp-Heat, is addictive, damages the Liver, and eventually the Yin. Traditional Chinese Medicine advocates the use of substances in so much as they balance. Anything that creates imbalance is to be avoided.

Exercise 3.16. Treating a Hangover

The following are some home remedies for alcohol intoxication:

1. Make a tea of Ge Hua (kudzu vine flower) and Zhi Ju Zi (hovenia dulcis fruit) for hangover or alcohol poisoning.
2. Drink watermelon juice (blend watermelon with a little water). Watermelon rehydrates, cools the body, and drains Damp-Heat.
3. Take milk thistle in tincture form long-term to protect and gently detoxify the Liver.
4. Daikon radish counteracts the Damp-Heat qualities of beer in particular.

Tools of Self-Exploration

In terms of plant spirit medicine, psychoactive plants talk so loudly and abrasively that even the densest human will listen. These plants (like ayahuasca, opium, belladonna, and iboga) have been used historically to open up the consciousness of initiates during religious ceremony. Their purpose in these circumstances is not to create dependency, but rather to give a strong enough experience, and to create a sufficient opening of consciousness, that the initiate may then hear the softer voices around him/her. Sometimes they are used on an ongoing basis in ceremonies to facilitate shamanic journeying.

Such plants warrant great respect as they are not gentle. They will abruptly take the user for a ride into the deepest parts of the psyche. It is an acceptable risk in many traditional initiations that some who attempt the journey will not make it back. Like the traditional vision quests, where initiates forgo food and water and weather the wilderness alone, this may not be appropriate for modern people.

Hallucinogenic substances will also have a different effect on a person who grows up with certain world views. Those with painful pasts or who are just looking for extreme experience may get more than they bargained for. Hallucinogens must be used with caution and require an experienced guide to assist with journeying.

Cacao

If you need a tool to access the hidden aspects of the psyche I recommend using ceremonial-grade, raw cacao. Her spirit is unique in that she first creates a loving, peaceful, heart-opening experience, after which one is invited to delve into the deepest aspects of the self. Her journeys may take one through remembering deep and painful experiences, or bring up aspects of the personality one would rather not face. However, there is a noticeable absence of fear. Cacao facilitates seeing these issues in a loving light and helps to dissolve them.

Ceremonial grade raw cacao has a much more powerful effect on the body than the chocolate available at the grocery store. For the first time, I recommend attending a raw cacao ceremony that will provide additional safety (it does act upon the physical heart and is very warming). After this it can be used during periods of self-healing. Even without ingesting cacao, one can connect with the cacao spirit. She is quite approachable.

As with cigarettes, cacao can also be used addictively. Its hot nature can cause Yin deficiency and inflame Heat conditions. When paired deliciously with dairy and sugar, it also generates Dampness.

Plant Spirits

It is not necessary to ingest plants to experience their awareness-opening abilities. Plant meditation is safe, powerful, and easily accessible. See the Resource section on page 392 for more. Each individual will develop his/her own associations when working with plant spirits. These are a few of my own:

Moxa (artemesia species) – These are powerful, warrior-like spirits. Their smoke is used to root out evil Qi in the body and can be used for spiritual protection.
Sage (particularly white sage) – Has a grandmotherly energy to her. More gently, yet

authoritatively, separates out elements that should not be there. Used for smudging. I like to keep a plant in my meditation area.
Lemon Verbena – A particularly cheerful and warm plant spirit. Her fragrance and tea are very healing to those needing emotional support.

Freedom and Addiction

Inebriants, like sexuality, hold tremendous power, which is why societies place so many restrictions on both. As with sexuality, repression of inebriants only intensifies their shadow aspect. Inebriants are a lesson in the healthy balance between boundaries (Metal) and freedom (Wood); stillness (Water) and activity (Fire).

Paradoxically, appropriate boundaries create a condition of safety within which greater freedom can be experienced. Within the proper context, inebriants have the ability to break old patterns and limited thinking. Without boundaries, inebriants open the individual to negative influences and experiences, and bind them in addiction. Excessive boundaries, as found in religious zealotry or the military, fosters the opposite extreme of hedonism and addiction.

PRACTITIONER SECTION: TREATING DRUG ABUSE[1]

New addiction begins with a Heart excess imbalance. This is the euphoria phase where the new addict is not content with normal levels of joy and stimulation which are naturally followed by a return to calm. The new addict gets locked chasing an overjoyous state. Chronic addiction and withdrawal becomes Liver Qi stagnation. The addict can no longer achieve previous levels of euphoria, yet he/she keeps trying. Eventually, the addict is simply avoiding the increasingly painful sober state. The shift from Heart imbalance to Liver imbalance varies according to the individual. This pattern is also true of non-chemical addictions such as sex, hoarding, gambling, etc.

In cases of chemical addiction, there will be additional injury to various organ systems. Opiate withdrawal, for example, causes Liver overacting on Spleen. During physical withdrawal, Liver excess will present. Long-term abuse of all substances weakens Kidney Yin, and eventually Kidney Jing.

Treatment of all addiction requires sedating excess Heart Fire and smoothing Liver Qi, in addition to treating other presenting patterns. There is always a factor of Shen disturbance. The key to treating addiction is to calm the Heart and Liver enough that the addict can face what he/she is running from. Until the question "What am I running from?" is answered, the addiction will continue in some form or another.

The nature of addiction is manipulation and it is very easy for caring practitioners to get reeled in. When treating addicts be compassionate yet detached. Let them prove themselves. Do not come to their rescue or allow them to shirk personal responsibility.

1. My knowledge of treatment of addiction comes from lectures with Dr. Steve Given at Yo San University, Los Angeles. He has written several articles on the subject including "Understanding Addiction According to Traditional Chinese Medicine." The Journal of Chinese Medicine 54/12.

There is a distinction between different types of inebriants. Milder inebriants have more opportunity for good in relation to their side effects. The stronger the inebriant, the more potentially dangerous it is.

Addiction

All people have a hole inside themselves that can only be filled by self-actualization. Many will try to fill this hole with distractions. In susceptible individuals, this easily becomes full blown addiction.

Addiction is characterized by a disturbance in Fire and Wood. There is a drive for overstimulation and freedom from reality. The healthy functions of the Heart: intimacy, vulnerability, and connection, are replaced with fear of intimacy, overstimulation, and disconnection. The healthy functions of the Liver: expansion and growth, give way to narcissism, an inability to take responsibility for one's actions, lack of regard for consequences, and escapism. Shen disturbance and Liver Qi stagnation are part of every addiction pattern, even when the addiction transfers from substance abuse to another form of addiction. When the Kidney Yin is damaged there will be constant agitation, disdain for stillness, and paranoia. Addictions eventually consume Kidney Jing, at which point there will be severe health problems. An extreme example is methamphetamine, which can weather an addict overnight.

Food Addiction

Food cravings begin as the body tries to balance internal weakness. A craving for sweets indicates Spleen Qi and Blood deficiency. A craving for salty foods indicates a Kidney weakness. Food addiction arises when there is an emotional need to nurture the self that is not being met. It can also be an attempt to literally stuff ones voice. Excess weight also functions as a physical buffer to the outside world. Treatment of food addiction requires treating the Shen, like all addiction, with an additional focus on the Spleen.

Marijuana (Huo Ma)

Marijuana is called the "fire herb" in Chinese, and true to its name, it has a very heating effect on the body. The seeds, Huo Ma Ren (hemp seeds), are moistening and Blood nourishing, and used widely for constipation. The leaves were used with mulberry leaves as a wash to promote hair growth. I have not seen literature on the medicinal use of the flowering buds of marijuana in TCM, which is the part of the plant containing higher concentrations of the inebriating THC. Most of my knowledge, rather, comes from my clinical practice in Southern California. It is the use of the buds for mind-altering experience that will be discussed here.

TCM finds itself in a unique position on the marijuana debate for legalization and safety of use. With its quest for balance, TCM prefers to keep difficult herbs on the periphery. Marijuana is one such complicated herb, and there are many herbs and therapies which replace its positive functions, without its side effects. The same cannot be said for Western Medicine, however, where medical marijuana has been substituted for harsher medications in the treatment of pain, nausea, and anxiety.

Occasional use at low dosages will not produce ill-effects and is most appropriate in Cold Damp conditions. Marijuana should be avoided in cases of excess Heat or Yin deficiency. Chronic use causes excess Heat to accumulate in the body, causing Blood and Yin to dry up. Wind conditions (spastic diseases), menstrual problems, gnawing hunger, and liver toxicity may develop.

Marijuana abuse disturbs the Shen in a unique way. There is often a sense of spiritual superiority and grandiosity associated with its use. It envelops users in a psychic fog making it difficult to connect with non-users. There is a degree of denial attendant to marijuana addiction that I have only found in thin sugar addicts.

Tobacco

Tobacco is used spiritually across the Americas and has been adopted by the African, European, and Native-American hybrid religions as well. Its primary purpose is to act as a bridge between human and spirit realms. Intention is everything, as always. Without spiritual intention, and mixed with chemicals, cigarettes are a powerful addictive substance. When used addictively, smoking depletes Yin and Jing and damages the delicate Lungs. Smoking cigarettes (or marijuana) depletes the Vitamin C in the skin quickly causing increased wrinkling.

Ban Bian Lian (lobelia) is an herb specifically used to stop smoking. In ex-smokers, fenugreek seed tea helps to expel toxins from the lungs. Take one teaspoon of powdered fenugreek three times a day in hot water between meals for several weeks. Eat moistening foods such as asparagus, Bai Mu Er (white cloud fungus), sweet rice, Asian pear, Hei Mu Er (black wood ear fungus), and black sesame seed to rebalance the Yin.

Table 3.1. Inebriants and Their Effects.

Inebriants	**Qualities**
Beer and Ale (Defined as fermentation of grain)	As a general rule, the darker heavier beers more strongly tonify Qi and Blood. Performing as an enjoyable nutritional supplement for our malnourished ancestors, they can easily create Dampness and Damp-Heat in the modern, over-nourished body.
Wine (Defined as fermentation of fruit, wines tend to have a slightly higher alcohol content.)	Wine is more warming and moving than beer and less so than hard alcohol. Wine also improves digestion. Red wine is more warming than white wine and often triggers symptoms in menopausal women and rosacea cases. In excess, wine damages the Yin and creates Damp-Heat.
Hard Alcohol	Strongest action to Move Blood and most often used as base for medicinal wines. Excessive use more severely injures the Yin and generates Damp-Heat.
Marijuana	Creates Heat in the body and depletes Yin. Lowers testosterone and disrupts hormonal cycles in women.
Tobacco	When used in ritual context, attracts positive energy to a ceremony. Creates excess Heat in the body and depletes Yin. Chemical additives toxify the Liver. Smoking dries up Lung Yin, and creates Lung Heat.
Amphetamines	Creates false Yang. Devastates Yin and Jing. May be associated with sex addiction.
Cocaine	Creates false Yang. Devastates Yin and Jing. Lung Qi deficiency.
Prescription Painkillers	Strongly unbalance the Liver.
Opiates (heroin, methadone and morphine)	Causes Liver and Spleen disharmony. Devastates Yin more intensely. Phlegm-Heat.
Hallucinogens (PCP, LSD, and mescaline)	Damages Kidney Yin and overextends Kidney Yang.

Physical Development

It is as important to develop the body physically as it is to practice Internal Alchemy. Whereas Women's Inner Alchemy mostly develops Yin Qi, physical exercise develops Yang Qi. Optimal physical development requires understanding the role of Yin and Yang as it relates to physical exertion. Yang Qi is designed for short bursts of energy and is unsustainable over long periods. Living things can maintain a Yin state indefinitely. This relates to physical development in that periods of intense, focused activity are balanced with longer periods of rest and recovery. This is readily observed in Nature. Even the most aggressive predator will spend most of its time sleeping.

View physical exercise as an enhancement of overall health. Most modern workout subcultures approach exercise in unbalanced ways. There is a trend towards extreme experience, rather than long-term vitality. Exercise should be focused on increasing the long-term health and vitality of the body. One should finish workouts feeling invigorated, not depleted.

The health of the Spleen, and overall digestive functioning, is key to physical development. Healthy, attractive muscular development depends on it. Lifting heavy objects uses Qi and Yang. Tonify the Spleen and Kidney Yang while training strength. Endurance requires Qi and Yin. Tonify Spleen Qi and Kidney Yin when training for endurance.

In all species in nature the female is pushed to develop her physical body comparably to a male. Engage in a variety of forms of physical movement. This allows the body to master opposite movement qualities: fast and slow, graceful and forceful. It is important to test the limits of strength, endurance, and flexibility. Put the body in positions where it has to trust its own instincts. These experiences activate the meridians (develop the neuroconnections) the way nature intended it to happen. This is the healthy development of the Wood element of the body and reduces the propensity towards Liver Qi stagnation that all adults have.

Exercise 3.17. Rules for Physical Development

1. Be sure to fully heal injuries. Make sure to seek appropriate help whenever your body alerts you with pain, immobility, or numbness. This could mean a massage or sitting in a hot tub when the muscles are sore, etc. Regular acupuncture and massage should be part of every athlete's regimen.
2. Rest when you are tired. Drop the intensity when you feel run down. Balance intense physical exercise with "soft style" movements such as Dao Yin, qigong, Tai Chi, restorative or Yin yoga, etc. These will save your joints (joint injuries end the careers of most athletes) and make sure channels are open and running. They will also restore energy.
3. For well-rounded physical development include strength, mobility, flexibility, nuance of movement, and focus/body awareness.

PRACTITIONER SECTION: PHYSICAL DEVELOPMENT

Sore Muscles, Minor injuries – Sore muscles and injuries are Qi and Blood stagnation. Take 2-4 capsules of Yunnan Paiyao. A little rice wine or shot of hard liquor will make it more effective.

Endurance – Endurance sports deplete Qi and Yin. Take San Qi (notoginseng) with Xi Yang Sheng (American ginseng) long-term, see formula page 226. San Qi will move the Blood, and Xi Yang Shen will tonify Qi and Yin. Take Shan Yao (Chinese yam) regularly in formulas and diet to preserve the Essence, and tonify the Spleen.

Muscle gain, improved Skin tone – Healthy muscle tone and taut skin are signs of healthy Spleen Qi and Blood. This is why animal protein works so well for building muscle and rejuvenating the skin. Be sure to optimize digestion (page 70, page 248) and take Qi and Blood tonics such as Bu Zhong Yi Qi Tang or Ba Zhen Tang.

Increase Strength - Heavy weightlifting taxes Spleen and Kidney Yang. If not balanced with stretching and mobility, it creates Qi stagnation, which retards strength goals. To increase strength, tonify Qi and Yang with herbs such as Lu Rong (deer antler), Ren Shen (ginseng), and mountain ant, taking care not to overheat. If you run hot it is safer to follow the guidelines for muscle gain. Open your channels through soft style stretching and mobility exercises such as Dao Yin or Yin yoga.

Cut Fat – If you need to get lean, be sure to include bitter tasting substances such as ku ding cha (drink with meals), bitter melon, watercress, and other leafy greens. For water retention eat Yi Yi Ren (Job's tears), red adzuki bean (recipes page 351), and drink cornsilk tea.

Surgery Protocol for Athletic Injury

Two days prior to surgery: take 2-4 Yunnan Paiyao capsules with alcohol 3x a day. Workout (non-traumatizing) up to the day before surgery (if in good physical form) or at least get movement. Set the intention of quick healing.

Take the little red Yunnan Payao pill right after surgery. Continue Yunnan Paiyao capsules, 3 x a day until healed.

Get moving as soon as possible. When wounds heal sufficiently start water therapy.

Alternate ice and heat. Use firm massage to improve circulation and prevent scar tissue. In acupuncture treatments, get jumping Qi and use electrostimulation. With joint injuries, needle Ashi points above and below joint and move closer to the joint as it heals. With musle injuries, needle the origin and insertion along with the local Ashi points.

Combine Yunnan Paiyao with herbs to tonify and speed healing: Gu Sui Bu (drynaria), Lu Rong (deer antler), Huang Qi (astragalus), Du Zhong (eucommia bark), and the formula Si Wu Tang.

When treating muscle injury, tonify the Spleen. When treating tendon and ligament injuries, tonify Liver Blood. For broken bones or fractures tonify the Kidneys.

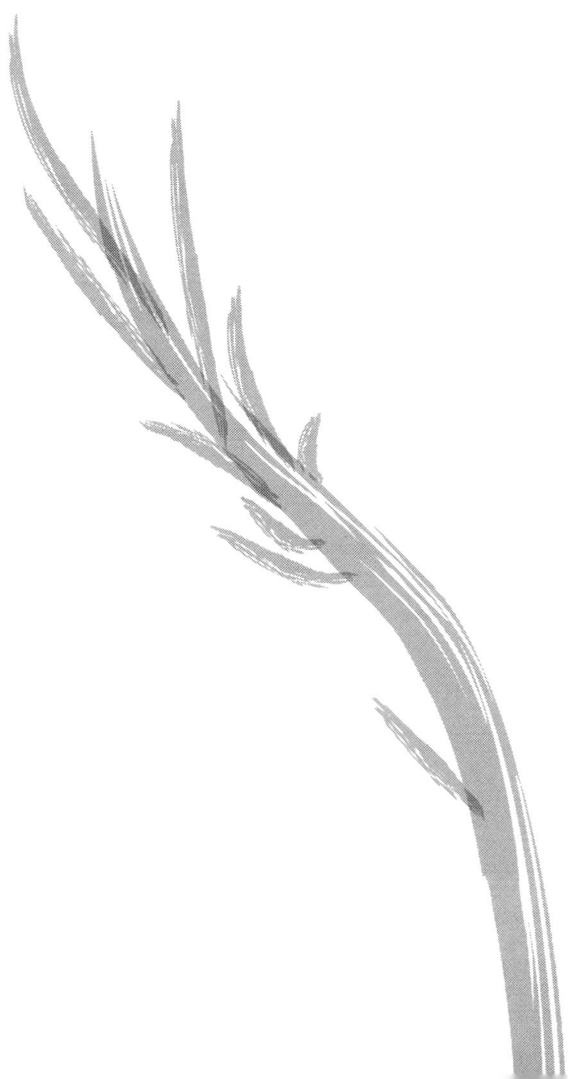

Chapter 4

Age 28

4 x 7, Tendons and bones become strong, the hair grows longest and the body is strong and flourishing.

四七，筋骨坚，发长极，身体盛壮；（28岁）

The 4th Cycle

Four x 7 begins the 4th Cycle in a woman's life. At the age of 28 the Earth Phase reaches its peak and a woman's body is at its physiological height through age 34. In this chapter we will cover the topics of pregnancy and postpartum care. Traditionally, this is considered the natural peek of a woman's physical vitality and the period that produces the healthiest and "smartest" babies, though many women will have babies much earlier and later.

DISCLAIMER

This chapter contains traditional knowledge from Taiwanese and mainland Chinese sources. I relay it here for its cultural and historical value as well as potential health value. Many health practitioners avoid treating pregnant and postpartum women. By providing this information I hope to give expectant mothers more choice on how to manage their health and that of their babies. Herbs and diet therapy should always be under the guidance of an acupuncturist. These practices are not necessarily supported by Western Medical practice. Always consult with your doctor.

Pregnancy

Traditional cultures understand that the health of the family begins with the health of the mother. Babies are created by the union of the Jing of both parents. Strong Jing produces vibrant, intelligent, talented children. The healthier a mother's Jing, the more she has to offer her baby. Further, the physical and emotional state of the mother during gestation and breastfeeding continues to greatly influence the constitution of the baby.

Chinese culture places emphasis on quality rather than quantity when it comes to children. This means both mother and father should be in optimal health and stability. Babies should be spaced apart by several years, as pregnancies close together weaken the Jing of the mother. Also, having fewer children, with more years between them, allows parents to focus more on each one. In this way, both children and parents benefit.

Pregnancy affects women differently. It depletes the Kidneys but conserves Liver Blood, as women do not have to replenish blood lost in menstruation every month. Women who are Liver Blood deficient often experience feeling strong and happy during pregnancy. On the other hand, women who are Kidney deficient can be pretty miserable during pregnancy, as vital minerals are leeched from them to feed the fetus. Understanding this can help women prepare better.

Traditional cultures also have elaborate postpartum traditions that continue for 30-40 days after giving birth. This is a necessary period of rest and recuperation that modern culture seems to have forgotten. Indeed, in Traditional Chinese Medicine, the postpartum period is considered one of the three "Golden Opportunities" to renew (or devastate) a woman's constitution. With all of the modern conveniences available today, many women are left haggard and permanently weakened after having children. This is absolutely unnecessary. You will want to read the section on Postpartum Recovery while you are still pregnant as you will need to make preparations in advance.

InVitro Fertilization (IVF) and Artificial Insemination (AI)

Western medicine has made it possible for parents to conceive in spite of natural blocks to fertility. If you and your spouse have difficulty conceiving naturally, it is still necessary for both of you to optimize your health. For women, this means maintaining a healthy weight, balancing your periods, eating an organic diet, learning how to quiet your mind, and getting eight hours of sleep each night. In fertility cases the pressure is typically on the woman, however, the quality of a man's Jing is equally important. Men must also maintain a healthy weight, achieve hormonal balance, eat an organic diet (particularly abstain from marijuana, beer, and hormone-laden dairy), and learn how to manage stress. Both parents should see an acupuncturist and live a healthy lifestyle for 3-6 months prior to fertility treatments. This will make for an easier IVF or AI process, increase the rate of success,[1] an

1. Paulus W, et al. Influence of acupuncture on the pregnancy rate in patients who undergo assisted reproduction therapy. Fertility and Sterility April 2002;77(4):721-4.

easier pregnancy, and a healthier mother and baby. You may be pleasantly surprised that you do not need medical intervention to conceive after all.

The number one cause of infertility I see in my practice is two-career couples trying to squeeze a child into their hectic, overworked lives. This is not ideal for the child or the parents. My Chinese TCM teachers would always say, "You need to make space for a child."[(2)] Many of us Westernized practitioners are reticent to say this to our patients, but it is absolutely the truth. You need to create a peaceful, happy opening in your life for a child to be born into. A child should be a conscious coming together of two people where there is enough time and space to enjoy the process.

Pregnancy Dietary Guidelines

Diet during pregnancy should be varied, whole food-based, with additional care to protect and nourish the Kidneys. Women can experience bone loss due to calcium depletion. With a limited supply of nutrients available in the body, preference always goes to supplying the fetus' needs, even if it is to the detriment of the mother. (There is an old wives' tale that says a woman loses a tooth per child.) Inadequate vitamin and mineral intake during pregnancy can lead to fetal maldevelopment and/or calcium depletion, bone density loss, premature senility, and even premature menopause in the mother.

During pregnancy, women's bodies also become more Yang (hot) and stagnant (the fetus is a form of stagnation in the body). This condition requires cooling and gently moving foods.[(3)] In addition to daily vitamin and mineral supplements, there are some additional recommendations.

Basic Rules of Eating During Pregnancy

1. Avoid coffee and black tea as they are heating and interrupt absorption of nutrients.
2. Eat calcium-rich foods liberally such as: bone broth (recipe p.342), dried fish,[(4)] organic milk, and seaweed.
3. Eat a protein-rich diet: include ample protein throughout the day to build Qi and Blood. The most challenging times to avoid animal protein are during pregnancy, breastfeeding, and menstruation.[(5)]
4. Eat vegetables 3 times a day: greens supply vital nutrients for the body and have a cooling and clearing function to clear excess Yang gently. This also helps prevent constipation.[(6)]

---

2. See Chapter 2, p.139.

3. Postpartum this is reversed, and the woman's body becomes Yin, requiring warming foods.

4. Eating dried fish, especially small fish, is encouraged in traditional Chinese culture to build calcium. In modern times, the benefits may be outweighed by the exposure of fish to pollution and heavy minerals. Choose fish carefully and avoid raw fish.

5. Interestingly, many women carrying daughters report craving a more vegetarian diet.

6. Use Mu Xiang Shun Qi Wan for pregnant women with constipation. It also works to wean people who are dependent on laxatives.

Traditional Beneficial Foods During Pregnancy

Lotus Root – Calms the Shen (nerves), promotes bowel movement, promotes metabolism, and eliminates gas.
Daikon Radish – Clears Phlegm and Heat. Improves digestion, eliminates gas, and increases absorption.
Chinese Cabbage, Cucumber – These are especially cooling vegetables. Vegetables as a group are cooling, detoxify, and increase metabolism.
Button and Shitake Mushrooms – Resolve Phlegm-Dampness. Safely moves stagnation.
Organic Chicken Gizzards – Improve digestion and absorption.
Shellfish – Used traditionally to calm the Shen (nerves) and stabilize the fetus. With toxicity issues may not be appropriate.

Foods Pregnant Women Should Avoid

Shrimp – Very Yang (hot-natured) and can trigger hormonal imbalance.
Liver – Expels blood from the uterus.
Raw Foods – Raw fish, salads, contain potential toxins and parasites.
Salty, spicy, burnt, or fried foods – Excess salt causes fluid retention, which is already an issue. Spicy and burnt foods create Heat, and a pregnant woman is already hot. Fried foods generate Dampness and Damp-Heat in the body.
Barley – Said to inhibit growth of fertilized egg.
Leeks – Said to affect the secretion of hormones.
Fruit with high sugar content – Such as watermelon, sugar cane, bananas. These destabilize blood sugar leading to weight gain and high cholesterol.

Spacing of Meals

Eat the heaviest, protein-rich meal for breakfast, the second largest meal for lunch, and a lighter, vegetable-based meal for dinner. Begin dinner by 6:30 pm. This allows for proper digestion and gives your intestines a rest. This is a general health guideline, but more important during pregnancy or any time you need special care. Optimal digestion means optimal nutrients available for the fetus.

1-3 Months

After conception, the Liver is the first thing to stagnate in the mother. It does so in order to block the release of Blood. This may cause increased tension, digestive complaints (such as morning sickness or constipation), and fatigue. These symptoms may also be caused by Kidney deficiency or Spleen weakness.

The first three months are the most unstable months of pregnancy. Avoid bicycling, spin class, and lifting more than 40 lbs.

PRACTITIONER SECTION: TREATING DURING PREGNANCY

Be particularly gentle during the first 3 months of pregnancy. You want to treat what the patient presents, just use gentler methods. Some things to note:

1. The very procedure of IVF produces some Blood Stagnation and taxes the Jing. These patients may present with Blood stagnation and Jing-deficiency symptoms throughout the pregnancy and postpartum period.
2. Swelling with numbness in the hands during pregnancy is Dampness and Liver Blood deficiency. Use Bu Zhong Yi Qi Tang with a high dosage of Fu Ling (poria) 30g. Needle Sp20 obliquely, Sp 9, and Sp5.(1)
3. To clean out the uterus, in case of inevitable miscarriage, take Sheng Hua Tang and follow the Postpartum Recovery protocol. Needle KD14, 18, ST28, 29, SP6, 12, 13, Ren 4.(2)

Using Herbs

Due to fear of litigation, many acupuncturists and herbal pharmacies avoid giving herbs to pregnant women, despite a long history of Chinese herbs being used in pregnancy. Should anything go wrong with the pregnancy there is no legal support for alternative therapies. I want to offer women the option to use herbs and acupuncture to treat conditions during pregnancy and avoid pharmaceuticals, even though many practitioners may not be able to offer this help due to legal fears.

Herbs to calm the fetus and stabilize pregnancy:
Bai Shao (white peony root), Bai Zhu (white atractylodes), Du Zhong (eucommia), Huang Qin (scutellaria), Sha Ren (amomi), Shu Di Huang (rehmannia), Xu Duan (dispsacus), Zi Su Ye (perilla leaf).

Herbs to dispel nausea during pregnancy:
Bai Bian Dou (dolichos nut), Huo Xiang (agastache), Sha Ren (amomi), Zhu Ru (bamboo shavings), Zi Su Ye (perilla leaf).

Herbs to stop uterine bleeding:
Ai Ye (mugwort), Bai Zhu (white atractylodes), Du Zhong (eucommia), E Jiao (gelatin), Sha Ren (amomi), Tu Si Zi (dodder seed), Xu Duan (dispsacus).

Bao Chan Wu You Fang is a classic formula for common pregnancy symptoms and to stabilize pregnancy.

Contradictions

Acupuncture points contraindicated during pregnancy (or used with caution):
GB21, LI4, UB31-UB34, SP6. Only moxa UB67 in case of breech positioning. Shallow needling on abdominal points.

See Chen, Chinese Medical Herbology, 1145 for a full list of herbs contraindicated during pregnancy.

1. Alex Tiberi. "TCM Pediatrics" (lecture, Pacific College of Oriental Medicine, San Diego, May 15, 2008).
2. Jane Lyttleton. *Treatment of Infertility with Chinese Medicine.* (China: Churchill Livingstone, 2004), 299.

Avoiding Morning Sickness

Morning sickness is a common symptom during the first trimester. Besides being uncomfortable, it can deplete mother and fetus of vital nutrients. Morning sickness is caused by Kidney deficiency, Spleen weakness with Dampness, Liver disharmony or all three.

Tricks for preventing morning sickness:

1. Prior to 7 a.m., while still lying in bed, have a few crackers or a piece of bread. Rest for an additional 20-30 min. Then get up and have breakfast.
2. Forget your diet. Eat whatever bland, simple, single food that sounds remotely appetizing. Often white bread or crackers are easiest.
3. Eat smaller, drier meals throughout the day. Have a snack every 2 hours or so.
4. If constipation and yellow urine occur, begin introducing soups or broths.
5. Take a tiny amount of ginger juice before meals.
6. Avoid pungent or triggering smells.
7. Soak feet in hot water every night. This grounds your energy and also helps sleep.
8. If these tricks do not work quickly, see an acupuncturist. If there is weight loss or severe vomiting, seek medical assistance.

PRACTITIONER SECTION: THE FIRST TRIMESTER

The Liver naturally stagnates after conception to block the release of Blood from the uterus. Needle Liver 8 and GB 43 during the first month to smooth this effect. Sun Simiao[1] recommended always tonifying and never sedating during pregnancy. The Qi of the mother needs to be present to nourish the fetus.

Treating Morning Sickness

The most common pattern for morning sickness is Chong channel dysfunction with rebellious Stomach Qi.

- Acupuncture: Use Pc 6, Sp 4, St 36, plus Kidney points such as KD7 and KD 27.
- Use the following herbs: Jiang Ban Xia (ginger processed pinellia), Sheng Jiang (fresh ginger), Fu Ling (poria), Bai Zhu (white atractylodis), Sha Ren (amomi fruit), Chen Pi (tangerine peel). If you need to use a patent, use Huo Xiang Zheng Qi Tang. Have your patient take the herbs in concentrate powder form. Add to 1 cup of water and take 2 tsp. every hour.
- Fu Qing Zhu advised the need to nourish Kidney to ground the Qi of the body. His famous anti-morning sickness formula; Shun Gan Yi Qi Tang:[2] Ren Shen (ginseng) 3-9g, Bai Zhu (white atractylodis) 9g, Bai Shao (white peony root) 9g, Dang Gui (Chinese angelica) 9g, Fu Ling (poria) 12g, Zi Su geng (perilla stem, to replace Su Zi, the fruit) 6g, Mai Men Dong (ophiopogonis) 9-12g, Chen Pi (tangerine peel) 6-9g, Sha Ren (amomi fruit) 3-4.5g, Shen Qu (medicated leaven) 6-9g. This can be used in deficiency cases and modified with the above herbs.

1. Sun Simiao (581(?)–682 A.D.) was a wellknown TCM doctor of the Sui and Tang dynasties.
2. Yang Shou-Zhong, trans. *Fu Qing Zhu's Gynecology*. (Boulder: Blue Poppy Press, Inc, 1995), 58.

4-6 Months

This is the most stable phase of pregnancy. Begin getting regular massages, increasing the frequency to weekly massages as you approach delivery. The second trimester is more forgiving and free of symptoms, yet keep in mind that as your belly grows you will need to make adjustments.

1. Take more frequent breaks. Avoid excessive sitting as it can create internal organ prolapse and low backache.
2. Begin using a belly band[7] as soon as your belly starts to protrude. This will protect your back and help save your abdomen from stretch marks. Be sure to keep your belly moisturized with avocado oil, Vitamin C, and Vitamin E-rich oils and balms.[8]
3. By the sixth month, refrain from picking up children or objects over 40 lbs.
4. By the seventh month, begin taking lukewarm, rather than hot, showers.

PRACTITIONER SECTION: MAKING THE BABY BEAUTIFUL

Needle Kidney 9 between the 2nd and 3rd trimester to make the baby beautiful. It brings more Yin to the fetus. Kidney 9 is also a general point for detox.

7-9 Months

Edema (water retention) and sciatica (hip and low back pain that can refer down the legs to the feet) are common towards the end of pregnancy. The growth of the fetus impedes blood and lymph flow to the lower extremities. Take the following steps:

1. Avoid prolonged standing.
2. Elevate your legs throughout the day.
3. Limit salt intake.

PRACTITIONER SECTION: THE THIRD TRIMESTER

Continue providing nourishing, gentle treatments. Edema and sciatica are the most common complaints during this time. Needle Sp5 to strengthen the Spleen and leech out Dampness. Needle ASHI points on the buttocks and use electrostimulation. Follow with prenatal massage.

Have the mother eat red adzuki beans, 60g or 1/4 cup dry beans, daily.

7. A belly band is a stretchy belt that wraps around your lower back and under your belly to provide extra support, relieving pressure on your ligaments, connective tissue, and skin. This guards against low back pain and stretch marks.

8. If you still get stretch marks, they should be treated while still red and vascular.

4. Eat foods to reduce edema: red adzuki beans, Huang Qi (astragalus) tea, or carp stew (recipes p.420).
5. Get acupuncture and prenatal massage weekly, especially during the last month of pregnancy.

9th Month and Delivery

Reading the old texts on childbirth, I am reminded of the precariousness of delivery and the first month postpartum, for both mother and child. We must treat this time with the respect it deserves by preparing the mother's body (and fetus') as much as possible before labor, and strengthening her and the newborn for the first month after birth.

The current trend in Western medical practice is to strictly define the due date and to induce if the baby is a week late. This may restrict your personal preferences as mother. I recommend getting a doula or midwife.[9] They will help support you through the process in a more personal and nurturing way as well as act as an advocate interfacing with hospital staff.

In addition to this, TCM has tips to facilitate the process. Fu Qing Zhu[10] recommended taking Hua Tai San (Slippery Baby Powder,page 366) regularly during the month before birth. It can be taken daily two weeks prior to projected delivery. Contrary to its name, Hua Tai San does not contain anything to make the baby slip out. Rather it prepares the mother (and baby) for a speedy delivery by strengthening Qi and Blood and calming the Shen. Natural labor requires a great deal of the mother's and baby's energy.

During the final month it is important to open up the hips and relax the muscles in the pelvic floor. Being relaxed and open will facilitate labor and lower the incidence of vaginal tears. Vaginal tears occur when the perineal muscles are too tight or the baby descends too quickly through the birth canal. These tears are not uncommon during vaginal delivery and they can be severe. Episiotomies are a medical intervention whereby a small surgical incision is made on the perineal muscles during the second stage of labor to make delivery easier and to avoid tearing. This incision is much easier to repair than a naturally occurring tear. The decision to have an episiotomy is heavily debated. If you choose not to have one, take extra precautions prior to delivery. One month prior to your due date, perform daily perineal massage to relax the muscles. Practice various forms of squatting motions to stretch out the muscles and tendons. Consider using a perineal dilator, which uses a balloon-like apparatus to incrementally open up the vaginal canal. Your doula or midwife will also have recommendations.

The day or so before the expected delivery, eat the Slippery-Baby congee (recipes page 367) to help

9. Doulas offer personal support leading up to and during birth and postpartum. They may offer massage, breathing techniques, herbal medicine, and act as an advocate during birth. A midwife acts as a primary care provider leading up to and during delivery. A midwife offers more individualized care than a traditional doctor but less so than a doula. Many women elect to have both.

10. Wellknown TCM gynecologist.

PRACTITIONER SECTION: FACILITATING LABOR

Acupuncture acts to support the natural process of childbirth. Traditionally, Ba Liao points in the sacral foraemen and GB 21 are needled and stimulated with electrostimulation. Additional points: ST12, Yin Tang, LI4, LV3, SP 6, ST 36, Pc 6, SP 4. Ear: Uterus, Shen Men, Abdomen, Sympathetic.

Checking Pulses for signs of impending labor

1. Check the pulse on both sides of the pregnant woman's middle finger. When you feel the pulse all the way to tip there are 1-2 days to delivery.
2. The delivery pulse on the wrist is superficial and rolling. It feels like it is jumping out of the skin.
3. Check the pulse on the belly button. Place your hand on belly button. Prior to delivery the pulse feels anxious, like the baby is separating from mother (which it is). When it feels empty underneath, like skin is separating from muscle, delivery will occur within 24 hours.

Breech Position

Use stick moxa on UB 67, daily or as often as possible until the baby turns.

promote labor and ease delivery. Get acupuncture and prenatal massage at this time to prepare the body for labor.

In cases of a scheduled C-section, take Red Date Tea (page 349) one week prior to surgery to mitigate the side effects of anesthesia and protect the Liver. Since you may need to ha ve an emergency C-section, it is a good idea to drink this tea anyway one week prior to expected delivery. It will also help to strengthen the mother in cases of natural childbirth. Continue taking Red Date Tea for one week post surgery.

As soon as the water breaks, honey water is traditionally used to speed natural childbirth.[11] Honey moistens Yin fluids, promotes uterine discharge, relaxes the muscles, and provides energy, which the mother will need. For women 36 or older, or those with more deficient constitutions, the Ren Shen Delivery Wine recipe is recommended in place of Honey Water. Ginseng has the added effect of greatly tonifying the Source Qi and boosting stamina, calms the Shen (nerves), and generates fluids. Do not take ginseng after delivery or for the first few weeks postpartum.

Recipe 4.1. Honey Water Recipe

Combine ½ cup of hot water with 2/3 cup of honey. Allow it to cool. Begin taking as soon as water breaks. It shortens labor and reduces pain.

11. Shuqi Zhuang. *Postpartum Recovery Program; a Manual of Rules and Recipes for the Postpartum Woman.* (Taiwan: Guang He Chu Ban She, 2005). ISBN 9578807015

Recipe 4.2. Ren Shen Delivery Wine[12]

Soak 10g Ren Shen (Chinese white ginseng), thinly sliced in ¼ cup of rice wine for 1 month prior to birth. Add 2/3 cup of honey and ½ cup hot water. Allow to cool. Begin taking as soon as water breaks. Drink during labor only. Avoid ginseng the first weeks after birth.

Recipe 4.3. Labor Induction Tea

If labor has stalled decoct 5-10 g of Qu Mai (dianthus). It moves the Blood and unblocks the bladder, bowels, and womb. It stimulates contraction of the uterus.

12. I have not had personal experience with it, nor do I know how safe it is to take alcohol during this time. Powdering the Ren Shen and making a strong tea with honey would extract less of ginseng's compounds but might be a safer alternative.

Postpartum Recovery

The second Golden Opportunity for a woman to shift the state of her health (for better or for worse) is the month following childbirth. What follows is a traditional version of Zuo Yue Zi, literally "sitting the month," and what is referred to in this book as Postpartum Recovery. It consists of diet and lifestyle guidelines for 30-40 days after giving birth. The plan is heavily influenced by Dr. Shuqi Zhuang, either directly from her books or through my teachers, and laywomen who were also influenced by her.[13] Recipes and other details are from my own clinical experience and modifications from my teachers.

What is Postpartum Recovery?

Postpartum Recovery is a system of diet and lifestyle guidelines to optimize a woman's recovery and long-term health after childbirth. Essentially it promises that your breasts will not sag, your body will not ache, and that your uterus and abdomen will return to normal size in record time. The three key components are rest, diet, and a list of practices and prohibitions. Postpartum Recovery should be carried out for 30-40 days after giving birth.

The concept of keeping the new mother warm, secluded, and rested is one that can be found cross-culturally, though it is a foreign idea in modern America. Today's society holds an unrealistic ideal that women should give birth, shed their weight gain immediately, and resume normal life, all on a hurried diet and limited sleep. Because of this unattainable standard many modern mothers never fully recover from having children. Instead, they suffer from lack of libido, weight gain, and hormonal imbalances for the rest of their lives.[14]

Postpartum Recovery is a part of Chinese and Taiwanese cultures, traditionally passed down from mother or mother-in-law to new mother, with new mothers generally staying at their relatives' home. Postpartum Recovery has been practiced at least as far back as the Song Dynasty (960-1279 AD). It is inconvenient for many modern Taiwanese mothers to stay with their relatives, who often work or live in other cities. For the past 30 years there has been a trend towards Postpartum Birthing Centers. The more affordable versions of these are located within hospitals. The private centers are more expensive, running a few thousand dollars a day, and also offer food delivery or babysitting services for lesser fees. These centers follow the Postpartum Recovery principles to varying degrees. More allopathically oriented centers discourage strict adherence to some traditional practices such as mothers not washing their hair for the entire period. You can find Postpartum Care centers in areas of the U.S. with large Chinese and Taiwanese immigrant populations (see Resources p.409).

13. Dr. Shuqi Zhuang is a well-known TCM doctor in Taiwan who specializes in postpartum care. She is considered "the" expert in many TCM and lay circles on traditional postpartum care.

14. I saw a special about Hassidic Jewish women in New York. I was taken by how healthy these women looked for their ages and after bearing so many children. This contrasted greatly with how exhausted many women I treat look after having one or two children. I later discovered that that they have strict menstrual and postpartum practices. These no doubt greatly contribute to the health and fertility of these women.

The Postpartum Recovery Plan presented here is clearly a product of Traditional Chinese and Taiwanese culture. Much of it will need to be modified for a Western audience. Just as many other Eastern practices like meditation, yoga, and acupuncture itself have been adapted for Westerners and modern culture, so can a postpartum tradition. Modifications are offered throughout the book. This section serves as a guideline that individual women can use to make their own choices. Postpartum Recovery is more than a cultural construct. It is a health practice, and one that is sorely needed at this time.

Who Needs Postpartum Recovery?

Anyone who becomes pregnant needs Postpartum Recovery. Whether the fetus comes to term or not, whatever manner of birth, whatever age or condition of the mother, the woman must replenish herself after the nurturing she gave prenatally.

There is a saying in TCM gynecology that "miscarriage is more serious than childbirth."[15] It is more important to undergo Postpartum Recovery if you miscarry or have an abortion. In cases of abortion, miscarriage, C-section, mothers with weak constitutions, difficult birth, or mothers over 35, an extended Postpartum Recovery period is in order. This consists of 40 rather than 30 days. The reasoning is these cases are all more traumatic on women. In the cases of miscarriage or abortion, the natural cycle was interrupted, and the body will suffer for not having completed it. The other circumstances represent women who have been weakened to a greater extent by giving birth. When in doubt, pamper yourself longer. It is always better to get slowly transition rather than rush back to your normal pace. Keep your reserves for when you need them. Ultimately trust your body to know when it is time to resume your normal level of activity. Use pregnancy and the time afterwards as a gift to remind yourself to listen to your body.

What Postpartum Recovery Promises

Women lose their health and appearance after having children mainly due to ignorance, an injustice I seek to right with the information in this chapter. Modern Western culture has forgotten the concept of depletion. We value pushing through and doing more, ignoring the fact that a woman's body is robbed of reserves and vitality during pregnancy and childbirth. This extends to the postpartum period where the ideal is of the "superwoman" who pushes out her baby and, only days later, has resumed her pre-pregnancy activities and body. Perhaps a few genetically fortunate women can accomplish this. Most women will recover beautifully IF supported. Postpartum Recovery promises a means to not only regaining your pre-pregnancy health and physique, but to surpass it. It provides the means to renew yourself, look younger, heal constitutional weaknesses, and balance your hormones.

Traditional culture insists that not following the Postpartum Recovery guidelines leads women to

---

15. Giovanni Maciocia. *Obstetrics & Gynecology in Chinese Medicine*. (Nanjing: Churchill Livingstone Press,1998), 60.

obesity, body aches, cold hands and feet, hyperpigmentation (dark spots), wrinkles, loss of libido, premature aging, and gynecological disorders later on in life.

General Guidelines

TCM states that pregnant women are Yang and postpartum women are Yin. Practically, this means that postpartum women must keep warm at all costs. They must eat hot foods (protein-rich) and avoid cold foods (raw foods, fruits, and vegetables). Rest, practices and prohibitions, and diet are the three basic components of the Plan.

The 3 Stages

Postpartum Recovery is divided into Three Stages. Stage 1 covers the first week postpartum. The focus is on gently clearing lochia[16] and residual toxins from the body. The first week is when the body is most vulnerable and prohibitions are strictest at this stage. Stage 2 is the second week postpartum, which supports returning the uterus and figure back to normal size. The remaining 2-3 weeks comprise Stage 3. The body is finally strong enough to tonify directly.[17]

Rest

Rest as much as possible the entire Postpartum Recovery. You are on self-imposed quarantine. Do not leave the house. Surround yourself with loving, supportive people who can do the cooking, maintain the household, and help care for your baby.

Of all the recommendations, this is the single most important and the hardest one for new mothers to comply with. The first two weeks spend as much time sleeping as you can bear. Pump your breast milk and get 10 hours of sleep a night. After two weeks you can increase activity around the house. However, never let yourself get tired during the full month. This admonition is for the newborn as well. He/she should be allowed to rest as much as possible. When mother and baby emerge into the world at the end of the first month they will do so strong and ready.

---

16. Lochia is the normal vaginal discharge after birth made up of blood, mucus, and placental tissue. It is important that these materials be discharged and the uterus be clean in order to avoid long-term gynecological problems. During C-section the uterus should be cleansed of these to speed healing.

17. Shuqi Zhuang. *Postpartum Recovery Program; a Manual of Rules and Recipes for the Postpartum Woman.* (Taiwan: Guang He Chu Ban She, 2005). ISBN 9578807015.

Practices

Communal Assistance

A key feature of Postpartum Recovery and its variants in various cultures is its dependence on family and friends. The husband should take the month off to oversee care. Extended family and/or friends should take turns running household chores and caring for the newborn. Not only does this allow for the greatest care of mother and baby, it places importance on bonding the new baby with the community. If family and friends are not available, consider hiring someone to assist with cooking, basic housework, and caring for the baby.

Regulating Lactation

Ideally, mothers should breastfeed for four months. Following the Postpartum Recovery plan will strengthen the mother and promote healthy milk production. From the first two weeks postpartum until you stop breastfeeding, eat milk-promoting recipes at least three times a week (page 355). These include ingredients such as carp, green papaya, peanuts, and pork trotters that build Qi and Blood in the body.[18] If there is still low milk production choose the appropriate milk-promoting formula (page 355) 1 cup 3 times a day for 3 days. When you wish to stop lactation, use the Roasted Mai Ya Tea (page 359). Drink 1 cup 3 times a day for 3 days.

Mastitis

Mastitis is an infection of the breast tissue and is a common postpartum malady. In TCM it is caused by Stomach and Gallbladder Heat Toxin or Qi Stagnation.[19]

PRACTITIONER SECTION: REGULATING LACTATION

To Promote Lactation, needle Ren17, Sp4, Pc6, ST36, LI4, LV3, Yin Tang. Give your patient Tong Gan Sheng Ru Tang (excess) or Tong Ru Tang (deficiency) (page 358).

To Stop Lactation, use Chao Mai Ya (roasted sprouted barley). Roasted substances astringe the milk. The combination of Chi Shao (red peony root), Dang Gui (Chinese angelica), and Chuan Niu Xi (cyathula root) promotes menses and discourages lactation.[1]

1. Shaoting Jing. "TCM Gynecology" (lecture, Yo San University, Los Angeles, May 1, 2003).

---

18. Breast milk is an extension of a woman's Blood.
19. Jiang Zheng. "TCM Gynecology." (lecture, Pacific College of Oriental Medicine, San Diego, January 20, 2007).

To prevent mastitis:

1. During pregnancy, Gua Sha (Figure 4.1) both breasts daily from the outside in towards the nipples. Either apply oil or place a piece of silk over the skin to avoid tugging the skin. Apply firm pressure and use a scraping movement until skin pinks up.
2. After childbirth, immediately begin massaging any nodules in the breast to soften them. This may be painful at first. Once the baby begins to nurse, the nodules will be dispersed.
3. At the first signs of inflammation or pain, make a strong decoction (60g) of Yi Yi Ren (Job's tears) and drink liberally.

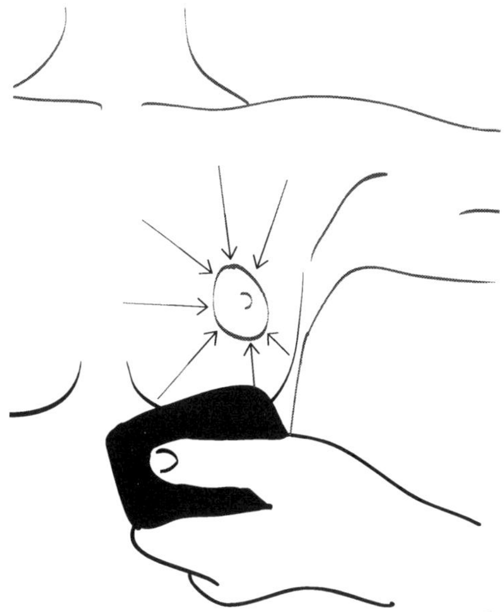

Figure 4.1. Gua Sha for Mastitis

Abdominal Binding

After giving birth, the abdomen and internal organs need help returning to their original places. Abdominal binding performs two functions. First, it minimizes the chances of organ prolapse and encourages the organs to go back to their rightful place. Second it helps the mother recover, and improve, her waistline. Without binding, that loose, puffy pooch may become permanent without a tummy tuck.

In cases of natural childbirth, begin the second day after giving birth. In case of C-section begin after the 6th day. Traditionalists insist that manually binding the abdomen is superior to manufactured postpartum girdles. Manually binding the abdomen requires assistance and more time. Many women prefer to buy a postpartum girdle. Numerous options can be found on the internet at a range of costs. Look for one you can tighten and that covers your full abdomen, starting under the breasts to your pubic bone. The girdle should be firm without much give. When using a postpartum girdle follow the same guidelines for abdominal binding. Be sure to continue to keep the belly moisturized.

Prescription for Six-pack Abs

Keli Lovejoy conducted field research with the Garifuna tribe in Orinoco, Nicaragua. They have a rich postpartum tradition which includes its own practices and herbal medicine. The women are known for their beauty and vitality. One day Keli came upon a woman, Maria Solis, fishing with the most amazing physique, including a little chiseled waist. She had heard this woman had nine children and was in her 40s. When Keli asked her what her secret was, Maria Solis smiled. Maria told her she wrapped her abdomen for 2-3 months after each child, "the longer the better." Maria also tensed her abdominal muscles for several repetitions daily, during pregnancy and after birth.

Manual Abdominal Binding Instructions:[1]

Traditionalists prefer manual binding to pre-made postpartum girdles. Both function to prevent prolapse of the internal organs and shrink the abdomen. The rules for manual binding are also the same. Manual binding requires assistance, making it inconvenient for most modern women.

1. **Dimensions:** Use a gauze bandage that will allow the skin to breathe, about 10.4 yards in length and 5.5 inches in width. You can use first aid wraps.
2. **Usage:** The binding is worn underneath the clothes, maintaining direct contact with the skin. Make sure you have alternate bandages in case they get wet.
3. **When to start:** In cases of natural childbirth: begin the second day after giving birth. In cases of caesarean birth: begin the sixth day. In cases of miscarriage: begin after the second day.
4. **Removal of binding:** The binding must be removed prior to the three main meals and refastened after eating. Wash yourself with a sponge after removing the girdle. For the first two weeks after giving birth, the binding should be worn 24 hours a day. If it gets loose, rebind and tighten it. After the third week the binding can be worn during the daytime only, and removed in the evening.
5. **Washing bandage:** Hand wash with gentle detergent and cold water and line dry.
6. **Method for binding:**
   a. Lie face up on your back. Bend your knees so that the soles of the feet lie flat on the bed. Place two pillows under your hips.
   b. Press down on your lower abdomen with both hands, massaging upwards, bringing the internal organs toward the heart.
   c. Use two (or three) rolls of gauze. The first is to bind from the pubic bone to the navel. This should take 12 rounds. For the first 7 rounds rise 1 inch each round, every round and a half make a slanting/oblique fold with the bandage in order to keep it from sliding, alternating side to side. For the last five rounds begin shifting up 1 1/2 inches with each round,

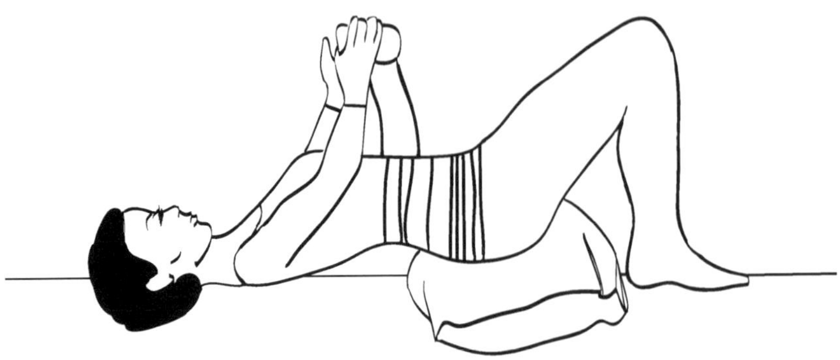

Figure 4.2. Abdominal Binding

1. Shuqi Zhuang. *Postpartum Recovery Program; a Manual of Rules and Recipes for the Postpartum Woman.* (Taiwan: Guang He Chu Ban She, 2005). ISBN 9578807015.

spiraling up, with a final round past the navel then use a safety pin to fix the binding in place.

d. The second roll is used to bind the upper abdomen. You may require a third bandage at first.

e. If you are very thin and your hipbones stick out, add padding to the lower abdomen, like a towel, before binding.

f. The bandages should be rolled up in a roll after removing to preserve the shape for later use.

Prohibitions

Avoid Cold Water

Avoid drinking or washing with cold water.

Reasoning:

Cold water internally is taxing on Stomach Qi and puts out the digestive fire. Cold water externally can easily cause Cold invasion.

Do Not Wash Your Hair

For the full 30-day postpartum period, do not wash your hair. Instead, use the Alcohol Wash Method. Make a mixture of equal parts 95% isopropyl rubbing alcohol and warm water. Add a few drops of essential oils for fragrance and antibacterial qualities.[20] Use a comb to part your hair and use a cotton ball to apply the alcohol and warm water mixture. Cover the entire scalp. Comb the hair afterwards. Be sure to thoroughly wash the comb with soap and water after each use. Use the Alcohol Wash Method daily, prior to one of your meals. Some women may prefer to braid their hair during this time.

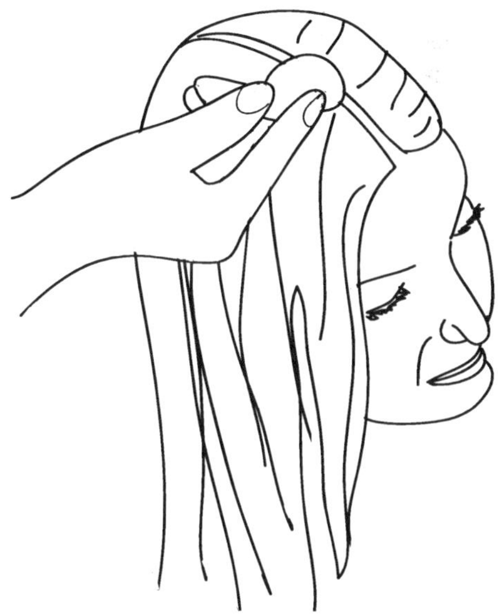

Figure 4.3. Alcohol Wash Method

Reasoning:
After giving birth the pores are lax and susceptible to

20. Citrus and rosemary essential oils help to cut oiliness. Clove, cinnamon, and other spice essential oils are antibacterial.

Cold invasion. Cold invasion in the scalp can lead to stagnation and blood congealing in the uterus. Alcohol astringes the pores.[21]

Modification:
Lessen the frequency of hair washing. Make sure the bathroom is warm. Immediately dry your hair. **Never** walk around with wet hair even if it is summertime.

Do Not Bathe

Do not bathe normally for the first two weeks postpartum. Instead use the sponge bath method below. At the beginning of the third week you can resume showering. Only after the full Postpartum Recovery (30-40 days) can you soak in a tub.

Method:
Mix warm water and rice wine in equal parts. Add 1 tbsp 95% isopropyl rubbing alcohol and one tbsp. of salt. Mix. Use a hand towel or sponge dipped in the mixture to wash yourself. For the genitals, use a strong green tea decoction, with salt and rubbing alcohol. The teeth and face can be washed normally, only be sure to use warm water. After washing yourself apply talcum powder to your abdomen before refastening the binding or postpartum girdle.[22]

Reasoning:
Again, the pores are lax postpartum and highly susceptible to Wind invasion. A bath in a tub is prohibited the entire Postpartum Recovery period due to the vulnerability of the genital region.

Modification:
The very idea of this will be too much for most women. To modify, shower, but do not soak in a tub. Take shorter, warm showers in a warm bathroom. Make sure to dry yourself thoroughly and do not leave the bathroom until your pores have returned to normal.

Maintain a Warm Ambient Temperature

Maintain an ambient temperature of 77-82 degrees F (25-28 degrees C) at all times, no matter what the season. Block or redirect air conditioning vents from blowing on you. Wear long pants, long sleeve, a cap, gloves, scarf, and socks at all times.

---

21. The use of alcohol as a bathing method seems at first peculiar. There is, however, a tradition in the West of alcohol used to astringe the pores on the skin and guard against Wind invasion. Famed American strongman Adolph Nordequest writing in 1905, made suggestions on how to safely take care of one's self after exercising and inducing perspiration. After using a dry towel to dry off completely, he advised readers to apply a solution of 95% alcohol, witch hazel, and arnica, which "not only [will] have the effect of closing the pores, but it will relieve sore muscles" - Viking. *Strength and Health; How Disease May be Successfully Combated by Physical Culture.* (New York: Richard K. Fox, 1905), 27. Accessed from www.Sandowplus.co.uk

22. The concept of the sponge bath is common to all postpartum recovery traditions in China. This washing solution recipe was taken from - Shuqi Zhuang. *Postpartum Recovery Program; a Manual of Rules and Recipes for the Postpartum Woman.* (Taiwan: Guang He Chu Ban She, 2005). ISBN 9578807015

Modification:
Maintain the temperature at 77-82 degrees F and avoid drafts. Cover up as needed. Do not allow yourself to feel cold.

Do Not Lift Weight or Climb Stairs

This means avoiding weightlifting and picking up anything heavy. Avoid going up and down stairs for the entire 30-40 days.

Reasoning:
There are two reasons. First, you need to conserve your energy. Second, straining can cause organ prolapse.

Modification:
Have your helpers do any lifting for you as much as possible. Avoid weight training for 30-40 days. Return to weight training very slowly and cautiously for six months after giving birth.

If you were athletic prior to giving birth and are in robust health, start with gentler versions of muscle control exercises, Pilates, yoga, and calisthenics for the first month. Do not overstrain. After the first month, begin to resume these exercises at regular intensity. Focus on maintaining function, strength, stimulating blood flow, and emotional well-being. Do not establish any new fitness goals beyond recovering your previous form for the first six months postpartum.

Avoid cardio exercises entirely the first month. Excessive strain and sweating can easily create Qi and Yin deficiency. Slowly resume cardio after the 30-40 days. Wait six months to resume intense cardio training.

Do Not Carry Your Baby

For the same reasons you should not lift weights. Have someone else carry and bathe the baby, preferably the father or other family member to encourage bonding.

Modification:
Have hired help or family members carry your baby for you as much as possible.

Lie on Your Side to Nurse

Lie on your side propped with pillows so that you are very comfortable. Have someone carry the baby to you.

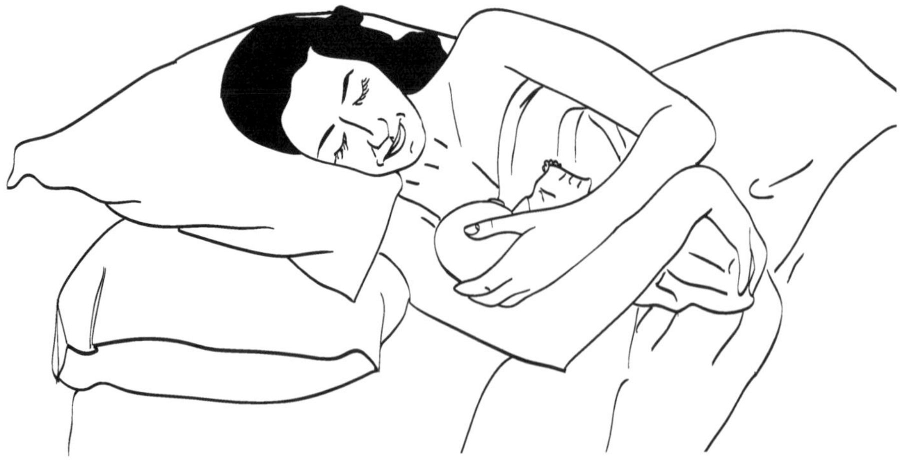

Figure 4.4. Proper Nursing

Do Not Shed Tears

There is a Chinese saying that "One teardrop from a postpartum woman is as valuable as 500g of gold." Traditionally, a postpartum woman should not be told of a relative passing or any other painful events. The husband should shoulder all burdens for her. A postpartum woman should smile often.

Reasoning:
The eyes are very vulnerable during the Postpartum Recovery due to Liver Blood deficiency.

Modifications:
This admonishment is likely not only about conserving body fluids and saving your eyes. Qi and Blood deficient individuals are more easily and deeply hurt by painful events. Take extra care to ensure you are surrounded by loving, supportive people (this is a good life strategy in general). Your helpers should buffer stress and challenges from you for the 30-40 days.

Do Not Watch TV or Read

Listen to relaxing music. Avoid watching TV or reading. If you do watch TV or read, take a break every 15 minutes to prevent eye strain. Make sure to massage your eyes daily.

Reasoning:
The eyes are dependent on healthy Liver Blood and Kidney Yin to function, both of which are deficient at this time. Take extra care of your eyes.

Eye Massage Techniques (Figure 4.5):

1. Use a warm wet towel compress on your eyes to begin.

2. Close your eyes. Use your thumb or middle fingers to press firmly working your way around the orbital bone.
3. Use your thumb knuckles to do a figure 8 pattern around your eyes.
4. Use both middle fingers to press from the center of the hairline out, working down to the temples.

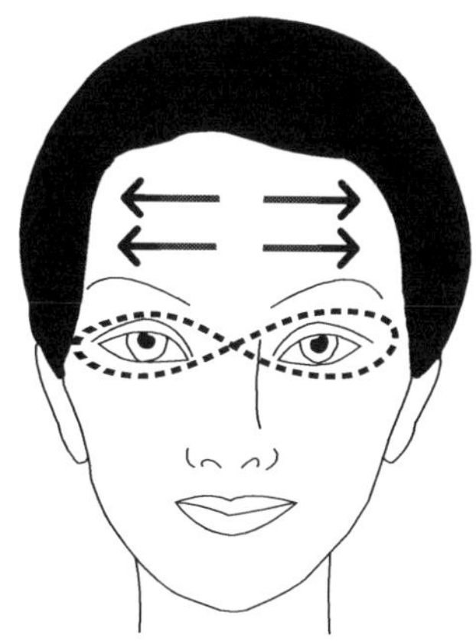

Figure 4.5. Eye Massage

Do Not Over Eat

You need to eat adequately to recover postpartum, especially if you are breastfeeding. However, be careful not to overdo it. Water retention easily converts to fat at this time.

Dietary Guidelines

The Postpartum Recovery diet is designed to rebuild a postpartum woman's health quickly. These guidelines are applied to all food made during the postpartum month.

1. **No Salt**
Avoid using salt to flavor foods. It will increase water retention and slow the process of discharging excess fluids from the body. A modification of this is to avoid salt while cooking and adding as little as you can when you sit down to eat. You will end up using less salt.

2. **Ginger (browned)**
Cook most of your food with browned ginger. That is, sauté the ginger until it develops a crunchy brown layer on both sides. Do not blacken, however. Charred herbs are used to stop bleeding, and we do not want to interrupt the discharge of lochia. The preparation of ginger is very important. Fresh ginger goes to the Lungs and Stomach. Browned ginger goes to the uterus. Dried ginger goes to the Middle Jiao, warming digestion.

3. **Rice Wine (No Water)**
Rice wine is used in all recipes postpartum.[23] Rice wine warms the body and moves stagnant Blood. Replacing water with rice wine was thought to be safer and to reduce water weight. Traditionally rice wine was home brewed. If you make your own you will want to allow 9 months - 1 year for aging, and optimally 5 years. Like any wine, rice wine gets better with age.

23. Chinese rice wine and sake are both made from rice but are very different in taste, alcohol content, and properties. Rice wine has a similar taste and alcohol content as sherry, but different properties.

Red rice wine, in particular, was used due to its added benefits of moving stagnant Blood and easing digestion (recipes page 336).

Tradition demands that postpartum women not drink any water for 1-4 weeks postpartum and make their beverages with rice wine. While moderate alcohol intake is fine while breastfeeding, I find this potentially unsafe for both mother and baby.

The modern adaptation is to use special Postpartum Water (Yue Zi Shui). To make Postpartum Water, rice wine is specially processed to remove the alcohol content to less than 1%. If you want to adhere strictly to postpartum rules, I recommend buying bottles of Postpartum Water and using it for all cooking and drinking. (see resources page 392).

A second option is to avoid cold drinks and excessive water intake. Add rice wine to dishes and simmer them uncovered for 30 min. to reduce most of the alcohol content. Rely on soups for most of your fluid intake.

A third option is to avoid cold drinks and excessive water intake. Take your water warm and sip throughout the day rather than overwhelming your body at one sitting. You can also make the Postpartum Recovery Tea (page 341) with water instead of rice wine and drink the tea as your daily liquid. Rely on soups for most of your fluid intake.

4. **Black Sesame Oil**
Use cold pressed, organic black sesame oil as your cooking oil. Black sesame seeds tonify the Blood and Kidney Yin.

5. **Special Foods for Each Stage**
Special foods are used during each stage to address special health issues. Red adzuki beans and Yi Yi Ren (Job's tears) clear Dampness and water retention. Fish is used as it is an easy way to assimilate protein.

During Stage 1, week 1, liver is eaten to both move and nourish Blood. During Stage 2, week 2, kidney is eaten to nourish the Kidneys and help contract the uterus. During Stage 3, weeks 3-4 /5, chicken is eaten to tonify Qi and Blood and support lactation.[24]

Additionally, there are foods to promote lactation (pork trotters, carp soup, green papaya) and generally nourish the body (red dates, longan berries).

6. **Placenta Encapsulation**
This is a modern take on an old practice. The placenta contains hormones and nutrients that can help speed postpartum recovery. It was traditionally eaten by postpartum mothers to help them recover hormonal balance. There are now practitioners trained in placenta encapsulation. This is a sanitary method by which the placenta is washed, dehydrated, and put into capsules to be taken throughout the first postpartum month. I recommend finding

---

24. Shuqi Zhuang. *Postpartum Recovery Program; a Manual of Rules and Recipes for the Postpartum Woman.* (Taiwan: Guang He Chu Ban She, 2005). ISBN 9578807015

someone who is trained in a safe method of doing this or becoming trained yourself. You will also need to make special arrangements during delivery to save your placenta (see resources page 392).

Vegetarian Options

Pregnancy, breastfeeding, and menstruation are the most challenging times to forgo animal products. Extra effort must be made to tonify the Blood. Besides diet, you will need to rely more heavily on herbal formulas. After the initial two weeks, replace Sheng Hua Tang with stronger Blood Building formulas such as Si Wu Tang modifications. See the Vegetarian Options section on page 359.

Preparation Options

There are a few options for getting your postpartum meals. If you are extremely lucky, you will have a family member, friend, or hired help to prepare meals for you. Most women do not have this option, however.

If you live close to a Chinese or Taiwanese immigrant community, you can arrange for a postpartum meal delivery service (see resources page 392). This is the easiest and most expensive option. These services often offer the option to pick up the meals frozen at a reduced price.

You can also prepare the recipes yourself ahead of time and freeze. This is the most economical and allows you to cook for your taste. I recommend freezing the recipes in the proper portions and organizing them by stage so you can easily take them out and heat them each day. You might need to purchase a small freezer for this.

The Postpartum Recovery Plan

Stage 1 - Week 1

Treatment Principle:
Detoxify the body and discharge lochia.

The focus of the first week is to gently discharge from the body the lochia and any residual contents from the womb. Water retention needs to be efficiently cleared as well. However, the body is also at its weakest, so extra care must be taken to conserve Qi and Blood.

Practices

1. Begin abdominal binding/postpartum girdle. In cases of natural childbirth, begin the second day after giving birth. In case of C-section begin after the sixth day. Maintain the binding/girdle day and night, removing only for bathing and meals.
2. Placenta Encapsulation procedure (if you choose).
3. Take Red Date Tea (page 349) if you had a C-section.

Prohibitions

1. Avoid cold water and cold drafts at all costs. Maintain an ambient temperature of 77-82 degrees F (25-28 degrees C) at all times.
2. Do not wash your hair (or do so less frequently and dry hair immediately.)
3. Do not take a bath (or take quick warm showers).
4. Do not lift any weight, climb stairs, or exercise beyond mild mobility and stretching (such as Dao Yin, or yin or restorative yoga)
5. Do not carry your baby. Lie on your side to nurse.
6. Only surround yourself with kind, loving people. Avoid anything that makes you sad or upset.
7. Protect your eyes. Limit TV viewing, reading or straining your eyes.

Rest

Get 10 hours of sleep a night (pump milk and have helpers feed baby to accommodate this). Rest the remainder of the day. Have others maintain the house and do the cooking.

Diet Schedule

Avoid cold foods and use as little salt as possible. Cook all foods and liquids with Postpartum

Water or a dash of rice wine. Traditionally, no vegetables are eaten the first two weeks postpartum because they are too cleansing. I recommend eating cooked, tonifying vegetables like carrots, green papaya, pumpkin, and beets. Eat your largest portions at breakfast and lunch, and smaller portions at dinner to support digestion.

Talbe 4.1. Stage 1 Sample Meal Plan (Recipes page 340):

Before Breakfast	Sheng Hua Tang
Breakfast	Choose an egg recipe or vegetarian option Postpartum Congee
Snack	Adzuki Bean Soup
Lunch	Choose a liver recipe or vegetarian option 1 small bowl of fish soup 2 small bowls of steamed vegetables 1 small bowl of Yi Yi Ren Rice
Before Dinner	Sheng Hua Tang
Dinner	Choose a liver recipe or vegetarian option 1 small bowl of fish soup 2 small bowls of steamed vegetables 1 small bowl of Yi Yi Ren Rice
Snack	Adzuki Bean Soup
Drink	Postpartum Recovery Tea, Red Date Tea

Stage 2 - Week 2

Treatment Principle:
Contract the internal organs, uterus, and pelvic cavity.

After much of the excesses have been discharged from the body, the focus of the second week is to contract everything back to its normal size.

Practices

1. Continue abdominal binding/postpartum girdle. Remove during meals and bathing only.
2. Continue taking placenta capsules.
3. Use moxa on lower abdomen.

Prohibitions & Rest

Same as Week 1.

Diet Schedule

Begin introducing green vegetables.

Table 4.2. Stage 2 Sample Meal Plan (Recipes page 350):

Before Breakfast	Sheng Hua Tang
Breakfast	Choose an egg recipe or vegetarian option Postpartum Congee
Snack	White Fungus and Red Date Soup or Peanut Soup
Lunch	Choose a kidney recipe or vegetarian option 1 bowl of fish soup 2 small bowls of steamed vegetables 1 small bowl of Yi Yi Ren Rice
Before Dinner	Sheng Hua Tang
Dinner	Choose a kidney recipe or vegetarian option 1 small bowl of fish soup 2 small bowls of steamed vegetables 1 small bowl of Yi Yi Ren Rice
Snack	Adzuki Bean Soup
Drink	Postpartum Recovery Tea

Stage 3 - Weeks 3-4/5

Treatment Principle:
Nourish, supplement, and renew strength.

After two weeks the body has been cleared of toxins enough to focus primarily on tonifying.

Practices

Continue abdominal binding/postpartum girdle. It can now be removed at night, during meals, and to bathe.

Prohibitions

1. Can start showering. Do not soak in a tub until after the 30-40 days.
2. Do not lift any weight or climb stairs. Depending on how well you have recuperated, you can slowly start to increase the intensity of your activities and add some yoga (no heated room or strenuous styles yet), calisthenics, and Pilates-type exercises. You are still focusing on mobility and firing the muscles to begin working, but without exertion.

Rest

Same as weeks 1 and 2.

Diet Schedule

Fruit can now be added to the diet. Stop taking Sheng Hua Tang and replace with a customized formula.

Table 4.3. Stage 3 Sample Meal Plan (Recipes page 353):

Before Breakfast	Blood-building Formula (given by acupuncturist) or Lactation formula p.373
Breakfast	Choose an egg recipe or vegetarian option Millet Congee or Oatmeal Fruit
Snack	White Fungus and Red Date Soup
Lunch	Choose a Chicken recipe or vegetarian option 1 bowl of Pig's Feet soup, Cod and Tofu Soup, or Green Papaya Soup 2 small bowls of steamed vegetables 1 small bowl of Stir-fried Rice
Before Dinner	Blood-building Formula (given by acupuncturist) or Lactation formula
Dinner	Choose a Chicken recipe or vegetarian option 1 bowl of Pig's Feet soup, Cod and Tofu Soup, or Green Papaya Soup 2 small bowls of steamed vegetables 1 small bowl of Stir-fried Rice
Snack	Adzuki Bean Soup
Drink	Postpartum Recovery Tea

What to Expect After Postpartum Recovery

Lochia can continue for up to three weeks after birth. Lochial discharge that continues after one month typically indicates an infection, which is treated fastest with antibiotics. Normal menstruation should return four months after giving birth. After vaginal delivery it takes one year or more for the Ren and Du channels to unite again. Practice vaginal exercises to speed this process (page 144).

After the first month postpartum, you may slowly return to regular life, but you must still recuperate your body. If you are breastfeeding, continue taking the Lactation-promoting Formula, Pig's Feet Soup, or Cod Soup as needed to keep milk plentiful. Eat chicken recipes regularly and follow a balanced diet. When you are ready to stop breastfeeding take the Roasted Mai Ya Tea (page 359). In order to restore (and improve) your breasts, use breast massage (page 139) and take an appropriate rejuvenating formula after you have finished lactating (page 226).

Slowly resume physical activity and exercise routines. Take six months to build yourself back up to your former shape, after which you can start setting new goals.

Chapter 5

Age 35

5 x 7, The Yang-ming channels begin to weaken, the complexion starts to wither and the hair begins to fall.

五七，阳明脉衰，面始焦，发始堕；（35岁）

The 5th Cycle

Five x 7 years begins the 5th Cycle in a woman's life. Between the ages of 35 to 41 years, Earth declines and goes into the Metal Phase. The Metal Phase is characterized by self-reflection and refining our gifts. Without intervention, the Jing will slowly begin to decline at this stage, correlating to a decline in hormones. The exact age of Jing decline will vary based on individual constitution and lifestyle choices. Live hard and party hard, and the Jing can get depleted as early as the twenties. On the other hand, following rejuvenation practices, such as the ones outlined in this chapter, can conserve the Jing well into older age. Now is the time to lay the groundwork for a healthy menopause. Doing so will delay menopause, greatly reduce menopausal symptoms, and minimize the need for bioidentical hormone replacement. Women can begin following these guidelines earlier, but everyone should start by age 35.

Unfortunately, it is becoming common for women to experience premature menopause (i.e. premature aging) at this time of their life. This is not the natural way. Seek the care of an

PRACTITIONER TIP: POSTPONING MENOPAUSE

Needle points below the knees for anti-aging. Specifically between the ages of 35-41, focus on strengthening the YangMing channels with needling and moxa. Patients can moxa their lower Stomach channel daily. Have your patient on 1-3g of powdered ginseng daily.

acupuncturist, make lifestyle changes (avoid overwork, irregular diet, excess dairy and sugar, and emotional stress), and practice daily rejuvenation to reverse premature menopause.

In Chapter 1 of the *Yellow Emperor's Inner Canon*, right after the sage Qi Bo describes the 7 Cycles of Jing for women and the 8 Cycles for men, he goes on to say that this is the way of "ordinary humans" who "tended to abuse themselves."[1] Qi Bo goes on to tell the Yellow Emperor that those blessed with good Jing or who lived a good lifestyle could easily extend their vitality by many years. Qi Bo talks further of several types of people: "immortals," "sages," and "naturalists." These were all mortals who had learned to live in tune with the Dao (natural cycles). These people were able to live into their 100s with youthfulness and vitality.

Traditional Chinese Medicine teaches us that how we live is a choice. Do not listen to society's ideas of how we should age. Use the information in the remaining chapters of this book to make your own choices. It is not that we must live a limited life after age 35. It is that we no longer have the luxury of living badly.

---

1. Maoshing Ni, trans. *The Yellow Emperor's Classic of Medicine*. (Boston: Shambala, 1995), 4.

Rejuvenation

At age 35 begin taking rejuvenating herbs and follow a restorative diet and lifestyle to boost the Jing (and hormone levels). Women should begin practicing proper skin care and facial regiments in their twenties. By age 35, begin Cosmetic Acupuncture and other rejuvenating treatments as it is easier to conserve than to reverse damage in the future. You can start rejuvenation treatments at any age, particularly if you are under great stress or after serious illness.

What follows are natural ways to build vitality and beauty. In TCM, beauty is a sign of health, and thus the foundation for beautifying the body is to nourish from within, to which external treatments are supplementary. Even the most advanced cosmetic surgery relies on the health of the skin and body for good results.

Diagnosing Your Skin and Face

Your skin is a primary diagnostic tool for the state of your internal environment. When using natural medicine, maintaining youthfulness is an extension of optimizing health. Exterior signs of aging correspond with internal changes.

Assessing Skin Thickness and Texture

Thin skin – Deficiency, Metal constitution
Thick skin – Strong constitution or excess Phlegm-Damp
Enlarged pores – Dampness, Wei Qi deficiency
Wrinkles – Qi Stagnation and Kidney Yin deficiency
Hyperpigmentation (dark spots) – Liver imbalance, Blood stagnation
Pallor, dullness, looks like the light is out – Blood deficiency
Redness – Yin deficiency with Heat or excess Heat
Loose skin, sagging, jowls – Spleen Qi and Yang deficiency
Cellulite – Spleen Qi Deficiency with Phlegm-Damp
Spider veins – Spleen Qi Deficiency with Phlegm-Damp and Blood Stagnation

Assessing Moisture Levels

Dry skin – Blood or Yin deficiency
Oily skin – Phlegm-Damp or Damp-Heat

Face Mapping (Figure 5.1)

1. **Line under eyes/upper cheeks** – Gallstones or Gallbladder Damp-Heat
2. **Dark or greenish circle around mouth** – Digestive weakness or food allergies
3. **Dark circles under the eyes** – Kidney deficiency or Blood stagnation
4. **Under eye puffiness** – Kidney deficiency
5. **Puffiness or droopiness of upper eyelid** – Spleen deficiency
6. **Fa Lin Lines (nasolabial folds)** – Sign of living your life with purpose. When too deep indicates over purpose or overwork
7. **Line under lips** – Lack of joy
8. **Lines around the mouth (smoker's lines)** – Over-nurturing others and under-nurturing the self; Yin deficiency
9. **Suspended dagger (vertical line between eyebrows)** – Anger
10. **Darkness and indentation on temples** – Escapism, addiction
11. **Wrinkles on sides of cheeks** – Grief
12. **Round nose** – gourmand (takes great pleasure in food and drink)
13. **Double chin** - Earth element sign, enjoys comfort and good food

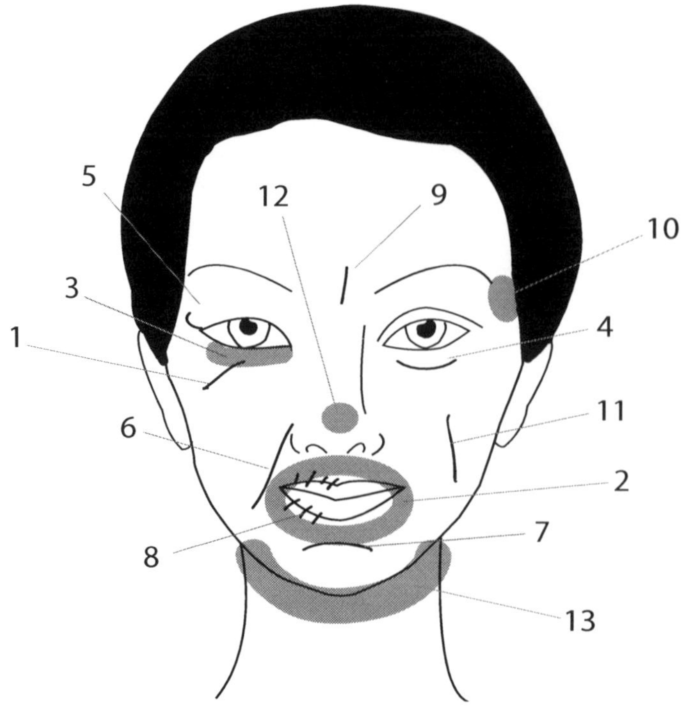

Figure 5.1. Face Mapping

Rejuvenating Lifestyle

These are simple steps to rejuvenate the body. Rejuvenation, because it involves the Kidneys, requires consistent nurturing over a long period of time.

Sleep

A teacher of mine used to say that not getting to bed before 10 each night "makes you stupid." Perhaps this is the blunt Chinese way to motivate people. Inadequate sleep will not only adversely affect brain functioning, it also causes premature aging and weight gain. The hours between 10 p.m. and midnight are the most restorative hours of sleep. It is best to retire when you feel a little tired, as going to bed exhausted weakens the Kidneys. Make sure to get 8-9 hours of uninterrupted sleep each night, as sleep deprivation also weakens the Kidneys. Also, go to bed and wake up with a smile. Another teacher of mine firmly believes this is the key to staying young. If you suffer from insomnia, see page 293.

Regular Relaxation

Emotional stress is the single biggest factor in pathology and premature aging. Worse still, it blocks inspiration and Divine connection. Learning to calm your Mind and emotions is the most important step to retaining your youth and vitality and achieving long life.

Most of life is outside our control and this naturally produces stress. Stress does not help us. Rather it scatters and disconnects us from ourselves by placing the focus on the chaos of the world. We can only begin to take control of our minds and emotions when we accept that the only thing we have control over is how we respond to life. We must make a daily commitment to practice relaxation techniques and to let go of negative events and people. When we feel overwhelmed, we must seek out friends to talk with or healers to help us relax.

To begin, plan daily relaxation. Daily meditation, breathing exercises, qigong, or yoga practice will shift the focus back to the present moment, the only time there is any power. Additionally, get regular acupuncture and massage to keep stress from building up in your body. These are tools to remind the Mind daily to be present.

If you cannot be present, kind, and at ease with yourself and others, you are doing more than you can handle. Do not overcommit and make every effort to remove stressful people and situations from your life. As you stop giving them your attention, they will move on somewhere else. Besides a routine dedicated to relaxation, it is important to break up the day with moments of being present. This is the most important practice, to stay in the present moment in a state of relaxation, while being aware of the world around. With practice, it takes more external disruption to upset inner peace.

Balanced Work

Overworking mentally, especially when straining on a computer, taxes Qi and Blood, and eventually Kidney Yin. Overworking physically, depletes Kidney Yang. Even if you are still young enough to test your physical limits, one day the reserves simply will not be there anymore. It is better never to reach this day. Overworking to collapse is a sure way to Chronic Fatigue Syndrome and Fibromyalgia. Beginning at age 35, keep regular hours, get enough sleep, and balance periods of overexertion with periods of rest.

Exercises that Exhilarate

Like partying all weekend, working the body to exhaustion is not a good long-term strategy, particularly beyond age 35. Maintaining youthfulness for life requires a shift from recklessness to awareness. Exercise must be carried out in a goal-oriented fashion, where superfluous activities are eliminated.

You cannot make your body more beautiful while you mistreat yourself. The mark of a good exercise routine is that your body moves better and has more vitality. This concept was shared by old-time American strongmen such as Adolf Nordquest, who was able to transform himself from a sickly child to a powerful man.

Exercise 5.1. Rules for Exercise

1. Warm up your joints prior to exercising with mobility drills. Finish your workout routines with stretching. These steps protect against injury and increase neuroconnections in the body.
2. Limit cardio to 45 min. Excessive cardio depletes your body and does more harm than good. If you enjoy running, do short 45-sec. sprints between walking.
3. Lift heavy weights 3 times a week, giving yourself ample rest in between. This builds muscle, strengthens bones and ligaments, and promotes fat loss.
4. Try to exercise between sunrise and sunset. This is Yang time when you should naturally be active. When the sun has set, it is time for rest.
5. Do not go to exhaustion. The ideal time to stop is when you feel energetic and alive. This will produce better aesthetic and health results.

Self-Concept

Actress Sophia Loren once said that the secret to her youthfulness was she kept perfect posture and she did not "make old people noises." What starts the process of aging is that we begin to think, feel, and act old. It is the expectation that by such and such age "I will be old." If we ignore the common level of consciousness, we will live a different reality. Have the expectation that you will live with vitality for the rest of your life; that rather than closing in on you, life will continue to expand.

See yourself as beautiful and healthy and take actions to affirm this daily. This becomes more important over the years because there is increasing social pressure to start behaving like an old person. Keep yourself manicured at all times, as if you were going to meet a new lover. Wear pretty underwear. Adorn yourself with clothes, accessories, and scents that make you feel beautiful.

This is not the same, however, as behaving childishly or dressing inappropriately. Wisdom and grace are natural gifts we acquire from living longer. We can integrate these while keeping up our curiosity, passion, and energy.

Rejuvenating Qigong Exercises

Continue the Inner Alchemy exercises and vaginal exercises in Chapter 3. These are additional exercises intended for cultivating youthfulness.

Exercise 5.2. Energetic Face Washing (Figure 5.2)

Perform after meditation or qigong exercise.

1. Warm your hands by rubbing them together.
2. Hover your hands close to your face, but do not touch your skin. Feel the heat from your hands.
3. Begin at the chin and move up the face, over the scalp and down the neck

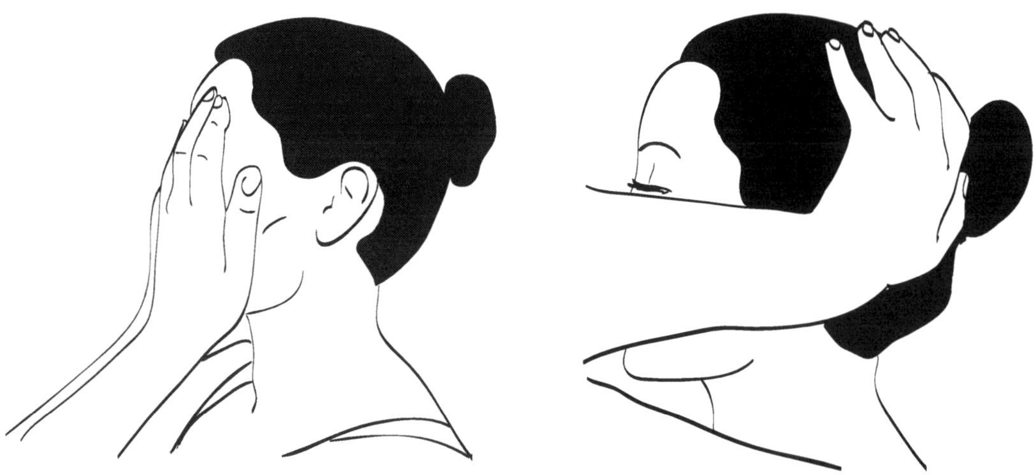

Figure 5.2. Energetic Face Washing

Exercise 5.3. Swimming Dragon (Figure 5.3)

Women's waists tend to widen in proportion to the rest of the body as female hormones decrease and Spleen Qi weakens. Several seated and standing versions of this exercise exist in different qigong traditions. They involve using a serpentine movement that mobilizes all the joints of the body. My teacher's teacher used this exercise to start her menses again so she could have a child. It also lubricates the joints, increases mobility, narrows the waist, and balances the hormones. Moving slowly allows you to tune your own energy. Perform 16 repetitions twice a day for maximum benefit.

1. Keep feet and palms together for the entire exercise. You will be using the hands to draw a figure 8, crossing the body at the throat, heart, and lower abdomen then back up again.
2. Bring the palms together to the right of the head, face turned to the left, hips sticking out to the left.
3. Cross the hands across the body at throat level to the left side of the body as the face and hips move to the right. Continue the figure 8 motion.
4. Cross the hands across the body at heart level back to the right side as the face and hips move back to the left. Continue the figure 8 motion.
5. Cross the hands across the body at the level of the lower abdomen to the left as the face and hips move to the right.
6. Work back up the body.
7. Perform 16 repetitions twice a day.

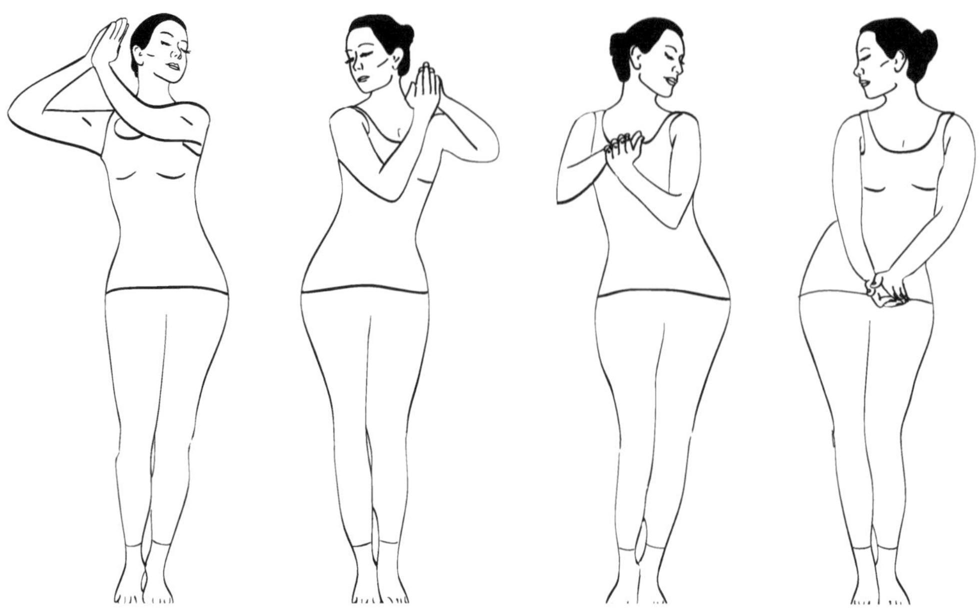

Figure 5.3. Swimming Dragon

Exercise 5.4. Hip Figure 8s (Figure 5.4)

Doing hip isolations rejuvenates the Kidneys, frees sexual energy, and keeps the joints of the lower body supple. Figure 8s can be performed by moving the hips in four directions: up, down, forward, and backwards. Practice moving quickly and slowly. To advance, practice doing them with a jade egg and initiate the movements from your vaginal muscles (Jade Egg Practice page 145).

Begin standing with feet shoulder width, tailbone tucked under, and spine straight. Be sure to move from the hips only, keeping the rest of the body as still as possible. The movements will feel choppy at first. Over time they will become smooth.

Up: Stick your hip out to the right. Then move the hip straight up and in. As you do this begin sticking your left hip out to the left, then straight up and in. Repeat 24 times.

Down: Stick your right hip out to the right, then straight down and in. As you do this begin pushing your left hip out, then straight down and in. Repeat 24 times.

Forward: Twist your right hip forward, then down. Twist your left hip forward and down. Re- peat 24 times.

Backwards: Twist your right hip backward, then down. Twist your left hip backwards and down. Repeat 24 times.

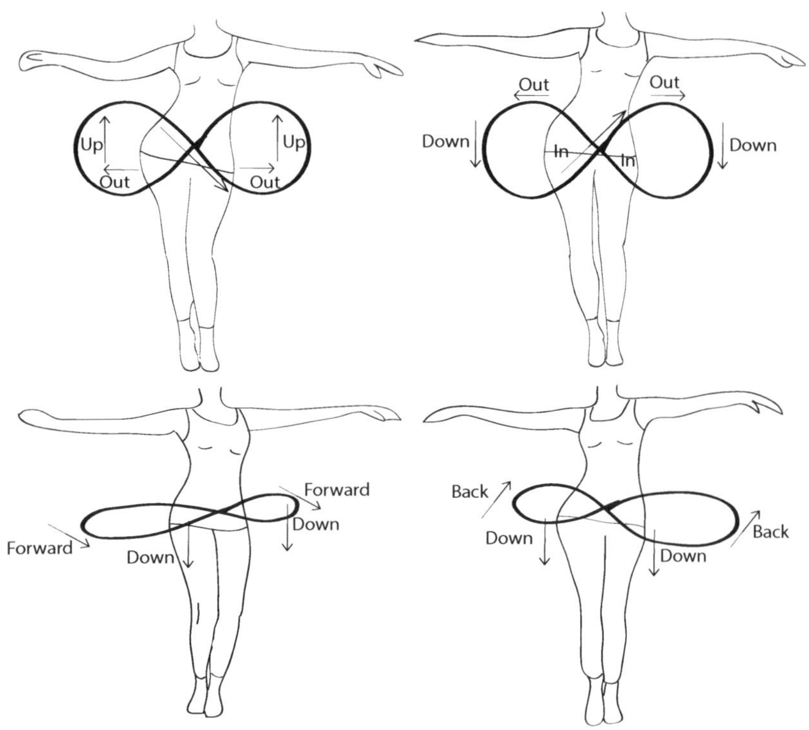

Figure 5.4. Hip Figure 8s

Exercise 5.5. Hip Circles (Figure 5.5)

These are also called omnis or Tahitian shimmy when done quickly.

Stand with the feet less than hip width apart. Tuck the pelvis under so the spine in neutral. Keep your back straight. A variation is to bend over and support your upper body by pressing down just above the knees.

1. Begin by sticking your hip out to the right, then to the front, then to the left, then back.
2. Smooth out the movement.
3. Repeat going opposite direction.
4. Perform 25-100 repetitions each side.

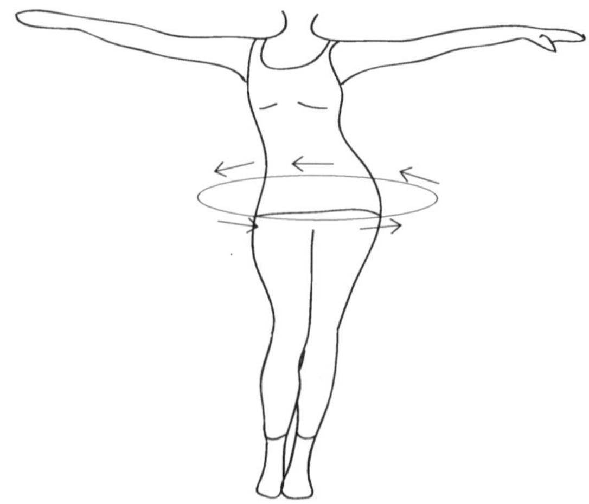

Figure 5.5. Hip CIrcles

Some daily opportunities to get present:

Engaging multiple senses helps you get present.

1. Connect with your plants in the morning when you water them. Feel how they come alive and start to chatter.
2. Become one with your dogs when you walk them. Notice the smells and sounds. Dogs are masters of observation, let them teach you.
3. Practice making eye contact and really listening to the people you come in contact with today. It is the wish of every living thing to be truly seen.

Anti-Aging Diet

Continue the health-promoting diet as introduced in Chapter 1. This includes eating the biggest meal early in the day, having dinner prior to 7 p.m., eating vegetables at each meal, avoiding excess sugar and carbohydrates, increasing good fats/decreasing bad fats, drinking warm drinks with meals, only drinking water 30 minutes before or after meals, not skipping meals, chewing thoroughly, enjoying food, and eating in a pleasant environment. It is important to get any weight issues under control now prior to hormonal changes.

Habits that Age:

1. Eating sugary, high carbohydrate foods.

2. Eating excess dairy products or cold foods.
3. Skipping meals.
4. Eating late at night.
5. Eating processed foods.

Beautifying Herbs

Longevity herbs can be taken regularly at any age. They should be taken with greater frequency after age 35. Expect to take tonic herbs for three to six months before you see significant results. Deficiencies in the body take far longer to correct than excess conditions. Draining treatments can quickly clear an excess case, whereas it takes regular supplementation over time for the body to rebuild itself.

Ren Shen (ginseng) has well-deserved fame as a premiere tonic. It has the potency of a serious herb and warrants extra respect. There are several types of ginseng, all of which boost energy, strengthen the hormones, and build immunity. Taken daily beginning at age 35, **ginseng will delay menopause and aging.**[2] If the stronger Qi tonifying action of Ren Shen is desired, it can be combined with Xi Yang Shen (American ginseng) or other Yin tonics to balance its heating and drying nature.[3] Dosage is 5-10g in decoction, or 0.5-1g per day powdered, as it is most commonly taken.[4]

Table 5.1. Comparing Types of Ginseng

Ginseng Type	Indications	Contraindications
Ren Shen **Bai Shen** **Chinese White Ginseng**	Tonifies Yuan (Source) Qi. One of the only tonics that will not tonify a pathogen, making it ideal to boost your energy during colds, infections, or cancer treatmentsupport. Best suited to Cold constitutions. Strengthens digestion. Increases strength and endurance. Tonifies Qi and Blood. Improves vision. Calms the Shen, improves memory. Anti-aging, regulates hormones. Boosts immunity, anti-cancer. Lowers cholesterol, normalizes blood sugar.	Warming. Can cause bleeding disorders, menstrual irregularity, and dryness. Avoid in Heat conditions. Contraindicated in high blood pressure. Generally contraindicated in children, unless very deficient. Monitor the dosage carefully. If any Heat or Dryness symptoms develop such as dry mouth or feeling warm, reduce the dosage. A tiny amount can still be therapeutic.

2. This action is strengthened by the addition of raw San Qi. See "Recipe 5.1. Vitality Formula" on page 226.
3. Yueying Li. "TCM Cosmetology." (lecture, Yo San University, Los Angeles, June 6, 2003).
4. John Chen. *Chinese Medical Herbology and Pharmacology.* (City of Industry: Art of Medicine Press, 2001), 837.

Ginseng Type	Indications	Contraindications
Xi Yang Shen **American Ginseng**	Tonifies Qi and Yin. Clears Heat. Generates body fluids. Qi tonifying (energy boosting) action is weaker than Chinese or Korean ginsengs. Best choice for perimenopausal women, Yin deficient or Heat conditions, and endurance athletes.	Most commonly used and safe for almost everyone. Balance with other herbs in cases of stagnation. Caution in Cold or Damp conditions.
Hong Shen **Chinese Red Ginseng**	Steamed Chinese Ginseng. Same actions as Chinese White Ginseng, with additional capacity to tonify Yang. Best suited to Cold constitutions.	Very Warming. Same concerns as Ren Shen, only stronger.
Hong Shen **Korean Red Ginseng**	Steamed Korean Ginseng. Same plant as Chinese ginseng; when grown in Korea produces a much more heating and Yang tonifying herb. Best suited to Cold constitutions.	Hottest ginseng. Same concerns as Ren Shen, only stronger.
Dong Yang Shen **Japanese Ginseng**	Same plant as Chinese ginseng; when grown in Japan produces a more gentle function. Tonifies Lung and Spleen Qi. Non-drying.	Balance with moving herbs for cases of mixed excess and deficiency.
Tai Zi Shen **Pseudostellaria**	Mildest. Best choice for children and the very weak. Tonifies Lung and Spleen Qi. Generates Body Fluids. Builds immunity and safe for use during illness.	Balance with moving herbs for cases of mixed excess and deficiency.
Ci Wu Jia **Siberian Ginseng**	Not a true ginseng. It is milder in effects than ginseng but has adaptogenic properties. Tonifies Spleen Qi and Kidney Yang. Calms the Shen. Often used for joint pain.	None
Dang Shen **Codonopsis Root**	Often called "poor man's ginseng" and is not a ginseng. Triple the dosage is used in recipes asking for ginseng. Tonifies Spleen and Lung Qi. Generates Blood and Body Fluids. Builds immunity and safe for use during illness.	Balance with moving herbs for cases of mixed excess and deficiency.

Wu Wei Zi (schizandra) is a premiere beauty and longevity tonic for women. It generates fluids, astringes the Kidney Yin and Jing, and calms the Shen. It contains all five flavors and nourishes the Jing, Shen, and Qi. The prevalent signs of aging in women are due to Lung and Kidney Yin fluid deficiency, which can happen abruptly with the drop in hormones during menopause. Wu Wei Zi is thus effective for many menopausal symptoms: night sweats, insomnia, wrinkles, vaginal dryness and atrophy, sallowness and thinning of the skin, and polyuria. Many modern women begin losing their Yin fluids far before menopause due to overwork, inappropriate lifestyle, and after childbirth. To prevent this Wu Wei Zi can be taken long-term from an early age. Taking Wu Wei Zi regularly generates sexual fluids, increases sensitivity in the genitals, and enhances Inner Alchemy practices and sexual cultivation. It plumps up, smoothes, and adds glow to the skin. Wu Wei Zi also calms and sharpens the Mind, strengthens eyesight, and cleanses the Liver. Avoid in exterior Wind conditions as it can bind the pathogen inside the body. Soak in water for several hours and rinse before cooking to reduce tannins (acidity). The seeds should also be crushed with a mortar and pestle prior to cooking to fully extract the active components.[(5)]

He Shou Wu (polygonum) can be taken long-term without side effects in a formula or alone as a tea. Nourishes Blood and Jing and is a key herb to rejuvenate the hair.[(6)] He Shou Wu also clears toxins, treats malaria, moistens the intestines, and lowers cholesterol. It is most often used in its prepared form.

Tu Si Zi (dodder seed) is a major longevity herb. It tonifies Yin and Yang, safely without heating or drying. Benefits the Jing, increases cognitive functioning, strengthens eyesight, and astringes excess urination and diarrhea.

Dang Gui (Chinese angelica) is one of the most used herbs, particularly in menstrual conditions or physical injury. Dang Gui nourishes Heart and Liver Blood as well as moves the Blood. It treats constipation due to Blood deficiency. Menstruating women should use Dang Gui throughout the cycle in formulas and recipes. In post-menopausal women, it should be featured in longevity formulas and recipes. It is often combined with Huang Qi (astragalus) to generate new Blood and beautify the skin.

Huang Qi (astragalus) raises Spleen Qi to treat prolapse and sagging conditions. It also strengthens immunity, tonifies the Spleen and digestive function, increases energy, and boosts Blood production. Huang Qi increases low hormones and rejuvenates muscle, skin, and breast tissue when used in formulas. Its raising function is so strong, however, it must be used with caution in cases of Yin deficiency or headaches.

Top 10 Chinese Superfoods

Additionally, there are foods we can eat regularly for their anti-aging qualities. They enhance brain function, beautify the skin, boost the hormones, and promote longevity. These foods appear regularly in Chinese Food Therapy.[(7)]They also help protect against deficiency in vegetarians or those who want to reduce meat intake.[(8)]

---

5. Featured in "Recipe 5.1. Vitality Formula" on page 226.
6. See "Beautifying the Hair" on page 236.
7. "To secure the body at the root, you must provide it with food. To rescue from the speed of disease, you must rely on medicinals." "Nurturing Life in Classical Chinese Medicine: Sun Simiao on Healing without Drugs, Transforming Bodies and Cultivating Life," The Journal of Chinese Medicine, accessed November 11, 2012, http://www.jcm.co.uk/product/catalog/product/view/10293/nurturing-life-in-classical-chinese-medicine-sun-simiao-on-healing-without-drugs-transforming-bodies-and-cultivating-life.
8. Sun Simiao specifically noted that cow's milk, black sesame seeds, and bee honey were "far better than meats."

Long Yan Rou, Gou Qi Zi, Sang Shen Zi are potent superfoods that can (and should) be eaten indefinitely without creating imbalances. Additional foods have positive and negative qualities that need to be kept in mind.

1. **Long Yan Rou** (longan berry) – Long Yan Rou beautifies the skin. It tonifies Spleen Qi and Heart Blood, aids cognitive functioning, and calms emotional issues. Long Yan Rou is ideal for students or those who do a great deal of mental work. It is excellent for the elderly, recovery from illness or emotional trauma, and postpartum or post-menses. Use for symptoms such as weakness, insomnia, worry, forgetfulness, and palpitations. Eat them fresh or dried in soups, congee, smoothies, trail mix, etc.
2. **Gou Qi Zi** (go ji berries) – Gou Qi Zi nourishes the Lungs, Liver, and Kidney Yin making it an ideal general anti-aging herb. It beautifies the skin and hair. It is excellent for symptoms of blurry vision, weakness of low back and knees, premature gray hair, infertility, dry cough, and steaming bone.[(9)] Gou Qi Zi can stimulate contraction of the uterus and should be used with caution during fragile pregnancies, but is ideal for postpartum and during menses. Eat them fresh or dried in soups, congee, smoothies, trail mix, etc.
3. **Sang Shen Zi** (mulberries) – Nourishes Liver Blood, Kidney Yin, and Body Fluids. Sang Shen Zi lubricates the bowels for constipation. It is used for symptoms of dizziness, blurred vision, premature gray hair, hot flashes, weakness of low back and knees, tinnitus, and insomnia. This is an excellent long-term tonic for women who tend towards Liver Blood deficiency and are depleted by their monthly periods. Eat them fresh or dried in soups, congee, smoothies, trail mix, etc.
4. **Hei Zhi Ma** (black sesame seeds) – Tonifies Liver Blood and Kidney Jing. Hei Zhi Ma lubricates the bowels for constipation. It is used for premature gray hair, insufficient milk in nursing mothers, blurred vision, and tinnitus. Brown sesame seeds go to the Spleen and also lubricate the intestines to treat constipation. Grind and use in soups, congee, smoothies, etc.
5. **(Hei) Da Zao** (black jujube date) – Is a Middle Jiao-focused herb. It tonifies the Spleen Qi and Stomach, nourishes the Blood, calms the Shen, and harmonizes potential toxicity of other herbs (with Gan Cao). Da Zao is used for fatigue, pallor, low appetite, muscle weakness, scanty menses, blurred vision, irritability, and emotional instability resulting in hysterical crying. It is used with raw ginger to harmonize the exterior. It has the ability to protect the Liver, and is recommended prior to and after surgery. Da Zao can create Dampness and heat in the body. Avoid in cases of yeast infection or intestinal parasites. Eat them fresh or dried in soups, congee, smoothies, baking, etc. Note: Da Zao and Hong Zao are the same fruit processed differently. Da Zao is blanched in boiling water and baked until the skin becomes black and shiny. It is also larger and has a smoky fragrance and taste. It is used more for Blood deficiency. **Hong (Da) Zao** (red jujube date) – It is smaller than Da Zao and red. Hong Zao is blanched slightly in boiling water and dried under the sun. It has the same properties as Da Zao. It is used more for Qi deficiency.
6. **Shan Yao** (Chinese Yam) – Tonifies both Qi and Yin, and is slightly astringent. Shan Yao is

9. Excellent for prostate inflammation. Take one handful daily along with pumpkin seeds.

Gifts of Having a Hive

Being in service to your own bee hive is much greater than the medicinal properties of the products they produce.

1. You learn to see your landscape through their eyes. You experience how certain flowers, the weather, water sources, environmental contaminants all affect their production.
2. It will multiply immensely the yield of your garden and fruit trees.
3. It teaches you gentleness and patience. Bees respond to subtle changes in your vibration. If you are not present and calm in your dealings with them you will get stung.
4. You are in service to a key part of nature. Bees were tied to goddesses and oracles in ancient times and have much to teach us about feminine power. The geometric structure of their homes, their sense of community, and their service to nature are all deep lessons.

used for fatigue, loose stools, vaginal discharge, respiratory weakness, frequent urination, and night sweats. This is a top herb/food for postpartum, post-menses, and perimenopause. Combine with Huang Qi (astragalus) for endurance athletes to boost energy and for diabetes to lower blood sugar. Eat raw as a salad, or add dried herb to soups and congee. Balance with Chen Pi (tangerine peel) or cooking spices in cases of Dampness.

7. **Mushrooms and Fungi** – There are numerous types of mushrooms and fungi that are useful in regular diet to prevent disease as they concurrently tonify deficiencies and clear excesses. **Ling Zhi** (reishi mushroom) is a mystical herb. It nourishes the Heart and calms the Shen, dispels Phlegm, and tonifies Qi and Blood. Ling Zhi strengthens immunity and inhibits cancer and tumor formation. **Hei Mu Er** (black wood ear fungus) moistens the Yin and Body Fluids. It is used for Blood Stagnation and Phlegm. Black wood ear helps dissolve fibroids and tumors. It also strengthens the Heart and decreases cholesterol in the blood. **Bai Mu Er** (white cloud fungus) moistens the Yin and Body Fluids. It is for thirst and dry cough. White fungus beautifies the skin and is often used in desserts.
8. **Bee Products – Honey** detoxifies the body and harmonizes the Liver. It is useful in the overworked, menstrual disorders, excess rich foods, constipation, stomach ulcers. Pasteurized or heat-processed honey moistens Dryness. Raw honey (comb honey) drys Dampness (edema, excess weight, Phlegm conditions). Raw honey contains pollen and all of its properties.[10] **Local bee pollen** is excellent for treating allergies and building immunity. For this purpose take regularly and continuously. For allergies take 1 tsp daily. For athletic endurance take 2-3 tsp daily. It decreases the need for animal proteins. **Bee Propolis** is a natural antiseptic that kills bacteria, fungus, and viruses. It is used for Heat Toxins in the body. Propolis is a resinous substance bees use to seal small holes and cracks in the structure of the hive. It helps to strengthen the hive and ward off diseases that could

10. Paul Pitchford. *Healing With Whole Foods; Oriental Traditions and Modern Nutrition.* (Berkeley: North Atlantic Books, 1993), 151.

attack in the crowded beehive workspace. **Royal Jelly** is a powerful rejuvenation tonic for both men and women. It decreases the need for animal proteins and is used to increase fertility.[11]

9. **Collagen-rich foods** – Ingest collagen-rich foods daily to rejuvenate the skin and joints. The best foods are bone broth made with connective tissue (page 328) and chicken feet/ pig's trotters (page 355). Collagen supplements can also be taken on a daily basis.
10. **The 5 Beans** – Different types of beans pertain to the different Elements and should be eaten regularly to balance the major organ systems. **Mung Beans** detoxify the Liver/ GallBladder system and clear Damp-Heat from the body. **Lima Beans** nourish the Lungs and beautify the skin. **Red Adzuki Beans** reduce edema and support Heart functioning. **Black Beans** tonify the Kidneys. **Soybeans** support the Spleen.

Food for Specific Actions

Moistening

White cloud fungus, asparagus, black wood ear fungus, sesame seeds, eggs, pork, Asian pear, dairy, soy products, millet, sweet rice, sardines or fish oil supplement.

Skin Beautifying

Seaweed (arame, kombu, wakame), avocado, cabbage, lima bean, great northern bean, oats, mango, Long Yan Rou (longan berries), Gou Qi Zi (gou ji berries), white cloud fungus.

Skin Hydrating and Brightening Soup

Shan Yao (Chinese yam) 100g (raw), 20g (dried)
Bai Mu Er (white cloud fungus) 20g
1 ½ cups of milk
honey to taste

Cook ingredients except honey for 20 min. Add honey and blend in a blender until smooth.[1]

1. Winnie. Juices, Teas, and Smoothies; 60 Ways to Great Health. (Henan Science and Technology Press, 2010). ISBN 978-7-5349-4542-7

Breast Rejuvenation

Green papaya, collagen-rich foods such as beef or pork trotters, chicken feet.

Increase Lactation

Adzuki beans, alfalfa leaf, black sesame seed, carrot, carp, shrimp, chicken, lamb, peanut, soybean, sweet potato, avocado, green papaya.

11. There have always been stories about beekeepers living long healthy lives which were attributed to the properties of the pollen, honey, royal jelly, or propolis. My experience is that these longevity benefits are in fact due to the process of keeping bees. To keep bees successfully and naturally requires being intune with the cycles of Nature, calming the emotions in their presence, and being in service to the tiniest of creatures.

Hair Beautifying

Seaweed (arame, hijiki,[12] wakame), black sesame seeds, black beans, blackstrap molasses, nettles, wheatgrass, He Shou Wu (polygonum), Gou Qi Zi (gou ji berries), walnuts. Avoid excess sweets.

Specific Beauty Remedies

Acne

Acne always involves Heat. This is often complicated with Qi and Blood deficiency (digestive weakness), Chong and Ren disharmony (hormonal imbalance) and Phlegm-Damp. Women in their 30s and 40s often develop acne on the chin, which relates to hormonal imbalance. Simple papules and pustules relate to excess Heat. Cystic acne indicates a deeper condition of Blood and Phlegm stagnation with Qi deficiency.

In terms of treatment, make sure to optimize bowel movements, as even minor constipation will increase Heat and toxicity in the body. Use cupping, running and stationary, on the back weekly. For marks that linger after acne breakouts or acne that is purplish take Yunnan Paiyao, 2 capsules 2 times a day. Skin problems always involve the Shen, so be sure to practice relaxation. Topically, use Vitamin A 1-3 times a week.

Flower Complexion Tea[1]

Jin Yin Hua (honeysuckle) 2g
Ju Hua (chrysanthemum) 2g
Mei Gui Hua (rose) 1g

Bring 2 cups of water to a boil. Remove from heat and add flowers. Steep 10 min. or longer. Use for minor acne conditions.

Dian Dao (Acne-clearing) Powder

This is a traditional acne treatment: Use powdered Da Huang (rhubarb) with Liu Huang (sulfur) at 1:1 ratio.

50 grams of powder can be added to 500g of jojoba oil and 160g bees-wax. Melt together over low heat and pour into containers to cool and store. Or simply mix the powder with water to form a paste and apply.

1. Winnie. *Juices, Teas, and Smoothies; 60 Ways to Great Health.* (Henan Science and Technology Press, 2010). ISBN 978-7-5349-4542-7

Acne-Clearing Diet:
Drink plenty of water and eat vegetables at every meal to flush out toxins and promote regular bowel movement. Yi Yi Ren (Job's tears) is one of the best foods to treat acne conditions. Eat a handful daily, cooked with grains, in soups, or in congee (see Clear Skin Congee #1 and #2 page 327). **Include** mung beans, dandelion greens, Zhen Zhu (pearl powder), and seaweed (5g)[13] daily in the diet. A mixture of mung bean powder, seaweed, and apple cider vinegar can be applied topically. **Avoid** heating or inflammatory substances: sugar, spices, garlic, alcohol, marijuana. Dairy and food sensitivities can be the triggers in some individuals.

12. The Japanese consider hijiki seaweed to be the strongest for increasing the health and fullness of the hair.
13. Seaweeds are particularly effective for cystic acne. Take Kun Bu (kelp) in pill form for one to three months to see results.

Hyperpigmentation (Dark Spots, Sun Spots, Cholasma)

Hyperpigmentation occurs more frequently in those with higher melanin production. The more a woman tans and the less she burns in the sun, the more predisposed she is to hyperpigmentation as she ages. Living in a dry, sunny climate also increases hyperpigmentation. Asians, Latinos, and lighter complexion African Americans are particularly susceptible. Hyperpigmentation occurs when the dermis is injured, as an inflammatory reaction, sun damage, and due to hormonal fluctuations (as occurs during pregnancy). Avoid sun exposure as much as possible and use an SPF of 30.

Skin Brightening Drink:

Blend 1 ½ inch round of Bitter Melon (cored) with a 3 inch slice of Honeydew melon with water to cover. Drink immediately. This is also helpful for acne and to cool off in the summer.

The key to treatment is to regulate Liver functioning internally. Take lemon and orange or a supplement regularly to increase Vitamin C in the body. Topically, use Vitamin C three times a week.[14] A key herb for hyperpigmentation is Zhen Zhu (pearl powder). Take pearl powder daily as a treatment and preventive for freckles, liver spots, cholasma, and general hyperpigmentation. Pearl powder clears acne, eczema, and non-healing sores. In addition to beautifying the skin, pearl powder calms the Heart and Liver for palpitations, insomnia, visual disturbances, eye disorders, and tension.

Beautifying Flowers

Flower teas are beautiful, fragrant, and pleasant tasting, as well as effective for a variety of conditions.

Table 5.3. Beautifying Flowers

Flower	Properties
Gui Hua **Osmanthus**	Improves complexion Boosts the immune system Clears Wind Heat - alleviates sore throat
Ju Hua **Chrysanthemum**	Clears Heat from the Liver - benefits the eyes, relieves eye pain, and improves vision Sedates Liver Wind - alleviates headaches and migraines Clears Wind Heat - clears fever
Mo Li Hua **Jasmine**	Moves Qi - reduces stress, improves circulation Resolves Phlegm - lowers cholesterol, aids in weight loss, clears Wind Heat

14. According to Dr. Richard Huber, creator of 302 Skincare, using Vitamin C more often causes the receptors in the skin to become saturated and leads to inflammation and diminished efficacy.

Flower	Properties
Mei Gui Hua **Rose**	Moves Liver Qi - relieves menstrual pain and PMS, improves blood circulation Improves complexion Harmonizes Liver and Stomach - relieves stomachache and belching
Tao Hua **Peach Flower**	Promotes weight loss Lightens and brightens the skin - prevents and treats melasma, freckles, dark spots
Luo Shen Hua **Hibiscus Flower**	Resolves Phlegm and Food stagnation - aids digestion, promotes weight loss, reduces cholesterol Regulates the Liver - improves circulation, lowers blood pressure, protects the Liver
Jin Yin Hua **Japanese Honeysuckle**	Clears Heat and Toxins - detoxifies, clears inflammation Clears Wind Heat - reduces fever, alleviates sore throat Clears Damp-Heat - infection in urinary tract or bowels
Xun Yi Cao **Lavender**	Calms the Shen - calms the mind, promotes sleep Smoothes Liver Qi - relaxes muscles, alleviates migraines, resolves depression

Anti-Aging Dietary Plan

With all cases of deficiency, follow the basic dietary guidelines on page 70, adding specific foods and recipes. If you are menstruating, be sure to follow the Menstrual Renewal Program page 97. As a general rule, raw foods cleanse excess from the body and cooked foods tonify deficiencies. The proportion of cooked foods should be higher the greater the degree of deficiency.

To guard against aging we want to tonify deficiencies as soon as we start to feel their symptoms. Yang deficient conditions are a progression of Qi deficiency. Yang deficient conditions contain Qi deficiencies with cold symptoms and added weakness of function. Qi and Yang deficiency are often tonified together. Similarly Yin deficiency is a continuation of Blood deficiency. Yin deficient cases will have Blood deficiency signs with Heat symptoms and added fluid deficiency signs. Thus, Blood and Yin are often tonified together.

Qi Deficiency

Symptoms:
Fatigue. Foggy-headed. Abdominal bloating. Loose stools. Poor appetite. Loose skin. Poor immunity. Muscle weakness.

Diet Plan:
Meals should be simple and easy to digest. Eat cooked foods and a higher proportion of grains. Eat

congee first thing in the morning, such as the one for Spleen Qi deficiency (page 327), and recipes containing Spleen tonic herbs such as the Student's Soup (page 330), regularly.

Include:
White rice, sweet rice, oats, chicken, beef, lamb, sweet potato, yam, winter squash, walnut, pungent cooking spices and herbs (clove, cinnamon, oregano, thyme, ginger, etc.).

Limit:
Salads, raw fruit, seaweed, brown rice, dairy, nuts, and cold temperature foods.

Exacerbated by:
Qi deficiency is often caused by poor eating habits, stress, worry, excess studying, excessive physical work, too much heavy weight-lifting or cardio, or excessive sports or dance. It can also be constitutional (Jing-related).

Lifestyle:
Eat regular meals, get adequate sleep, and manage stress.

Yang Deficiency

Symptoms:
Qi deficient symptoms with addition of: inability to control bladder or bowels properly resulting in nocturia, urinary or fecal incontinence, leukorrhea, cock's crow diarrhea.[15] Infertility. Frigidity. Desire to sleep all the time. Cold. Low backache. Knee weakness. Poor memory.

Diet Plan:
Long cooking and roasting food. Grain-based diet with alcohol, spices, and warming foods added. Eat Forbidden Congee or Congee to Astringe the Kidneys (page 327) several times a week. Take a small cup of Du Zhong Wine every night (page 374).

Include:
Bone broth, yams, sweet potato, rice, oats, lamb, beef, chicken, salmon, kidney, walnut, chestnut, black beans, ginger, onions, garlic, Gou Qi Zi (go ji berries).

Limit:
Salads, dairy, and cold temperature foods.

Exacerbated by:
Kidney Yang deficiency is often caused by excessive physical work, too much heavy weight-lifting, or excessive sports or dance. Extreme physical environment and exposure to cold as in deep sea diving. Sexual activity before or during puberty damages the Kidney. It can also be constitutional (Jing-related).

15. This poetic term refers to chronic loose stools that wake you up first thing in the morning. In this case it is not related to heat or food poisoning.

Lifestyle:
Take saunas, hot stone massages. Avoid swimming in cold water.

Blood Deficiency

Symptoms:
Pallor of skin, tongue, and nails. Look like the "light is off." Fatigue. Dizziness. Dry stools or constipation. Emotional and physical sensitivity. Timidity and lack of confidence. Neediness. Insomnia, anxiety, and palpitations.

Diet Plan:
Eat a higher proportion of animal products (20-30%) and green vegetables (40- 50%). Eat at least half the diet cooked. Take Rejuvenation Recipes (page 368) several times a week.

Include:
Bone broth, beef, chicken, pork, liver, pork trotters, eggs, black beans, beets, carrots, leafy greens, rice, Long Yan Rou (longan berries), Gou Qi Zi (go ji berries), mulberries, black sesame seed, blackstrap molasses, wheatgrass, seaweed, spirulina. Be sure to follow the Stage 3 diet plan, particularly Dang Gui Chicken (page 353).

Avoid:
Excessive salt and sugar, raw foods, and pungent foods.

Exacerbated by:
Excessive care-taking. Lack of sleep. Overwork, especially staring at a computer screen. Deficient diet. Stress. Excess working out (especially during period).

Lifestyle:
Take special care during menses and post-menses when Blood is depleted.

Yin Deficiency

Symptoms:
Dryness. Heat in the head, palms and feet. Restless. Night sweats. Heat comes from within (steaming bones). Excessive sexual desire. Tinnitus. Constipation. Low backache. Knee weakness. Poor memory.

Diet Plan:
Include some raw foods to clear heat. Eat soups, plenty of vegetables, and drink water. High quality dairy to moisten dryness. Eat 50% vegetables to hydrate and animal products (20-30%). Take a Yin-nourishing Congee (page 327) and Rejuvenation Recipes (page 368) several times a week. Diet should both add moisture and astringe fluids.

Include:
Moistening: bone broth, seaweed, spirulina, Shan Yao (Chinese yam), millet, oats, wheat, good quality dairy, eggs, black beans, pork, pork kidney, duck, sardine, oyster, mushroom, seeds & nuts (sesame, chia, hemp, walnuts, almonds, chestnuts, etc.), Gou Qi Zi (go ji berries), mulberries, blueberries, blackberries, Bai Mu Er (white cloud fungus), Hei Mu Er (black wood ear fungus).

Astringing: yogurt, citrus, vinegar, tomato, Wu Wei Zi (schizandra).

Avoid:
Heating and drying foods like coffee, spices, alcohol, and garlic.

Exacerbated by:
Kidney Yin deficiency is typically caused by chronic emotional stress and mental overwork, drugs and medications, extreme emotional environment, severe febrile disease, or excessive cardio workouts (sweating). Sexual activity before or during puberty also damages the Kidneys. It may also be constitutional (Jing-related).

Lifestyle:
Avoid excessive exercise (fluid loss) particularly hot-room yoga, sauna, spin, and competitive sports. Include more rest. Avoid overwork. Take special care during menses and post-menses when Yin is depleted.

Chinese Herbal Formulas for Anti-Aging

The key to looking youthful and vibrant is a steady supply of Qi and Blood. When there is Blood deficiency, the skin lacks glow and we feel easily overwhelmed. Blood deficiency also makes us feel unattractive and undermines our confidence. Taking care of others consumes Blood as does monthly menses. Blood production starts with digestion, which is why proper diet and herbs to tonify Spleen Qi are so important.

To reverse deficiencies of Qi, Blood, Yin, or Yang, take herbal formulas for 3-6 months. You will gradually notice a return of vitality such as increased glow, moisture to skin, and feeling stronger. Some women, due to constitution or lifestyle, will need to take a rejuvenation tonic regularly all the time. Others can return to a normal healthy lifestyle. Formulas ideally are customized to the individual. There are few herbs that can be taken long term. Even these herbs should be stopped or alternated periodically (every 3 months or so).

The formulas presented here will boost Qi and nourish Blood as well as tonify the Kidneys.

Recipe 5.1. Vitality Formula

70% Ginseng (American, Chinese, or Korean or combination)

30% raw San Qi (notoginseng)
1 pinch Da Huang (rhubarb)

Powder the herbs individually. Combine the first 2 herbs in the following ratio: Ginseng 70% to raw San Qi 30%. Take 1 tsp. first thing each morning in hot water, adding a tiny bit of Da Huang.

Tonifies Qi (and Yin if using American Ginseng), moves the Blood, and gently detoxifies. This formula is used for Heart Disease and Stroke prevention. It is also an excellent long-term anti-aging formula and can be used to postpone menopause. Choose the appropriate ginseng based on your constitution (page 215). To strongly and safely tonify Qi, use American Ginseng with Chinese Ginseng.

Recipe 5.2. Sheng Mai San

1-2g Ginseng (American, Chinese, or Korean or combination)
2-4g Mai Men Dong (ophiopogon tuber)
1g Wu Wei Zi (schizandra)

Powder the herbs individually. They can be bottled at the above ration or individually. Take at the advised dosage: Daily dosage first thing in the morning in hot water.

Tonifies Qi and Yin. More appropriate for dry skin, wrinkles, menopausal symptoms. To strongly and safely tonify Qi, use American Ginseng with Chinese Ginseng.

Recipe 5.3. Hormone-Boosting Formula #1[16]

Dang Shen (codonopsis) 15g, Dang Gui (Chinese angelica) 9g, Bai Shao (white peony root) 12g, Bai Zhu (white atractylodes)12g, Dan Shen (salvia root) 15g, Tao Ren (peach kernel) 9g, Yin Yang Huo (epimedium)12g, Nu Zhen Zi (privet fruit) 15g, Han Lian Cao (eclipta) 12g, Sheng Di Huang (raw rehmania) 12g, Tu Si Zi (dodder seed) 15g, Fu Ling (poria) 15g, Chen Pi (tangerine peel) 9g, Gan Cao (licorice) 6g.

Decoct the herbs (page 330). This formula is very versatile, treating Qi, Blood, and Kidney deficiencies. At the same time, it is neither cloying nor drying, making it appropriate for patients who are too Damp to handle stronger tonics or too Yin Deficient to handle Huang Qi (astragalus).

Recipe 5.4. Hormone Boosting Formula #2[17]

Huang Qi (astragalus) 30g, Shan Yao (Chinese yam)18g, Bai Shao (white peony root)15g, Tu Si Zi (dodder seed) 15g, Yin Yang Huo (epimedium) 15g, Sheng Di Huang (cooked rehmannia) 15g, Fu Ling (poria) 9g, Huang Bai (phellodendron) 6g, Mu Dan Pi (tree peony root) 6g, Zhi Zi (cape

---

16. Modified from formula given to the author by Dr. Yueying Li. (Yo San University Clinic, Los Angeles, June 26, 2002).

17. Modified from formula from Jiang Zheng. "TCM Gynecology." (lecture, Pacific College of Oriental Medicine, San Diego, November 2, 2006).

jasmine fruit) 6g, Yin Chen Hao (artemesia) 6g, Mai Men Dong (ophiopogon tuber) 6g, Sha Ren (amomi) 3g, Chen Pi (tangerine peel) 3g.

Decoct the herbs (page 330). This is formula builds the hormones, strengthens Spleen Qi and Kidney Yin. For patients with Yin Deficiency/Yang Rising, omit or severely lower Huang Qi and use Dang Shen 30-60g.

Recipe 5.5. Jade Screen Formula

Huang Qi (atragalus)
Fang Feng (ledebouriella root)
Bai Zhu (white atractylodes)

Powder the herbs individually and combine in equal proportion. Take 1 tsp. first thing every morning. Tonifies the Wei Qi and expels Wind. This formula specifically strengthens immunity. It also tightens the pores.

Beautification Rituals

Techniques for Rejuvenating the Face[18]

Be sure there is some slick to the skin when performing the massage so as not to drag the skin. Use a cleanser or moisturizer to make the skin surface more slippery. These techniques can also be applied to the body.

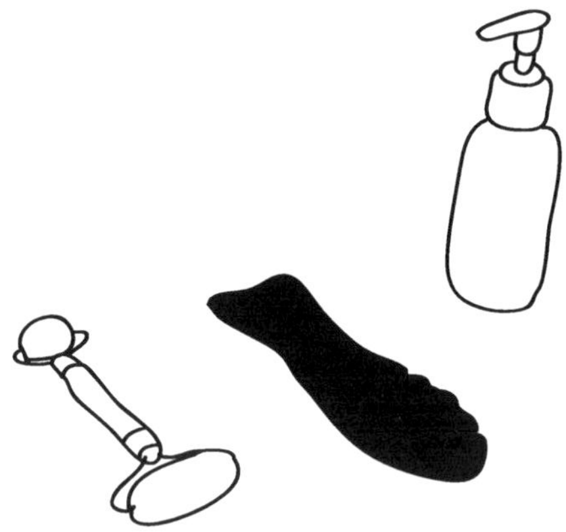

Figure 5.6. Beautification Tools: Jade Roller, Gua Sha, Oil

Pinching (Figure 5.7)
Starting at the neck, use your thumb and index finger to pinch along imaginary lines, working up the entire face and neck. Work firmly, grabbing the tissue. Always work up and out.

Slapping
Starting at the neck, slap the skin working up. Make sure to focus under the chin, cheeks, and jaw line.

Hot and Cold
Alternating temperatures strongly increases blood circulation and lymphatic flow. Hot and cold therapy on the face can consist of a warm wet towel followed by jade rollers kept on ice.

Jade Rollers (Figure 5.8)
Jade stone has the property of increasing Yin. They are naturally cool, but you can intensify this action by keeping them on ice. Roll the entire face for one min. after applying moisturizer at night. It increases Qi and Blood circulation to the surface of the skin and guards against wrinkles.

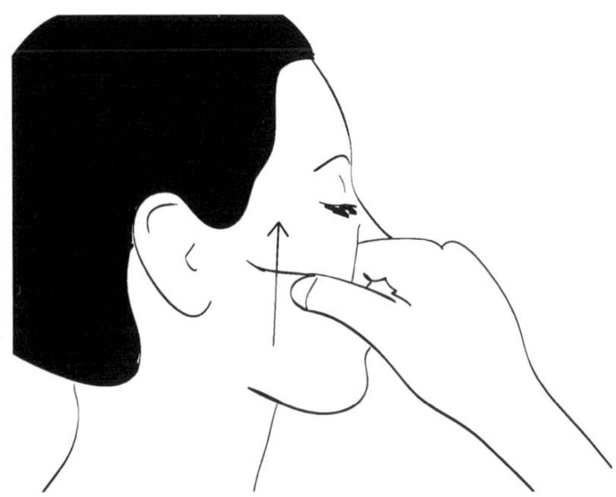

Figure 5.7. Pinching

Gua Sha (Figure 5.9)
Decongests the skin and increases circulation. This is a scraping technique that is best performed with a specially shaped horn. Apply a thick layer of moisturizer or wetted cleanser.[19] Work making little horizontal and vertical movements back and forth. Performed properly the skin will pink up. If there is a lot of congestion it will be uncomfortable the first few times.

18. Based on conversations with "Valesca" in 2011, who taught me the pinching, slapping, and honey exfoliation techniques.
19. Dr. Yueying Li recommended placing silk over the skin and performing Gua Sha over it.

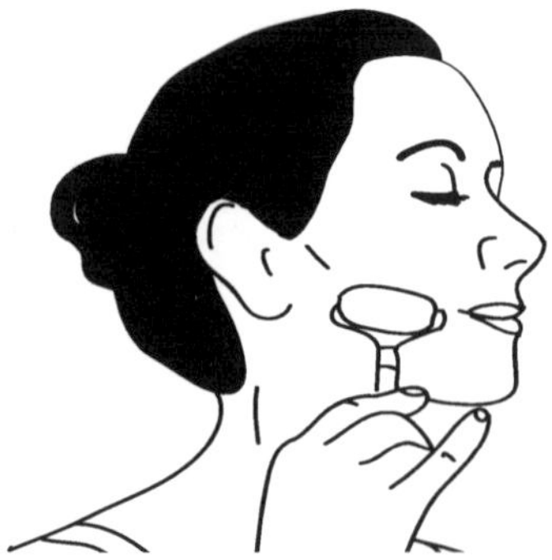

Figure 5.8. Jade Roller

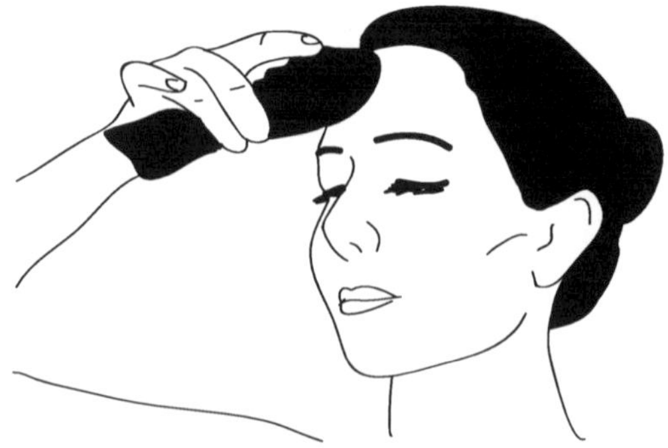

Figure 5.9. Gua Sha

Rejuvenating the Body

The techniques used on the face also can be used on the body: Pinching, Slapping, Gua Sha, Jade Rollers. Exfoliation and hot and cold stimulation are the same principle on the body as on the face, only more intense.[20] Korean culture has a wonderful body rejuvenation ritual. At least once a month, women go to special bathhouses where they do circuits of hot and cold therapy, soaking, along with an intense scrub.

Body Exfoliation Ritual

If you do not have access to a Korean bathhouse, you can reproduce this technique at home. Ideally once a week or at least once a month, do the following ritual to keep your skin (and internal organs) healthy:

1. Shower and thoroughly scrub yourself. You can use a loofah, sugar scrub, or exfoliation mitts.
2. Take a hot bath with herbs or essential oils.
3. Take a quick cold rinse in the shower.
4. Apply extra-moisturizing oil or lotion.

Body Lotion Bar

160g beeswax, 500g oil (jojoba, avocado, shea butter, etc), 40g of herbs (optional), 1 tsp essential oil (optional).

Heat ingredients except for essential oils over medium heat until liquefied and well mixed. Remove from heat and add essential oils. Strain and pour into molds to cool. Use on your hands and feet at night with gloves and socks.

20. Honey exfoliation is too mild for the body. Sugar Wax, made of caramelized sugar, honey, and lemon juice, is used for hair removal. It also has a similar effect on the skin of the body as honey exfoliation has on the face and is used with the same flicking motion as honey. It thoroughly removes dead skin, stimulates collagen and elastin, and leaves skin glowing.

Topical Skin Treatments

Topically, be sure to hydrate the skin nightly. Every night apply a thick layer of moisturizer to the face. Use pure, thick Vitamin E oil over eye cream at night. The drier the climate or the skin, the more important this is. In the case of acne conditions, test moisturizers to find one your skin tolerates.

The following are examples of homemade masks that can be used as skin treatments for conditions as indicated. These can be used with powdered Chinese herbs to make a thick paste.

Anti-Aging

Indications:
Wrinkles, Thinning Skin, Sagging, Dull Complexion

Treatment Principle:
Nourish Qi and Yin. Increase microcirculation.

Herbs:
Royal Jelly, Ren Shen (ginseng), Zhen Zhu (pearl powder), Huang Qi (astragalus)

Mask Base:

- Orange mask: 1 cup carrot or pumpkin, 2 egg yolks, juice from 1/2 lemon
- Yogurt mask: 1 tbsp yogurt, 1 tbsp honey, 1 tbsp powdered oats
- Honey mask: 1 tbsp honey, 1 egg yolk, 1 tbsp olive oil, 2 drops essential oil

Essential oils:
Carrot seed, Frankincense, Rose (cooling), Lavender, Rosehip, Patchouli, Geranium (ideal for menopausal women), Rosewood

Hyperpigmentation

Indications:
Dark Spots, Cholasma

Treatment Principle:
Balance Liver. Move Blood.

Herbs:
Zhen Zhu (pearl powder)

Mask Base:
- Yogurt & Lemon mask: 1 tbsp yogurt (or kefir), juice from 1/2 lemon, 1 tbsp honey, contents of 2 capsules of Vitamin E
- Milk mask: 1/2 cup cow's milk, 1/2 apple or mango, 1/4 cup oats
- Lemon and Yolk mask: juice of 1/2 lemon, 1 egg yolk, 1 tbsp honey, 1 tbsp olive oil

Essential Oils:
Helichrysum italicum, Mandarin, Lemon, Blue Tansy

Clearing Complexion

Indications:
Acne

Treatment Principle:
Clear Heat. Resolve Phlegm Obstruction. Move Blood.

Herbs:
Huang Lian (coptis), Da Huang (rhubarb), Liu Huang (sulfur)

Mask Base:
- Carrot and Egg mask: 1 carrot, 2 eggs
- Yogurt and Orange mask: 1 tbsp yogurt (or kefir), juice of 1/2 orange, 1 tbsp powdered oats
- Mung Bean mask: 1/4 cup milk, 1-2 tbsp mung bean power
- Algae and Clay mask: 1/2 cucumber, 1 tbsp soaked seaweed, 1/4 cup aloe gel

Honey Exfoliation Ritual

This treatment stimulates collagen and elastin, increases circulation, and exfoliates dead skin. Use once a week or as needed. It is contraindicated in rosacea or irritated skin.

1. Wash face and dry.
2. Warm less than a dime-size amount of honey between you fingers. Spread it on your face a little at the time.
3. Begin pressing and popping off, always moving upwards (Figure 5.10). The honey will turn white as it collects dead skin. Your skin will pink up.
4. Rinse with cold water and moisturize.

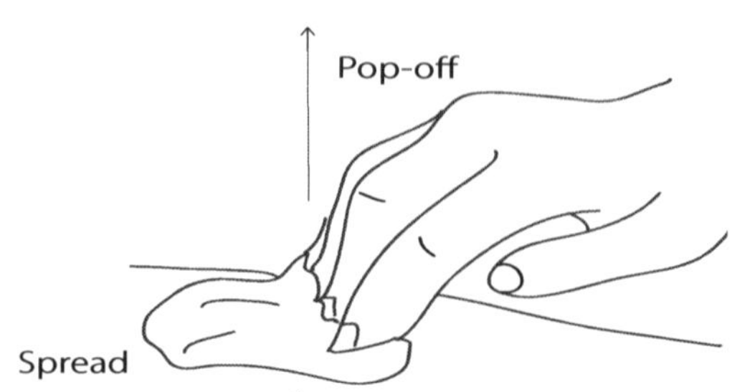

Figure 5.10. Honey Exfoliation

Essential Oils:
Neem, Tea Tree, Frankincense, Roman Chamomile, Rosewood

Calming

Indications:
Rosacea, Irritated Skin

Treatment Principle:
Clear Heat. Gently Hydrate.

Herbs:
Mu Dan Pi (tree peony root bark), Ju Hua (chrysanthemum)

Mask Base:

- Aloe and Cucumber mask: 1 tbsp aloe gel, 1/2 cucumber, 1 egg, 1 tbsp wheat flour, 1 tbsp honey
- Milk and Potato mask: 1/4 cup milk, 1 potato, 1 egg

Essential oils:
Avoid fragrances.

Specialty Treatments for Eyes

Soak cotton pads in one of the following recipes and use as a 10 minute compress on the eyes:

- Vinegar cucumber eye mask: 1 tsp white vinegar, 1/2 cucumber, 1 egg - lightens dark circles and eliminates puffiness
- Ju Hua (chrysanthemum) tea - calms redness, irritation and puffiness

Breast Rejuvenation

After I recovered from the initial shock of being flashed by a 60-year-old woman, I was struck by the fact that she had the most beautiful breasts I had ever seen. She was a Russian esthetician, "Valesca," working in our clinic. She had flawless porcelain skin and a warm, girlish charm. She was always trying to tell us "girls" how to take care of ourselves; to keep ourselves young. Apparently she did not think we were listening and needed some proof.

It was yet another example in my life that much of what we call aging is in fact a lack of wisdom on how to care for ourselves. I begged her several times to write a book, as she knows much more than she was able to share with me in the workplace. Earlier I listed her massage techniques for the face. Below I list her massage technique for the breasts.

Healthy ideals of beauty relate to an optimum internal balance. The firmness and fullness[21] of the breasts are an indicator of the strength of Spleen Qi and Blood and hormone levels. The fact that so many women lose firmness of their breasts after childbirth and breastfeeding is a testament to the fact that women are not recovering their health after having children.

Women can lose the fullness in their breasts due to stress, overwork, and even heartbreak and then attribute it to "aging." Aging is a catch-all category for all manner of commonly occurring pathology. A combination of diet, breast massage, and Chinese herbs can help regain the breasts in two months. Following these directives will lift and firm the breasts, though not necessarily increase cup size.

Breast Massage Protocol

Whereas the breast massage exercises in Chapter 3 are focused on Internal Alchemy, these are focused on rejuvenating the tissue. I recommend performing both sets of exercises daily. If performed correctly the skin will pink up. This indicates sufficient blood flow to the skin. Apply oil to the breasts when doing the following exercices:

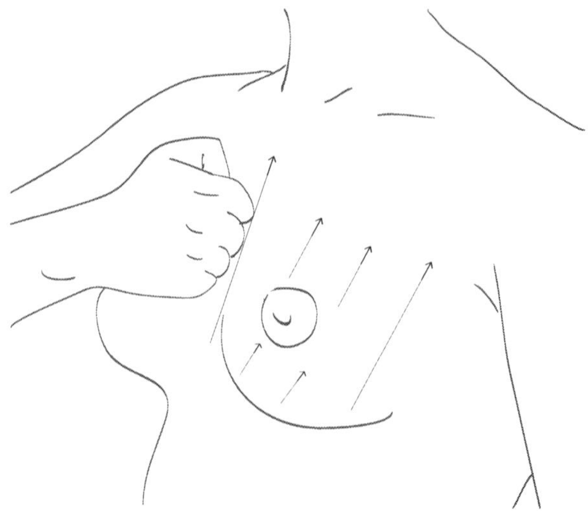

Figure 5.11. Knuckling

Knuckling[22]
Make loose fists. Use your knuckles to massage working up the lines shown in Figure 5.11. Work deeply until the skin pinks up. It will be borderline painful at first as there will be more stagnation (like deep tissue massage.) To affect the deeper tissues that you want to get to, you have to be a bit aggressive.

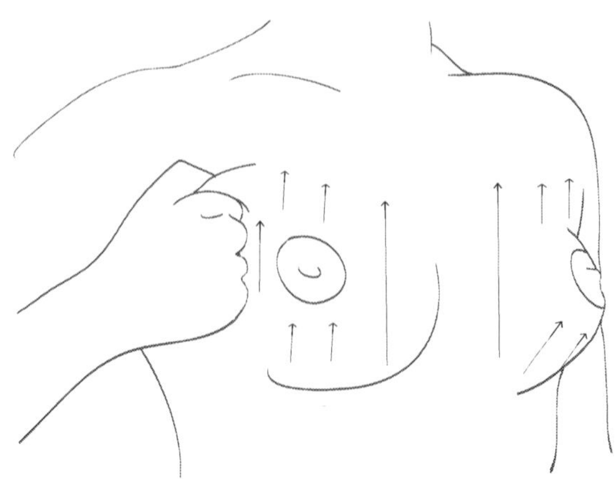

Figure 5.12. Pinching

Pinching
Next use your thumb and index finger to pinch up the lines shown in Figure 5.12. Again work deeply, really grabbing the tissue. Always work up.

Slapping
Slap the breast tissue working up. Valesca also advocated using a rolled up towel for this. She

21. Breast rejuvenation does not drastically affect cup size unless a woman is under-developed or lost mass due to childbirth or illness.

22. These techniques will prevent and treat fibrocystic breasts and other accumulations.

was amply endowed and perhaps it works better for women with larger breasts.

Breast Massage Oil

1/2 cup Jojoba oil

1 tsp Evening Primrose oil

1 tsp Rosehip oil

15 drops carrot seed oil

5 drops each: cypress, ylang ylang, geranium, lavender essential oils

Hot and Cold

Valesca recommended using ice on the breasts. Hot and cold therapy will greatly increase circulation and flush out waste material from the cells.

Attitude

I have noticed that women who radiate beauty, delight in and appreciate their own bodies. The breasts are made to nourish babies on a physical plane, and energetically are an extension of the heart. They deserve time and attention. Perform the breast massage daily and wear pretty bras. There is a bit of controversy over this, as some Inner Alchemy practitioners advocate no bra to strengthen the tissue and others recommend always having support. I personally advocate wearing pushup bras on a regular basis.

Because most of us rarely see other women naked, all we have as reference are the surgically augmented breasts we see portrayed in the media and entertainment industry. A beautiful, sexy person is a fully embodied person. The more we become comfortable moving energy through our bodies, the more confident and beautiful we become. This attitude change is a process, so be patient. Social control and consumerism are based on keeping us feeling inadequate. Everyone has their own lies to undo.

PRACTITIONER SECTION: BREAST REJUVENATION

In addition to diet and herbs, there are several techniques that help firm the breasts. However, in our litigious, prudish society you may not want to include breast rejuvenation in your practice.

Apply topical herbs. Combine Si Wu Tang with Huang Qi (astragalus), Wang Bu Liu Xing (vaccaria seeds), Jie Geng (platycodes). Add the ground raw herbs (not concentrate) to jojoba oil at 5% by weight. Bring to a boil then let sit for 1 month. Apply this to the breasts when performing breast massage or during treatment. Or simply make a strong decoction, soak some 4x4's and apply as a compress for 10 min.

Needle points to strengthen Qi and Blood and open the Chong: like St 36, Sp 6, 4 doors, Pc6/Sp4. ST 41 is particularly important to strengthen the ST channel. Needle local points: Ren 17, PC 1, St 18, St 15. Ren 17 is most important to bring Qi into the area. Be sure to activate the needle. Insert and needle up. Pull the needle out slightly and needle down. Pull the needle out slightly and needle right. Pull the needle out slightly and needle left. Moxa around the area. Electro-stimulation can be used on these points (this technique requires deep insertion). Ultrasound will firm the skin and drive the herbs in. Microcurrent can be used at the end using an upward motion.

Chinese Herbal Formulas to Restore and Maintain the Breasts

It is helpful to eat green papaya and collagen-rich foods (such as pig's trotters or collagen supplements) weekly in addition to taking herbs. Any Huang Qi (astragalus)-based Spleen tonifying formula will work, like Bu Zhong Yi Qi Tang or Gui Pi Tang. These can be taken in pill or tincture form. A caution: there are many Yin Deficient women who cannot handle Huang Qi (astragalus) or only when well-balanced in a formula. Without sufficient Yin to anchor them, the herb scatters their energy and they will experience symptoms such as headaches and agitation.

Recipe 5.6. Tong Ru Dan

Ingredients:
Ren Shen (ginseng) 30g, Huang Qi (astragalus) 30g, Dang Gui (Chinese angelica) 60g, Mai Men Dong (ophiopogon tuber) 15g, Mu Tong (aristolochia) 0.9g, Jie Geng (platycodi) 0.9g.

Decoct the herbs (page 330). The effects of this formula vary on the timing. After childbirth this formula promotes milk production. Taken other times it helps fill out sagging breasts due to low hormone. Traditionally these herbs are cooked with two pig's trotters (pig's feet) or ox tail, with peanuts. I personally do not appreciate this combination and prefer to decoct the herbs separately and make a pig's trotter soup (page 355) eaten on the same day.

Beautifying the Hair

The shine and luster of the head hair is traditionally related to the condition of the Kidneys. However, other factors such as poor nutrition, Blood deficiency, excess Heat, and particularly stress, have a big impact on the health of the hair. The health of the Liver has much to do with the "life" and vibrancy of the hair. This is why women with hormonal imbalances suffer from bad hair days around their menstruation or particularly stressful times. The general rule for hair health is the same as for all rejuvenation: stimulate circulation and nourish simultaneously.

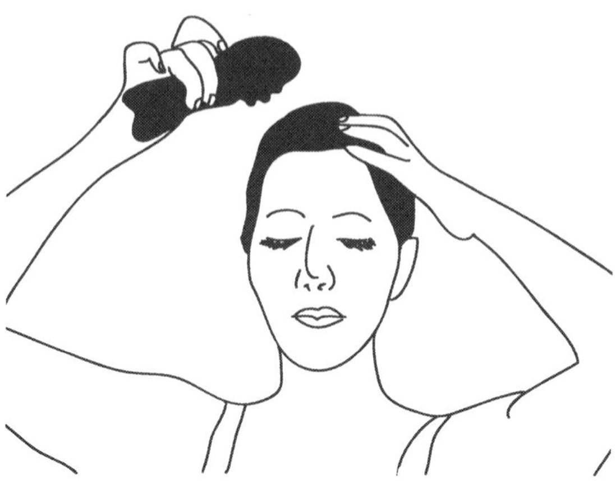

Figure 5.13. Gua Sha

Increasing Circulation

If the hair is in good condition, it is enough to brush the hair in every direction for 20-50 repetitions as part of the evening ritual. This will maintain the health of the hair, foster good mental functioning, and calm the mind. For those with textured hair who do not want to break the curls, use a large Gua Sha tool with teeth (Figure 5.13). Firmly "comb" your hair with it until the scalp tingles.

In cases of hair loss or to stimulate new growth, use a seven-star needle (plum blossom needle) or dermaroller .5-1.5 mm once a week with a topical growth stimulator. (Figure 5.14) Use the seven-star needle or dermaroller along the Du channel of the neck and upper back as well. Finish with a massage of the scalp, neck, and shoulders.

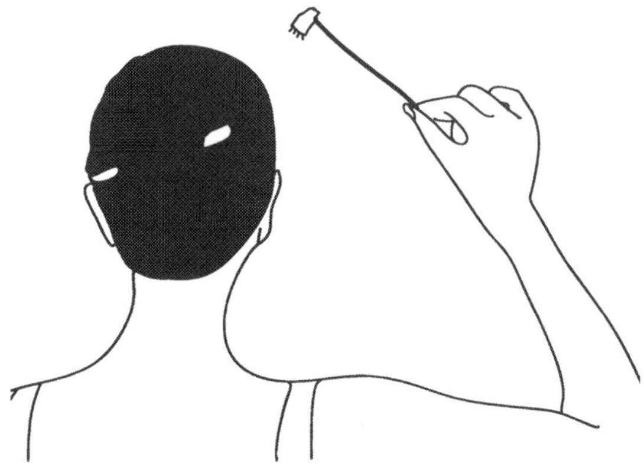

Figure 5.14. Seven-Star Needle

To increase hair length, the ends must be protected. Use a weekly mask made of coconut or olive oil, 1 egg yolk, and rosemary essential oil. Leave on for 30 min.

Nourishing Internally

Following the recommendations for anti-aging listed earlier in this chapter will also nourish the hair. Excess sugar and poor quality salts in the diets cause hair loss. Stress and over thinking will cause hair thinning. Additionally, Wind or Heat toxins in the body can cause rapid hair loss. In case of hair loss use He Shou Wu (polygonum), walnuts, and black sesame seeds daily in the diet and in herbal formulas. For deficiency cases of hair loss, use Qi Bao Mei Ran Wan, a classic formula for hairgrowth. For Liver excess cases, use Long Dan Xie Gan Tang.

Topical Hair Growth Tincture:

Ingredients:
Sheng Jiang (fresh ginger, finely chopped) 40g, Ce Bai Ye (platycladus leaves) 20g, Han Lian Zi (eclipta seeds, crushed) 20g, Huo Ma Ren (hemp seeds, crushed) 20g

Soak ingredients in 100 mL 75% isopropyl rubbing alcohol or hard liquor for 1 week . Apply the tincture to the entire scalp. Use a seven-star/plum blossom needle or 0.5-1 mm dermaroller to stimulate the scalp. Finish by massaging the scalp and neck.

Hair Growth Oil:

8 ounces Emu oil

15 drops each: basil, lavender, thyme, rosemary, ylang ylang, lemon essentials oils.

Mix and apply daily. Follow with scalp massage.

Recipe 5.7. Hair Growth Formula[23]

Ingredients:
Huang Lian (coptis) 6g, Huang Qin (scutellaria) 9g, Mai Men Dong (ophiopogon tuber) 6g, Dang Gui (Chinese angelica) 12g, Sheng Di Huang (raw rehmania) 12g, Sha Ren (amomi) 3g, Bai Shao (white peony root) 9g, Chuan Xiong (ligusticum) 6g, He Shou Wu (polygonum) 15g, Gou Qi Zi (go ji berries) 15g, Gou Teng (uncaria) 8g, Ju Hua (chrysanthemum) 8g.

It addresses the major causes of hair loss: Blood deficiency, Heat in the Blood, Liver Wind, and Kidney deficiency. It addresses mixed patterns, which are the most common. It is especially helpful in younger people with stress and overwork.

Recipe 5.8. Hair Darkening Formula - Qi Bao Mei Ran Wan

Ingredients:
He Shou Wu (polygonum) 15g, Fu Ling (poria) 10g, Niu Xi (achyranthes) 8g, Dang Gui (Chinese angelica) 12g, Gou Qi Zi (go ji berries) 12g, Tu Si Zi (dodder seed) 15g, Hei Zhi Ma (black sesame seed) 8g, Bu Gu Zi (psorelea) 8g.

Grind into a powder. Mix 9g of powder with honey to form pills. Take 1 pill 2 times a day with hot water.

This is a classic hair darkening formula for Liver Blood and Kidney Yin deficiency cases. It can also be decocted.

Recipe 5.9. Er Zhi Wan

Ingredients:
Han Lian Cao (eclipta leaves) 15g, Nu Zhen Zi (privet fruit) 15g

Decoct the herbs. Tonifies Liver and Kidney Yin for premature gray hair, dizziness, low back weakness, and tinnitus. It is gentle and safe.

23. Adapted from a formula by Dr. Huabing Wen, conversation, May 2002.

Cosmetic Surgery Recovery

If you elect to have cosmetic surgery to reverse the signs of aging, preparing your body prior and nurturing yourself after surgery speeds recovery time and enhances the results of cosmetic procedures. This protocol is indicated for surgical procedures, laser, or intense peels.

One week prior to the procedure, take Red Date Tea (page 349) or Date & Wood Ear Tea (page 372) twice a day. This protects the Liver from anesthesia (and Toxins) and helps recover Qi and Blood afterward. Take Qi and Blood tonics such as Gui Pi Tang or Ba Zhen Tang to strengthen your body. Take this with Yunnan Paiyao, 2-3 capsules, two times a day to optimize Blood circulation.

After the procedure, take the small red Yunnan Paiyao pill. Until you are healed, take 2-3 Yunnan Paiyao capsules, two times a day to speed wound recovery and prevent infection. Continue taking Qi and Blood tonics to boost the health of the skin.

Topically, Yunnan Paiyao powder can also be applied to wounds to speed wound healing and minimize scarring. In cases of deep lasers or peels on large areas use a compress made of diluted colloidal silver soaked in gauze and apply twice daily for 10 minutes at a time.

Get at least 10 hours of uninterrupted sleep a night while you are recovering. Eat cooked, easy to digest, nourishing foods. Take Qi-building Congees in the morning (page 327). Recipes from all Stages of the Menstrual or Postpartum Recovery Programs are appropriate such as Pork Trotter Soup (page 355). Take a collagen supplement daily to promote healthy connective tissue and skin formation. If appropriate, get acupuncture and massage to promote healthy circulation.

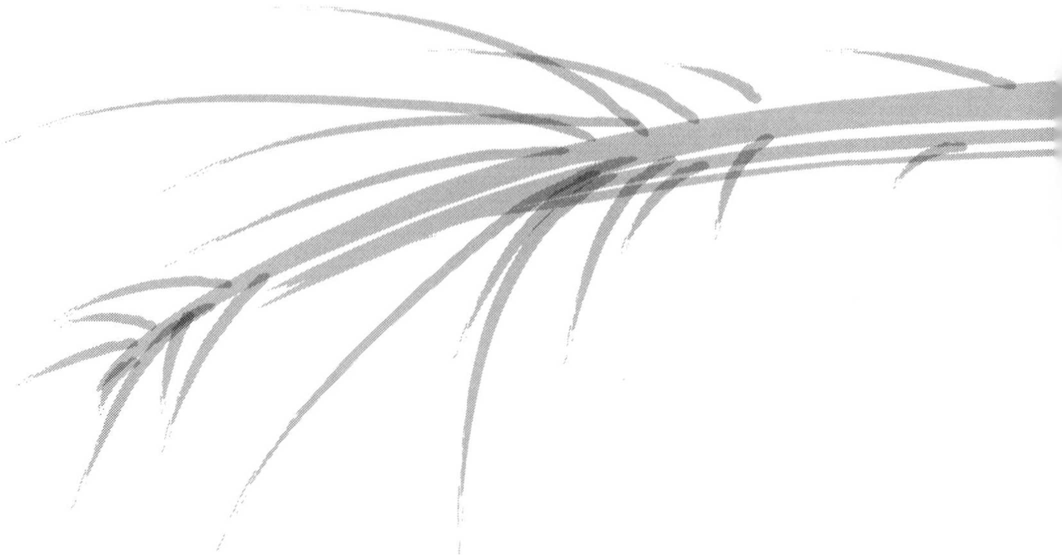

Chapter 6

Age 42

6 x 7, The three Yang channels are weak, the face darkens and the hair begins to turn grey.

六七，三阳脉衰于上，面皆焦，发始白；（42岁）

The 6th Cycle

Six x 7 years begins the 6th Cycle in a woman's life. Between the ages of 42 and 48 the Metal stage continues. A woman's true nature surfaces and this is the phase when her life choices begin to show. There is a saying in Chinese Face Reading "until 40 your face is what you inherited from your parents. After 40 it is your own."[1] After age 40, our faces begin to tell the tale of the predominant expressions we held, our battle wounds, and our internal strengths and deficiencies.

The passage at the top of this page from the Yellow Emperor concerning the 6th Cycle sounds bleak, but Chapter 1 of the ancient text explains that this is our destiny only if we choose to abuse ourselves and live outside of the Dao; the natural rhythms of the universe. We are constantly given opportunities to change the course of our lives.

Traditional Chinese Medicine advises no more strenuous exercise from this stage on. What this means in practical terms varies according to the individual. The body now has fewer reserves and there is no longer a buffer of protection from overexertion. Our bodies also need extra energy to repair. Workouts should be done with either less intensity or shorter periods with more recovery time between them. End workouts feeling exhilarated rather than wiped out. At the same time, it is necessary to exercise regularly to maintain strength, mobility, flexibility, and coordination. The tendency to lose these abilities with age is a consequence of disuse. This is a time to begin acting wisely and efficiently.

1. Patrician McCarthy. "Chinese Face Reading." (lecture, Yo San University, Los Angeles, February 3, 2003).

Perimenopause Preparations

Premature menopause is a popular term these days whereby women's hormonal levels begin to drop prematurely, sometimes as early as the early 30s. Though some women rejoice, thinking it just means an early end to their periods, this correlates to Jing deficiency and premature aging. It should be treated immediately.

Although the drop in hormones that precedes menopause can begin between 35-48 years old, the "normal" age is at 41 or 42.(2) This means that in Cycle 6, premenopausal symptoms might begin to surface. There are cases, such as my grandmother, who did not experience symptoms until her 50s and stopped bleeding at nearly 60 years old. Menopause in a healthy woman is a smooth process with some episodes of hot flashes and dryness symptoms. The transition, however, also triggers latent imbalances. This is why so many women develop a litany of symptoms; it is the karma of our life choices.

The three organs that govern a woman's hormonal functioning are the Kidney, Spleen, and Liver. The Kidney and Spleen both tend to decline at this stage, but the Liver remains the focal organ until menstruation has ceased. Though a decline in Kidney Jing is the root of menopause, the Liver is implicated in much of the drama of menopause such as hot flashes, night sweats, irritability, homicidal tendencies, etc.(3) Stress, a disorder of the Liver, greatly accelerates aging and menopause.

In the 6th Cycle, continue the rejuvenation regiments from Chapter 5. In addition, this is an excellent time to rid your body of excesses, though these detox methods can be used at any age. Clearing these excesses is key to a smooth menopause and later years.

PRACTITIONER: POSTPONING MENOPAUSE

Use mainly acupuncture points below the knee as soon as perimenopausal symptoms begin, or preventively beginning in the early 40s. Include Pc 6 and Sp 4 contralaterally as well. Hot stone massage is also very helpful as it tonifies the Kidneys and moves Blood. Use formulas, particularly with ginseng, and diet therapy to tonify KD Jing and Yin, and clear Heat. This can delay menopause for years.

2. Shaoting Jing, "TCM Gynecology" (lecture, Yo San University, Los AngelesMay 1, 2003).
3. Hua-bing Wen, "Case Studies" (lecture, Yo San University, Los Angeles, May 27, 2004).

Detoxification

In modern Western culture detoxification has become an obsession akin to religious zealotry, complete with self-inflicted suffering, fabricated sins and constant guilt. This is used to balance the opposite extreme of gluttony and unconscious eating that is rampant in our society. Extreme dietary restriction and overeating actually foster each other. When our regular eating is balanced, detoxification takes on a much gentler nature. TCM's approach to detoxifying the body is one of creating balance.

Detoxification refers to clearing, discharging, and moving techniques used to rid the body of excess patterns. The degree of excess in the individual in relation to the degree of deficiency is what determines the strength of treatment. When applied to cases of excess, and to those strong enough to handle the treatment, fasting, colonics, and raw food diets will greatly improve one's health. These same detox techniques, applied to a deficient individual, will devastate Spleen Qi, and can also weaken Blood, Yin, and Yang. Many people injure their digestion, immunity, and vitality with excessive or inappropriate detoxing. The majority of people do best with a harmonizing approach. A stronger detox method (juice fasts, colonics, raw foods) for a few days may be necessary for excess cases with stronger constitutions after which a more gentle approach or nourishing regimen can follow. Most people do best on a longer, gentle detox that supports their Spleen Qi.

Strong Detoxification

Appropriate for:
History of drug and alcohol abuse. Hot natured, excess energy, red inflammatory conditions. No signs of weakness or deficiency.

Foods:
Raw food only, algae supplements, vegetable juice or water fasts.

Extra Treatments:
Colonics or enemas. Extreme hot and cold therapy: intense, extended sweating with ice baths.

Harmonizing Detoxification:

Appropriate for:
Digestive weakness: bloating, loose stools, tired after eating.

Chronic colds or infections.

Foods:
Eat 50-60% vegetables, mostly cooked. Include detoxifying foods: Yi Yi Ren (Job's tears), mung beans, red adzuki beans, dandelion greens, purslane.

Extra Treatments:
Massage. Mild sauna, steam room, milder hot and cold therapy. Include Spleen tonics and digestive herbs.

When designing a detox program, the first step is to clarify your goals. In my experience "detox" is most often code for five things: "I'm constipated," "I want to lose weight," "I feel horrible and want to change," "I feel sluggish and want more energy," and "I want spiritual purification." Then there are those who want to cleanse an organ system due to a specific ailment. This chapter focuses on harmonizing methods of detoxification to address these concerns, including: correcting digestive imbalances, clearing specific excesses, and a sample detox plan.

Top 10 Detoxifying Foods

Fasting is not the only way to clear toxins. Certain foods, eaten on a regular basis, will gently clear toxins from the body without injuring the Spleen (digestion). These foods tend to be clearing, cooling, and drying. They should be eaten sparingly in those who are underweight, have deficient or dry conditions, or in children. Also, vegetables as a group, and to a lesser extent fruits, are detoxifying.

1. **Lu Dou** (mung beans) – Clears Heat, Summer-Heat, and Heat Toxins from the body.They treat pesticide and heavy metal poisoning, as well as herb or drug overdose.Therapeutic dosage is 15-30g per day. Balance with warming spices in Cold conditions.
2. **Chi Xiao Dou** (red adzuki beans) – Clears edema (water retention) from the body, promote urination, tonifies the Spleen, detoxifies, and moves the Blood. They also strengthen the Heart. Red adzuki beans are ideal for excess weight, during postpartum, during menses, and to clear skin conditions. Therapeutic dosage is 10-30g per day. Avoid in Dry or underweight conditions.
3. **Bai Bian Dou** (hyacinth beans) – Is a very safe herb to tonify Spleen Qi, clear Damp, clear Summer-Heat, and detoxify. Bai Bian Dou is used for fatigue, nausea, vomiting, diarrhea, vaginal discharge, and lack of appetite. It treats excess alcohol intake, food poisoning, and ingestion of toxins. It is also effective against morning sickness. Therapeutic dosage is 10-30g per day.
4. **Seaweeds** – Are cooling and moistening, regulate water metabolism, detoxify the lymphatic system, dissolve Phlegm, and soften hardness. Seaweed treats every type of swelling: inflammation, nodules, tumors, edema, excess weight, and cystic acne. Seaweed is used to treat constipation, hyper- and hypo-thyroidism (dosage dependent),[(4)] and water retention. **Kun Bu** (kombu or kelp) is the seaweed strongest in these properties and is most often used in medicine, but any seaweed will do. Different seaweeds have different mineral

---

4. See discussion in John Chen. *Chinese Medical Herbology & Pharmacology*. (City of Industry: Art of Medicine Press, 2004), 715-716.

profiles making them ideally suited for different conditions. Therapeutic dosage is 5-15g per day. Algae as a group are more cooling and clearing than seaweed.

5. **Green Tea** – Is the unoxidized leaf from the *Camelia chinensis* plant. It is cooling, clears Dampness (particularly from the intestines), and harmonizes digestion. Like all forms of tea, it removes fats from foods and should not be taken with fat soluble supplements. Always drink tea with meals; on an empty stomach it can weaken Spleen Qi.
6. **Ku Ding Cha** (bitter nail tea) – Clears Wind Heat, clears Heat Toxins, harmonizes digestion, and transforms Phlegm. Ku ding cha is not of the tea family, but like oolong and puerrh tea, it removes fats from foods, lowers cholesterol, and helps reduce high blood pressure. Ku ding cha, however, is more effective for weight loss and has a stronger detoxifying effect. Use 1-2 "nails" in a cup. It can be re-steeped several times, 1-2 min each time. Ku ding cha is extremely bitter. Always drink with meals; on an empty stomach it can weaken Spleen Qi. Do not add stevia or any other kind of sweetener. The bitter taste is necessary for detoxification.
7. **Yi Yi Ren** (Job's tears) – When used raw, dries Dampness, clears Heat from the body, and reduces edema and swelling. Add ginger and tangerine peel to increase these effects. When dry-fried prior to cooking, it tonifies the Spleen. Most often recipes use half raw and half dry-fried Yi Yi Ren. It is used as diet therapy in many modern diseases such as cancer, rheumatoid arthritis, and candida, as well as during menses and postpartum. Add daily to soups and congees.
8. **Daikon Radish** – Improves digestion, clears Phlegm and Heat, and is diuretic. Daikon is mild tasting and excellent for stagnation of food, Phlegm-Damp, and Heat. Eat ½ inch slice of raw daikon three times a day after meals to aid digestion and reduce bloating. Daikon can also be pickled (which produces a strong smell), juiced, or cooked in soups. Lai Fu Zi (daikon radish seed) is an excellent digestive herb.
9. **Bitter Melon** – Clears Heat and Summer-Heat. True to its name, bitter melon is extremely bitter. Removing the seeds and white core and soaking in water prior to cooking removes some of its bitterness. It is generally anti-viral and anti-bacterial. Bitter melon balances the excessive sweetness of the modern American diet.
10. **Mushrooms and Fungi – Shitake Mushroom** (like all mushrooms to varying degrees) decreases cholesterol in the blood, boosts immunity, and clears excess mucus and Heat. **Hei Mu Er (black wood ear fungus)** moistens the Yin and Body Fluids. It is used for Blood Stagnation and Phlegm. It helps dissolve fibroids and tumors.[5] Strengthens the heart and decreases cholesterol in the blood.

5. Paul Pitchford. *Healing with Whole Foods: Asian Traditions and Modern Nutrition.* (Berkeley: North Atlantic Books, 2003), 354.

Optimizing Digestion

Yin Fire

Li Dongyuan,[6] in his Pi Wei Lun (Treatise on the Spleen an Stomach), was the first to explain the complexity of disease patterns present in chronic digestive (and most chronic disease) patterns under the umbrella term "Yin Fire." Yin Fire is a disease process that begins with Liver Qi stagnation and Spleen Qi deficiency (or Liver overacting on Spleen). This creates many potential disease patterns that, over time, combine and reinforce each other. Dampness is easily created by a weakened Spleen over time leading to Damp-Heat. If stagnation is more salient, this leads to Excess Heat, which may also in time combine with Dampness. Other imbalances complicate the pattern: Blood and/or Yin deficiency, Phlegm accumulation, Blood stagnation, and Heart and Kidney Disharmony. Yin Fire is a critical concept because it explains the complicated nature of treating chronic digestive and health issues

Typical lifestyle profile for Yin Fire:[7]

1. poor or irregular diet
2. emotional stress
3. excess use of medications
4. sedentary lifestyle

Next we will address how to optimize digestion (synonymous with strengthening the Spleen and soothing the Liver) to build the proper foundation for the Cycles that follow. During the transition of menopause, the Liver transfers its position as the primary actor to the Spleen. After menopause the Spleen becomes the number one source of health or disease, depending on its state of balance. Balancing digestion now creates eases the transition through menopause and post-menopause. These principles are of course helpful at every age.

Later we will address the different forms of stagnation and how to treat them. All disease patterns must be addressed concurrently. Remember that no matter the stagnation patterns, the foundation is always a healthy Spleen and smooth flowing Liver Qi. Treatment is always to optimize digestion and strengthen the Spleen in addition to clearing excesses.

6. Li Dongyuan (1180-1252 A.D.), creator of the "Earth school" which focused on strenthening and balancing the Spleen and Stomach as the basis of treating disease.

7. MacLean refers to Yin Fire as Primary Pathological Triad (PPT) and gives an excellent explanation in his book. Will MacLean, *Clinical Handbook of Internal Medicine: The Treatment of Disease with Traditional Chinese Medicine: Vol 2: Spleen and Stomach.* (Sydney: University of Western Sydney, 2002), 912.

Exercise 6.1. Abdominal Exercises

Pick one of the following abdominal exercises and perform daily on an empty stomach:

Abdominal Massage (Figure 6.1)

Begin either standing or lying down. Abdominal massage can be performed with oil on bare skin or over clothes. Make a loose fist with one hand and cup your other hand over it. Firmly press into your abdomen. Begin to circle around the belly button covering the whole abdomen. Continue 100 times, moving clockwise if you were looking down at your stomach. Perform in the morning and/or evening. If you have loose stools, use an open palm to circle gently and slowly in a counterclockwise direction.

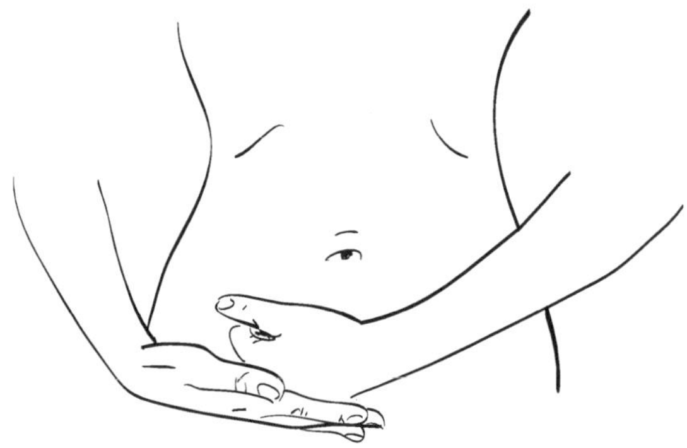

Figure 6.1. Abdominal Massage

Moving the Belly in 3 Directions (Figure 6.2)

This is a part of Earth tonification in 5 Element Qigong.[8] Practice visibly rolling your belly.

1. Try to ripple your belly vertically down, from your ribs down to your pubic bones. Only use your abdominal muscles. Do not move your spine.
2. Repeat going the opposite direction, moving up from your pubic bone to your ribs.
3. Repeat moving horizontally, from one side of your waist to the other. Then back the other way.

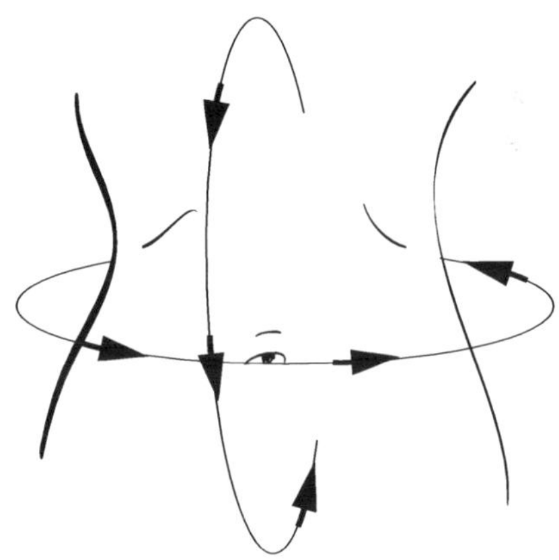

Figure 6.2. Moving in 3 Directions

This belly dancer's trick will help get you started. Lie down on your back and prop yourself up on your elbows. Make sure your abdomen is relaxed. Place a coin on your upper abdomen and use whatever abdominal movements necessary to flip the coin down the abdomen.

8. Daoshing Ni. "5 Element Qigong". (qigong class, Yo San University, Los Angeles, September 9, 2002).

Abdominal Vacuum (Uddiyana Bhanda) (Figure 6.3)

This is a tricky exercise at first, but worth the effort. It greatly strengthens the organs, disperses stagnation, and regulates all types of digestive disorders.

1. Stand with feet slightly apart. There are 2 options on posture. Begin with the first:
   a. Bend the knees. Round the torso forward. Rest hands just above the knees. Rest all the upper body weight on the hands so that the abdomen is completely relaxed. Beginners can press firmly with the palms against the very tops of the thighs to naturally hollow out the abdomen.
   b. Once the abdominal vacuum has been mastered with a rounded torso, practice the move standing upright with the hands on the hips.
3. Inhale deeply through the nose. Exhale forcibly and quickly through the nose. Con- tract the abdominal muscles to expel all air out of the lungs. Relax the abdomen.
4. Expand the ribcage without inhaling. This automatically pulls the abdominal muscles and organs up into the thorax, hollowing the abdomen. Alternately, slowly pull the navel up and in towards the spine.
5. Hold for a few seconds. Then slowly release. Breath normally for a few breaths. Repeat a few times.
6. To progress, add a abdominal circles from the previous exercise during the abdominal vacuum.

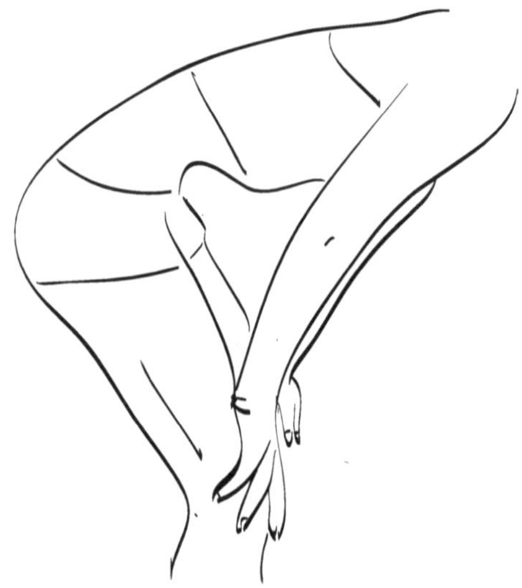

Figure 6.3. Abdominal Vacuum

Regulating Bowel Movements

The condition of the bowels is a key indicator to the health of the digestive tract, making them a good starting point for diagnosis.

Defining Normal Bowel Movements

Normal means one to two bowel movements a day. They should feel complete (no feeling like there is more left), formed (neither hard nor soft), no straining, almost odorless, and no excessive wiping.

Stool Diagnosis

Spleen Deficiency with Dampness

Symptoms:
Initial discharge of hard stool followed by loose stool or loose stools, abdominal distention (bloating), borborygmus (gurgling sound in the intestines), flatulence (gas), poor appetite.

Diet:
Follow Phlegm-Damp resolving diet page 260.

Lifestyle:
Eat regular meals. Get 8 hours of sleep each night.

Formulas:
Xiang Sha Liu Jun Zi Tang or Xiang Sha Yang Wei Tang, + Mu Xiang Shun Qi Pian

Damp Phlegm in Intestines

Symptoms:
Mucous, Loose stools, abdominal fullness, nausea.

Diet:
Follow Phlegm-Damp resolving diet page 260.

Lifestyle:
Eat regular meals. Get 8 hours of sleep each night.

Formula:
Huo Xiang Zheng Qi Tang

Liver Qi Stagnation

Symptoms:
Hard pellets, upper abdominal distention, flatulence, irritability, moodiness, constipation.

Diet:
Follow Qi Stagnation resolving diet page 258.

Lifestyle:
Practice relaxation daily such as meditation, tai chi, and soothing styles of qigong or yoga. Exercise is helpful, but avoid competition and extremism.

Formulas:
Shu Gan Wan + Mu Xiang Shun Qi Pian

Liver Overacting on Spleen

Symptoms:
Symptoms affected by varying moods, Alternating dry and loose stool in irregular pattern, borborygmus (gurgling sound in the intestines), upper and lower abdominal distention (bloating), flatulence (gas), irritability, fatigue, poor appetite.

Diet:
Follow Qi Stagnation resolving diet page 258.

Lifestyle:
Practice relaxation daily such as meditation, tai chi, and soothing styles of qigong or yoga. Exercise is helpful, but avoid competition and extremism. Eat regular meals.

Formulas:
Jia Wei Xiao Yao San + Mu Xiang Shun Qi Pian

Food Stagnation (improper eating)

Symptoms:
Partially digested food in stools with rotten odor, excessive gas, belching, abdominal distention (bloating).

Diet:
Follow Food Stagnation resolving diet page 260.

Lifestyle:
Eat small, simple meals.

Formulas:
Bao He Wan or Mu Xiang Shun Qi Pian

Food Stagnation with Spleen Qi deficiency

Symptoms:
Sour stools in children.

Diet:
Follow the Children's Diet page 52.

Lifestyle:
Give children regular, easy to digest meals.

Formulas:
Bao He Wan + Si Jun Zi Tang

Cold in Spleen and Stomach

Symptoms:
Loose, shapeless stools, cold in abdomen. May be a fishy odor.

Diet:
Follow Phlegm-Damp resolving diet page 260.

Lifestyle:
Eat regular hot, cooked meals. Avoid exposure to Cold. Get 8 hours of sleep each night.

Formula:
Li Zhong Tang

Spleen and Kidney Yang Deficiency

Symptoms:
Completely undigested food in stools, backache, cold limbs, fatigue, abundant pale urination, urgent bowel movement in early morning (cock's crow diarrhea).

Diet:
Follow Yang tonifying diet page 224.

Lifestyle:
Eat regular hot, cooked meals. Avoid exposure to Cold. Get 8 hours of sleep each night.

Formulas:
Si Shen Wan

Blood or Fluid Deficiency

Symptoms:
Very dry, hard stools, constipation.
Diet:
Include seaweed, nuts, seeds (hemp, flax, sesame, and chia). Follow a Yin tonifying diet page 225.
Lifestyle:
Eat soups and congees and drink plenty of water.

Formulas:
Yi Xue Run Chang or Ma Zi Ren Wan

Excess Heat

Symptoms:
Foul odor or dry stools, constipation.

Diet:
Follow a Heat clearing diet page 263.

Lifestyle:
Eat high raw vegetable diet.

Formula:
Huang Lian Su Pian

Damp-Heat in Large Intestine

Symptoms:
Mucus, tenesmus (rectal heaviness), borborygmus (gurgling sound in the intestines), thirst with no desire to drink, may be diarrhea or constipation or alternating.

Diet:
Follow Damp-Heat clearing diet page 265.

Lifestyle:
Practice relaxation daily such as meditation, tai chi, and soothing styles of qigong or yoga. Exercise is helpful, but avoid competition and extremism. Eat regular meals.

Formula:
Huang Lian Su Pian

Dysentery

Symptoms:
Pus and bloody stools

Diet:
Eat simple, bland foods including congee.

Lifestyle:
Seek medical attention.

Formulas:
Xiang Lian Wan or Ge Gen Huang Qin Huang Lian Tang

Constipation

Constipation is defined as less than one complete bowel movement per day. Ideally, an equivalent volume exits the body as goes in each day, and the belly is flat. This is not the case with constipation. It can be caused by a variety of factors including stress, poor diet, and medication. **Note:** colonics are a purging treatment appropriate only for excess cases. Use them with caution and moderation. Colonics can injure the Spleen in patients with mixed or deficient patterns.

Preventive Remedies:

1. Take a cup of warm water upon rising in the morning.
2. Go for a walk or do yoga first thing in the morning.
3. Perform abdominal massage daily.
4. Eat high fiber whole grains and vegetables.
5. Take probiotic foods or drinks with meals.

Differentiation of Constipation Patterns

Liver Qi Stagnation

Symptoms:
Stress, toxic Liver, depression, irritability, hormonal imbalance.

Remedy:
Course the Liver:

1. Take warm water with lime juice first thing in the morning.
2. Take warm water with 1 tbsp each, apple cider vinegar and raw honey, first thing in the morning.
3. Eat seaweed soup.
4. Take the formula Mu Xiang Shun Qi Pian.

Blood, Yin, and/or Fluid Deficiency

Symptoms:
Anemia, pallor, loss of blood or fluids, elderly or convalescing.

Remedy:
Moisten the Bowels:

1. Take 1 tbsp. of one of the following mucilaginous seeds: chia seeds, hemp seeds, flaxseeds, or sesame seeds; two times a day.
2. Grind 1 tbsp white or black sesame seeds. Mix with 1 tsp honey and warm milk (or water) first thing in the morning.

3. Cook a few prunes in coarse-ground whole grain cornmeal and eat for breakfast.
4. Use the formula Yi Xue Run Chang for pure deficiency. Use Ma Zi Ren Wan for mixed deficiency and excess patterns.

Excess Heat

Symptoms:
Inflammation or redness symptoms, irritability, agitation.

Remedy:
Purge Heat from the Intestines:

1. Take 0.5-1g powdered Da Huang (rhubarb) in warm water first thing in the morning.
2. Take the formula Da Cheng Qi Tang if severe with dry stools. Take Xiao Cheng Qi Tang if less severe.

Diarrhea

Diarrhea is defined as three or more loose or liquid bowel movements per day. Loose stools even once a day can be treated with the following methods.

Differentiation of Diarrhea Patterns

Spleen Qi Deficiency

Symptoms:
Chronic loose stools, fatigue especially after eating.

Remedy:
1. Add Lian Zi (lotus seed), Qian Shi (fox nut) to congee and soups.
2. Cook with nutmeg.
3. Use the formula Jian Pi Pian with meals for 3-6 months.

Liver Overacting on Spleen

Symptoms:
Stress, related to menstrual cycle.

Remedy:
1. Stress-relieving activities: meditation, qigong, yoga, acupuncture, massage.
2. Take the formulas Jia Wei Xiao Yao San + Mu Xiang Shun Qi Pian

Spleen Qi Deficiency with Dampness

Symptoms:
Abdominal bloating, loss of appetite, fatigue especially after eating, nausea, general heavy sensation, foggy-headed.

Remedy:
1. Avoid dairy, sugar, cold, and raw foods.
2. Cook with ginger and warming spices (avoid excessively spicy food).
3. Take the formula Ping Wei San. When symptoms lessen, take Jian Pi Pian with meals for 3-6 months.

Damp-Heat

Symptoms:
Abdominal bloating, foul smelling stools, sticky or loose stools, burning in the anus, thirst with no desire to drink, oily skin, acne.

Remedy:
1. Avoid alcohol, spicy foods, fatty foods, and dairy.
2. Take the formula Lian Po Yin or Xiang Lian Wan.

Stomach Flu

Symptoms:
Sudden turmoil (acute vomiting and/or diarrhea), cold symptoms.

Remedy:
1. Take the formula Huo Xiang Zheng Qi Tang every 3-4 hours.
2. Make simple soups with chicken, rice, and vegetables.

Food Stagnation

Symptoms:
Undigested food in the stools.

Remedy:
1. Take 1 tsp of powdered Mu Xiang (aucklandia) in warm water.
2. Take the formula Bao He Wan.

Kidney Yang Deficiency

Symptoms:
Cock's crow or daybreak diarrhea, undigested food in stools, feel cold, fatigue.

Remedy:
1. Avoid dairy, sugar, cold, and raw foods.
2. Take the formula Fu Zi Li Zhong Wan.

Bowel Regulating Detox

This diet can be used for extended periods of time without injury. It concurrently clears excesses while strengthening digestion.

1. Take a pinch of powdered Da Huang (rhubarb) in hot water first thing in the morning or last thing before bed at night. Vary the amount until there is no digestive upset. If there is any gurgling, cramping, or discomfort in the abdomen, lower the dosage. Da Huang in larger doses is a potent purgative, Blood mover, and powerful detoxifier. In tiny dosages it very gently cleanses the digestive tract and acts more like a tonic. (A patient of mine shed a sheath of muck that was lining her intestines after taking Da Huang daily in microdoses for two months.)
2. Take homemade probiotics daily. These may include dairy or water kefir, cultured vegetables, yogurt, kombucha, beet kavaas, etc. (recipes page 331). Coconut water kefir is particularly popular currently. Homemade probiotics also contain digestive enzymes.
3. Eat simple meals. A diet consisting of 50% vegetables is a gentle way to detox all excesses from the body. Avoid sugar, fruit juice, and white bread. White basmati rice is sometimes more appropriate for detoxification than brown rice, as it is easier to digest and less heating.
4. In cases of Spleen deficiency (unstable blood sugar) or excess weight (slow metabolism), eat every 3-4 hours. That is three main meals with 2-3 snacks.
5. Take an appropriate formula to strengthen the Spleen, calm Liver, etc.
6. Drink Bone Broth daily (recipe page 328).
7. Eat daikon radish and burdock root. They can be eaten raw, juiced or added to tea or soups. Daikon radish cleanses Phlegm-Damp from the entire digestive tract and removes abdominal bloating. Burdock root cleanses the Liver system and the fiber cleanses the intestines.
8. Add a greens formula to add additional vegetables into your diet.

Bowel Cleanse Detox Plan

Table 6.1. Bowel Detox Plan

Before Breakfast	Drink 1 cup of warm water with a pinch of powdered Da Huang (rhubarb).
Breakfast	1. Spleen Tonic Congee (page 327) – first food to reach the stomach. 2. Lean protein (¼ the meal) – lean cut of meat, fish, or meat substitute 3. Salad, steamed or stir-fried vegetables (½ the meal) – greens, mushrooms, broccoli, turnips, celery, carrots 4. Whole grain cooked cereal or sprouted grain bread (¼ the meal) – choose from rice, buckwheat, oats, millet 5. Probiotic drink or food
Snack	Protein shake
Between Meals	Drink 1 cup of warmed Daikon Radish Soup (page 366)
Lunch	1. Lean protein (¼ the meal) – lean cut of meat, fish, or meat substitute 2. Salad, steamed or stir-fried vegetables (½ the meal) – greens, mushrooms, broccoli, turnips, celery, carrots 3. Probiotic drink or food
Snack	Seaweed Miso Soup
Between Meals	Drink 1 cup of warmed Daikon & Burdock Drink
Dinner	1. Bone broth-based soup 2. Salad, steamed or stir-fried vegetables (½ the meal) – greens, mushrooms, broccoli, turnips, celery, carrots 3. Probiotic drink or food.

Types of Stagnation & Excesses

The following are the different kinds of accumulations that occur in the body causing disease. Use the diet and remedies with the bowel cleanse detox diet described previously or the detox plan later on. It is not always immediately clear whether symptoms are caused by stagnation or deficiency. A key indicator of stagnation or excess conditions is that physical movement or skipping a meal makes the symptoms better temporarily. Removing physical stagnation also acts to cleanse the corresponding emotional state.

(Liver) Qi Stagnation

The Liver is the "general" of the body in that it mobilizes the body's defenses and is the primary detoxifying agent for everything that enters the body. In an increasingly toxic environment, the Liver carries a heavy burden. Additionally, the Liver is the first organ system to respond to the emotional stresses of modern life. The Liver naturally wants to expand and grow. When we have unfilled desires it causes Liver Qi stagnation; which is why it is called the "disease of adulthood" as to live in society we must learn to delay gratification. Thus, the majority of people experience Liver Qi stagnation off and on.

Symptoms:
Muscle tension, especially in the upper back and neck. Abdominal distention (bloating). Alternating constipation and loose stools. Irregular periods. Breast soreness. Moodiness. Irritability. Anger or depression. Stress. Frequent sighing.

Biomedical Diseases:
Stress. Liver organ dysfunction.

Emotional Aspect:
Unfulfilled desires. Feeling stuck, blocked, or stifled by outer circumstances. Resentment. Anger. Repression.

Causative/Aggravating Factors:
Stress. Hormonal imbalance. Liver toxicity caused by medications, drugs, alcohol, or environmental toxins. These symptoms may also be aggravated during a detox treatment or regimen when excess toxins are released into the system.

Diet Plan:
Avoid extremes. Eat less and avoid eating when upset. Eat 50% vegetables. Include mildly pungent foods to help move the Qi. Include the sour flavor to heal the Liver.

Beneficial Foods:
Mustard greens, tomato, onion family, garlic, ginger, curried dishes, mint, citrus, vinegar, sprouted grains, cabbage. A little coffee or red wine is also effective.

Avoid:
Processed food (pizza, potato chips), cold foods or drinks (ice cream, beer, juice), too many salads, and excess spicy foods.

Lifestyle:
1. Physical movement and exercise, but avoid extremes and competition.
2. Progression on a goal or project.
3. Massage, acupuncture, energy work, qigong, meditation, and yoga are very effective.

Formulas:
Shu Gan Wan or Jia Wei Xiao Yao San

Blood Stagnation

Blood stagnation is the result of either a trauma or a complication of another stagnation.

Symptoms:
Pain after an injury. Stabbing or intense pain. Dark, purplish circles under the eyes.[9] Dark complexion. Menstrual cramps relieved by passage of clots.

Biomedical Diseases:
Tumors. Sites of traumatic injury. Stroke.

Emotional Aspect:
Long-standing depression or insomnia that develops years after a trauma and does not resolve. Trapped trauma.

Causative/Aggravating Factors:
Long-standing Liver Qi stagnation. Physical trauma. Unresolved emotional trauma. Cold foods or environment.

Diet Plan:
Follow the Qi stagnation-relieving diet. Eat 50% vegetables. Include pungent and warming foods to help move Qi and Blood.

Beneficial Foods:
Hei Mu Er (black wood ear fungus), eggplant, seaweeds, white pepper, red adzuki bean, garlic, ginger, Shan Zha (hawthorn berry), mustard greens, onion family.

9. Can also be Kidney deficiency, in which case there will also be pronounced puffiness.

Avoid:
Processed foods (pizza, potato chips), cold foods or drinks (ice cream, beer, juice), too many salads, spicy foods.

Lifestyle:
1. Physical movement and exercise.
2. Application of heat (if not acute, inflamed injury).

Formula:
Yunnan Paiyao

Food Stagnation

Symptoms:
Abdominal distention. Gas. Belching. Foul-smelling stools.

Biomedical Diseases:
Indigestion.

Causative or Aggravating Factors:
Consuming food in excess of the strength of Spleen Qi's ability to digest it. Either excessive rich, greasy, or hard to digest foods; too much food; or digestive weakness. In case of Qi deficiency, follow Qi deficiency diet page 52 and take herbs to strengthen.

Lifestyle:
1. Eat smaller portions.
2. Eat regular, simple meals.

Formula:
Bao He Wan

Phlegm and Dampness

Phlegm-Damp is the most prolific type of accumulation and the most challenging to resolve. The terms Phlegm and Dampness refer to the congestion of body fluids in different manifestations. Phlegm is used to refer to the Upper Jiao (Lungs), mental impairment (as in misting the Mind, foggy thinking, irrational behavior) and in certain channel pathology. Phlegm produces an enlarged tongue body. Dampness refers to the Middle and Lower Jiaos (mucus and bloating in the digestive tract, cloudy and dribbling urination). Dampness shows itself on the tongue as a thick, greasy coating.

When the Spleen Qi is weak there is limited Qi in the body. During the digestive process, this limited

Remedy for No Appetite in the Morning

No appetite in the morning is a sign of Dampness. Make the following congee (rice soup) and eat first thing in the morning:

Add 1/4 cup Cang Zhu (atractylodes), 1/8 cup raw Yi Yi Ren (Job's tears), 1/8 cup dry-fried Yi Yi Ren (Job's tears), and ½ cup white rice to 5 cups of water. Cook in a rice cooker or crock pot overnight. Eat 1 small bowl first thing in the morning for 1 month.

Qi is diverted to break down food, leaving the rest of the body without energy. The body is unable to properly break down the food, assimilating the vital and discharging the unusable. This produces Phlegm and Dampness; a turbid, sticky, clogging substance that gets lodged in the areas you are most vulnerable. This can manifest as sinus issues, excess weight, body aches, mental impairment, chronic cough, high cholesterol, masses, and other symptoms.

Because the root of Phlegm-Damp is weak digestion, some find temporary relief through fasting. There is a short-term experience of mental clarity and increased energy.[(10)] However, fasting will weaken the Spleen further, creating more tendency to produce Phlegm and Damp. This is the pathology of rapid weight loss followed by increased weight gain, or yo-yo dieting. Clearing Phlegm-Damp requires strengthening the Spleen with diet and aromatic herbs, while eliminating rich, Phlegm-Damp-producing foods. Diet, lifestyle, and treatments must be continued for several months to resolve.

Symptoms:
Heaviness. Foggy-headedness. Lethargy. Joint aches and stiffness. Edema (fluid retention). Sinus congestion. Lung congestion. Loose stools, diarrhea, or mucus in stools. Leukorrhea (vaginal discharge). Cloudy urination. No appetite in the morning. Excess fat or flabbiness.

Biomedical Diseases:
Obesity. Cellulite or flabbiness, even in thin people. Varicose and spider veins. High cholesterol. Autism. Cysts. Polycystic Ovarian Syndrome (PCOS).[(11)] Tumors and masses.[(12)]

Emotional Aspect:
Ruminating. Not letting things go. Feeling stuck. Old habits and stubborn negative thought patterns. Can impair mental functioning and cause irrational behavior.

Causative or Aggravating Factors:
Largely food-related. Eating excessive amounts of cold, greasy, heavy, sweet, or salty foods.

10. Many anorexics begin with Spleen Qi deficiency. They initially feel better when they do not eat and continue to fast indefinitely.

11. Kidney Yang deficiency is also part of PCOS. Eliminating sugar and Damp-producing foods is key to treatment.

12. Cancer is a complex condition involving Phlegm-Damp, Heat Toxin, Blood Stagnation always with an underlying deficiency.

Dairy. Simple carbohydrates. Processed foods. Cold, damp environments. Weak digestion. Poor or irregular diet. Stress.

Diet Plan:
Include hot, pungent, or bitter foods. Eat 50% cooked vegetables and lower amounts of carbohydrates and animal protein. Eat cooked, warm foods and drink (steam-frying is a preferred method).

Beneficial Foods:
Daikon radish, red radish, pungent greens (arugula, watercress, mustard) ginger, herbs and spices, hot pepper, onion family, lettuce, celery, red adzuki beans, buckwheat, rye, basmati rice, turnips, tea. Combine pungent or bitter foods with dairy and sweets to neutralize their effects. For example, tea with a fatty meal, meat with turnips or arugula. Eat sprouted grain breads only. Sprouting grains renders them more digestible and less Damp-promoting.

Avoid:
Cold temperature foods and drink. Even good quality cold drinks such as orange juice are very Phlegm-producing. No late night meals or junk food. Limit soy products, dairy, wheat, sweets, eggs, nuts, white flour, and beer.

Lifestyle:
1. Exercise is crucial to improve lymphatic flow. It is important to break a sweat and heat the body daily.
2. Acupuncture and massage.

Formulas:
Xiang Sha Liu Jun Zi Tang, Xiang Sha Yang Wei Tang, or Ping Wei San

High Cholesterol

Excess cholesterol is a combination of Phlegm-Damp and impaired microcirculation. Statin drugs have many serious side effects such as Liver damage, muscle pain, and inhibiting sexual functioning. They also do not address the underlying cause.

Diet Plan:
Follow the Phlegm-Damp-clearing diet above. Excess sugar is a huge culprit. Cut out simple carbohydrates, sugar, soda, and fruit juice. Avoid fried or greasy foods.

Beneficial Foods:
Grapefruit, celery, hibiscus flower, Hei Mu Er (black wood ear mushroom), shitake mushroom, lime juice, apple cider vinegar, Shan Zha (hawthorn berry), Jue Ming Zi (cassia seed), red rice yeast (contains natural statins). Drink oolong or puerrh with Ju Hua (chrysanthemum), or ku ding cha with meals. Take Date and Wood Ear Tea page 372 daily.

Lifestyle:
Regular exercise is crucial to improve circulation.

Formulas:
Yu Jin Jiang Ji Yin

Shan Zha (hawthorn berry) is very effective but its sour taste can hurt some people's stomachs. Jue Ming Zi (cassia seed) tea or the Date and Wood Ear Tea are often tolerated better.

High Blood Sugar Remedy

Where high blood sugar is due to digestive weakness using the following remedy: Take 1 tbsp of apple cider vinegar after each meal. Be sure to rinse teeth after ingesting vinegar or citrus juice as it can damage tooth enamel.

Excess Heat

Symptoms:
Can be constitutional Yang person with minimal symptoms. Strong body odor. Constipation. Loud voice. Strong personality. Gets red easily. Acne or rashes. Inflammation.

Biomedical Diseases:
High blood pressure. Inflammatory diseases. Ulcers.

Emotional Aspect:
Anger. Irritability. Repressed emotions.

Causative or Aggravating Factors:
Hot, dry, or pungent foods and spices. Alcohol and coffee. Hot environment.

Diet Plan:
Include cool, bitter, moistening foods. Excess Heat conditions do very well on a vegetable-based diet typical of western-style cleanses. Cooking should be limited to steaming, soups, and light stir frying. Eat plenty of raw foods and vegetable juices.

Beneficial Foods:
Bitter melon, vegetable juices, sprouts, most vegetables, soy products, mung bean, yogurt, seaweed, dandelion greens, pear, apple, eggplant, lemon, tomato, watermelon, cucumber, celery, green tea.

Avoid:
Stimulants: alcohol, chocolate, spices, and coffee. No lamb or chicken. No garlic, it is very heating.

Lifestyle:
1. Cool environment. Avoid saunas, heated room yoga.

Heat-clearing drink:

Blend 1 ½ round of deseeded bitter melon + 1/8 of a honey dew melon with water in the blender. Also makes a great summer drink.

2. Practice relaxation daily.
3. Avoid stress and competition.

Formulas:
Yu Jin Jiang Ji Yin, Long Dan Xie Gan Tang

Ulcers

Ulcers are an indication of Stomach Heat in Traditional Chinese Medicine.

Diet Plan:
Eat soft, wet foods such as those listed below. No pungent foods. Raw foods may be too harsh.

Beneficial Foods:
Congees made with rice, barley, millet, or oats. Yogurt, cucumber, cabbage, banana, avocado.

Avoid:
Stimulants: alcohol, chocolate, spices, and coffee. No lamb or chicken. No garlic, it is very heating.

Lifestyle:
1. Practice relaxation daily.
2. Avoid stress and competition.

Formulas:
Huang Lian Su Pian, Hai Piao Xiao (cuttlefish bone)

High Blood Pressure

Caused by Liver Yang Rising, which is a combination of Heat and Yin deficiency in varying ratios.

Diet Plan:
Follow Heat clearing diet. Include heavy minerals such as calcium and magnesium supplements.

Beneficial Foods:
Bitter melon, vegetable juices, sprouts are very helpful. Vegetables, soy products, mung bean, yogurt, seaweed, dandelion greens, pear, apple, eggplant, lemon.

Avoid:
Stimulants: alcohol, chocolate, spices, and coffee. No lamb or chicken. No garlic, it is very heating.

Lifestyle:

1. Practice relaxation daily.
2. Avoid stress and competition.

Formula:

Tian Ma Gou Teng Yin

Latent Heat Toxin

Latent Heat Toxins are the residue of toxic Heat that the Righteous Qi (immune system) was able to subdue but not completely remove from the body. These toxins become trapped in the body, resurfacing when immunity becomes impaired. Latent Heat Toxins are implicated in several diseases including: cancer, herpes (simplex and zoster), autoimmune disease, rheumatoid arthritis, psoriasis, yeast infections, and even acne. There are a number of ways to obtain latent Heat Toxins. Typically these are bacteria, viruses, or environmental toxins that were able to penetrate deep enough to take up residence. On a psycho-spiritual level they relate to old griefs, wounds, and resentments that were never completely healed. Use the Cancer clearing diet page 272.

Damp-Heat

Symptoms:

Lethargic. Strong body odor. Sticky, foul-smelling stools. Yellow vaginal discharge. Red, itchy, fluid filled skin conditions. Purulent (pus-like) discharge from the ears. Bitter taste in the mouth.

Biomedical Diseases:

Gallstones. Kidney stones. Leukorrhea (vaginal discharge). Herpes simplex and shingles. Hepatitis. Eczema. Jaundice. Urinary symptoms.

Emotional Aspect:

Resentment. Ruminating. Rage. Festering. Feeling stuck.

Causative or Aggravating Factors:

Poor diet. Excess greasy, rich, or difficult to digest foods. Long-standing digestive weakness.

Diet Plan:

Eat 50% vegetables, less carbohydrates and meat, low fat, no fried foods. Include cooling foods to

Yu Mi Xu (cornsilk) Tea

Cornsilk tea clears Damp-Heat from the Liver/Gallbladder and Kidney/Urinary Bladder systems. It is a mild herb and is most effective when the first symptoms of urinary discomfort are felt. Also drink in hot weather to cool off the body.

Take a large handful of dried cornsilk. Rinse and put in a pot.

Cover with water and simmer for 30-45 min. Allow to cool.

Strain and discard the cornsilk.

Drink warm as a tea, refrigerate and drink as iced tea, or add 1 cup to your water bottle and drink throughout the day. If caught early enough cornsilk tea will drive out minor infections.

clear Heat and some pungent flavors to disperse Damp. Increase raw foods and vegetable juices to the degree Heat is predominant. Include more cooked foods to degree Dampness is predominant.[13] Bitter foods are effective, even in small amounts.

Beneficial Foods:
Bitter melon, daikon radish, arugula, watercress, ku ding cha, mung beans, adzuki beans, Yi Yi Ren (Job's tears), cranberry juice, cranberries with orange peel, watermelon, tea, shitake mushrooms, seaweeds, most vegetables, asparagus, lemon, watercress, lettuce, radishes, burdock root (gobo), turnips. Eat sprouted grain breads only. Sprouting grains renders them more digestible and less Damp-promoting.

Avoid:
Garlic, spices, coffee, chocolate, alcohol, vinegar, nuts, dairy, fatty meats, avocado, banana, white flour, sweets, junk food. Limit salt and sugar.

Lifestyle:
1. Physical exercise. Avoid competition or overheating.
2. Practice relaxation.

Gallstones

Gallbladder inflammation (cholecystitis) and gallstones (cholelitheasis) are very common conditions in modern society. In the U.S. the allopathic intervention is to remove the organ rather than resolve the underlying imbalance; what TCM defines as Liver and Gallbladder Damp-Heat. Removing the Gallbladder adds stress to the Liver and impairs the ability to digest fats. Removing the organ also does not resolve the pattern pathology. Many patients will develop pain or other symptoms in the Gallbladder channel after gallbladder removal. They may be unable to digest fats or suffer from chronic loose stools. Emotionally, gallbladder removal adversely affects courage and discernment. There are times when an emergency surgery has to be done. If there is time, however, follow the steps below to dissolve stones and bring the Gallbladder back in balance.

Symptoms:
Inability to digest fats, upper abdominal bloating, puffiness under the eyes (see page 276 Figure 5.1), alternating chills and fever. During acute attack there is intense pain worse with pressure. The pain can start under the left lower ribs (pancreas area) and spread to under the right lower ribs (gallbladder area). The pain can also refer to the upper back and scapula area.

Diet Plan:
For one month follow the Damp-Heat clearing diet: 50% vegetables, less carbohydrates and meat, low fat, no fried foods. Follow Gallstone detox program below.

---

13. A gentle cleansing method appropriate for most people is to follow Dr. Robert and Shelley Young's alkalarian diet (authors of *The PH Miracle*). He has several books and two cookbooks providing a specific meal plan. You can also modify by adding some grains and meats if you are more deficient. I disagree with Dr. Young about following this diet indefinitely.

PRACTITIONER SECTION - GALLSTONES

Customized formulas are important in these cases to balance the strong action of the stone dissolving herbs. Patents such as Qing Dan Hua Shi Pian or Li Dan Pills are more effective than Western remedies but not as effective as the raw herbs or herb concentrates. These treatments do not need to be harsh to be effective. I find them more effective in formulas that concurrently harmonize the underlying condition.

Daily acupuncture during acute attacks is ideal: Needle GB 34 on the right with Dan Nang Xue with electro-stimulation. Needle ASHI points in the upper abdomen, LV 14, Ren 12, GB 40, GB 41, SJ 5, Yin Tang. Teach your patient to massage GB 34 daily.

Beneficial Foods:
Eat plenty of leafy greens, apples, pears, burdock root. Drink Liver Cleansing Broth with lime juice throughout the day (page 373). Take Yu Mi Xu (cornsilk) tea liberally.

Lifestyle:
Find ways to move your body gently every day.

Formulas:
See formula below, Qing Dan Hua Shi Pian, or Li Dan Pian.

Recipe 6.1. Gallstone Dissolving Decoction

The patent Qing Dan Hua Shi Pian or Li Dan Pills can be used, however the raw herb decoction is more effective.

Ingredients:
Hua Shi Cao (orthosiphon) 15g, Hai Jin Sha (lygodium spores) 15g, Jin Qian Cao (lysimachia) 30g, Yu Jin (curcuma) 6g, Yin Chen Hao (artemesia scoparia) 10g, Huang Qin (scutellaria) 9g, Chai Hu (bupleurum) 9g, Bai Shao (white peony root) 9g, Zhi Shi (aurantis) 6g, Dang Shen (codonopsis) 15g, Mai Men Dong (ophiopogon) 6g.

* Ji Nei Jin (chicken gizzard) - powder separately and add 1-2g of powder to cup of decoction before drinking.

Decoct herbs (page 330). Take 1 cup 2-3 times a day between meals. Take for 10 to 20 consecutive days prior to attempting a Gallbladder Purge. In cases of large gallstones, patients must be under the supervision of a health care provider, as large stones can become stuck during a flush creating a potentially serious situation.

This formula is contraindicated in pregnancy. In more deficient constitutions be sure to take Spleen tonics in pill form with meals (like Bu Zhong Yi Qi Tang or Jian Pi Wan). After the purge take a formula to harmonize the Liver such as Jia Wei Xiao Yao San for 3 months.

Recipe 6.2. Gallbladder Purge

Ingredients:
Wei Ling Xian (clematis) 15g, Gua Lou (tricosanthes)15-30g, Da Huang (rhubarb) 1- 6g, Mang Xiao (Epsom salts)1-6g.

1. Cook first two herbs with the Gallstone Dissolving decoction. Add Da Huang during last 5 min of cooking. Stir Mang Xiao after straining the decoction.
2. Adding these herbs to the Gallstone Dissolving Formula purges stones from the gallbladder. In cases of acute gallbladder attack, indicating a stone stuck in the biliary duct, add these herbs right away. In severe pain, add Yan Hu Suo (corydalis) 15g. In cases where there is no pain, take the Gallstone Dissolving Formula alone for 10-20 days to shrink the stones before adding the Purge Formula. The Purge Formula will cause loose stools. To reduce this effect, lessen the dosage of the last two herbs. Do not take the Gallbladder Purge formula long-term. Discontinue after stones have passed (they are iridescent green and float to the surface of the toilet).

Urinary Tract Infection (UTI) and Kidney Stones

Both are indications of Damp-Heat in the Urinary Bladder and Kidneys.

UTI Symptoms: Burning urination. Urgency to urinate. Dribbling urination. Lower abdominal heaviness and pain. If the infection progresses to the Kidneys: kidney pain (under lower ribcage in the back), fever and chills, pain down the insides of the leg.

Kidney Stone Symptoms: Same symptoms as for UTI, plus: very intense pain in back, kidney area, and/or down the insides of the legs. Fever and chills. Kidney stones are extremely painful, but are easier to treat and faster to resolve than gallstones. After taking the Kidney Stone Clearing Formula, jump up and down for a minute or so.

Diet Plan:
Stay hydrated. Eat cool, bitter, moistening foods. Cool environment. Cooking should be limited to steaming, soups, and light stir frying.

Beneficial Foods:
Adzuki beans, mung beans, asparagus, plenty of water, cornsilk tea, cranberries and cranberry juice (pure unsweetened) liberally.

Formulas:
For UTI, the homeopathic Urinary Aid (cystitis) from Professional Complementary Health Formulas,[14] is very effective. For Kidney stones use Kidney Stone Clearing Formula. In both cases take Yu Mi Xu (cornsilk) tea liberally.

---

14. http://www.professionalformulas.com

Recipe 6.3. Kidney Stone Clearing Formula

Ingredients:
Hua Shi Cao (orthosiphon) 15g, Hai Jin Sha (lygodium spores) 15g, Jin Qian Cao (lysimachia) 30g, Shi Wei (pyrrosia) 10g, Che Qian Zi (plantago seed) 10g, Chuan Mu Tong (akebia) 5g, Ze Xie (alisma) 10g, Hua Shi (talc) 10g, Qu Mai (dianthus) 5g, Du Zhong (eucomia) 10g, Xu Duan (dipsacus) 10g.

* Ji Nei Jin (chicken gizzard) - powder separately and add 1-2g of powder to cup of decoction before drinking.

Decoct herbs (page 330). Take 1 cup 2-3 times a day between meals. Fifteen min. after taking the decoction, stand on the last step of a staircase and jump to the floor 15 times. Take for 10 to 20 consecutive days until stones have passed. Take an appropriate Kidney tonic such as a Liu Wei Di Huang Wan modification for three months after passing the stones to strengthen the Kidneys.

Liver, Gallbladder, and Kidney Detox Plan

This plan clears Damp, Heat, and Toxins safely. It specifically detoxifies the Liver, Gallbladder, and Kidneys. It can be used for acne or inflammatory skin conditions, toxicity from pesticides, heavy metals or drugs, excess weight, liver or gallbladder disorders, kidney disorders, candida, and chronic digestive disorders.

The purpose is to detox safely, without weakening the body. In asymptomatic cases it can be done for one week, ideally in the spring, but any season as necessary. In cases of gallstones or kidney stones, follow this plan until the stones have passed.

The most important factors are the herbal formulas, the lemon juice or vinegar, and Liver Cleansing Broth. Be sure to drink the citrus or vinegar water through a straw to protect your tooth enamel. Mung beans, Bai Bian Dou (hyacinth bean), and red adzuki beans detoxify the body. Take 5g of Kun Bu (kelp) seaweed a day. Add to soup or, if there is an aversion to seaweed, take in capsule form. It dissolves Phlegm-Damp and detoxifies the body, as well as boosts thyroid functioning.

Table 6.2. Liver, Gallbladder, & Kidney Detox Plan

Before Breakfast	Mix 1 tbsp of lemon or lime juice or apple cider vinegar in warm water.
Breakfast	1. Drink 1 cup warmed Liver Cleansing Broth with meals. (page 373) 2. Lean protein (¼ the meal) – lean cut of meat, fish, or meat substitute 3. Salad, steamed or stir-fried vegetables (½ the meal) – greens, mushrooms, broccoli, turnips, celery, carrots 4. Whole grain cooked cereal or sprouted grain bread (¼ the meal) – choose from rice, buckwheat, oats, or millet

Snack	Fruit: apple, pear, pineapple, or cranberry (can be made into protein shake); or Vegetable Soup
Between Meals	Gallbladder Dissolving Formula or Kidney Stone Clearing Formula
Lunch	1. Drink 1 cup warmed Liver Cleansing Broth with meals. 2. Lean protein (¼ the meal) – lean cut of meat, fish, or meat substitute 3. Salad, steamed or stir-fried vegetables (½ the meal) – greens, mushrooms, broccoli, turnips, celery, carrots
Snack	Seaweed miso or vegetable Soup
Between Meals	Gallbladder Dissolving Formula or Kidney Stone Clearing Formula
Dinner	1.Drink 1 cup warmed Liver Cleansing Broth with meals. 2. Mung bean soup or vegetable soup 3. Salad, steamed or stir-fried vegetables (½ the meal) – greens, mushrooms, broccoli, turnips, celery, carrots

Summer-Heat

Symptoms:
Sensitivity to wind, lethargy, feeling hot, thirst, headache, and dark scanty urine.

Biomedical Diseases:
Heat stroke.

Causative or Aggravating Factors:
Hot summer weather.

Diet Plan:
Cooling, moistening foods and drinks.

Beneficial Foods:
Bitter melon, mung bean soup, cucumber, He Ye (lotus leaf) tea, Yi Yi Ren (Job's tears), watermelon, cornsilk tea, Bai Bian Dou (hyacinth bean).

Avoid:
Stimulants: alcohol, chocolate, spices, and coffee. No lamb or chicken. No garlic, it is very heating.

Formula:
He Ye (lotus leaf) Tea

Environmental Toxins

Pollution, pesticides, and the general lack of respect with which humans treat the Earth have imbued our food supply and environment with toxins. Our health is tied to the health of the environment. They cannot be separated. When Nature thrives and is vibrant, and we live in harmony with it, we thrive and are vibrant. It is that simple. There are short-term remedies to clear excess toxins from the body. However, long-term health requires a change in awareness of everyday people in making the world less toxic.

Diet Plan:
Eat organic, non-genetically modified, humanely and consciously raised foods.

Beneficial Foods:
Mung beans, seaweed (kombu), Bai Bian Dou (hyacinth bean), Yi Yi Ren (Job's tears), bentonite clay.

Lifestyle:
Become active in the environmental movement.

Formulas:
Xiao Feng San – external rashes

Recipe 6.4. Cleansing the Smoker's Lungs

This simple remedy can be used for clearing any lung toxicity, and is used after quitting smoking to remove accumulations from the Lungs:

Take 1 tsp. powdered Hu Lu Ba (fenugreek seeds) in warm water three times a day for 1-3 months.

Recipe 6.5. Heavy Metal Poisoning Formula

Lu Dou (mung beans) 30-60g, Fang Feng (ledebouriella) 15g, Gan Cao (licorice) 6g.

Recipe 6.5. Pesticide Poisoning[15]

A Chinese study used the following formula to successfully treat pesticide poisoning: 500g powdered mung beans, 60g of salt, 2,000ml of water. Soak for several minutes and strain. Make and drink 3 times in one day.

15. Zhe Jiang Zhong Yi Zha Zhi (Zhejiang Journal of Chinese Medicine) 1965; 7:7.

Anti-Cancer Foods

Cancer treatment is a specialty within Traditional Chinese Medicine that cannot be openly practiced in the U.S. Cancer is considered a combination of Blood stagnation, Phlegm obstruction, and latent Heat toxin that proliferate due to a major deficiency in the body. Treatments address all four patterns concurrently with special herbs.[16]

In addition, there are dietary and herbal measures to build the body's defensive Qi that help fight active cancer, keep it in remission, or prevent it altogether. The top tonics are Dong Chong Xia Cao (cordyceps) 5-10g a day, Ling Zhi (reishi mushroom) 1-3g a day, and Ren Shen (ginseng) 1-3g a day. These should be taken daily and typically in powder or pill form as separate herbs due to their expense. Cordyceps is particularly indicated for Lung cancer.

Diet Plan:
Eat organic, non-genetically modified, and unprocessed foods.

Beneficial Foods:[17]
Green or oolong tea, daikon or red radish, tomatoes, watermelon, pears, water chestnuts, mushrooms, Hei Mu Er (black wood ear fungus), Ba Mu Er (white cloud fungus), red adzuki beans, Lian Zi (lotus nut), Yi Yi Ren (Job's tears), Shan Zha (hawthorn berry), pepper, vinegar, light salting, small amounts of wine.

To soften masses: crab, jellyfish, seaweed, mussels, clam, sea cucumber, abalone.

Lifestyle:
1. Practice daily relaxation.
2. Enjoy physical exercise.

Formulas:
Strong tonics taken daily such as cordyceps, reishi mushroom, and ginseng.
Strong toxin clearing, Blood moving, Phlegm resolving formulas.

Excess Weight

Excess weight is challenging to treat because it involves making fundamental lifestyle changes. There may be food addiction, depression, vitamin/mineral deficiencies, hormonal imbalances, side effects from medications, or chronic illness complicating the situation. Short-term extreme diets invariably injure the Spleen leading to more Dampness (read fat) long-term.

Excess weight is by definition a proliferation of Dampness and Phlegm in the body. Permanent weight loss requires changing the constitution. Thus, the main strategy is to dry it up in one of

16. See Chen, *Chinese Medical Herbology*, 1095, for a list of herbs commonly used for cancer treatment.

17. Will MacLean, *Clinical Handbook of Internal Medicine: The Treatment of Disease with Traditional Chinese Medicine: Vol 2: Spleen and Stomach.* (Sydney: University of Western Sydney, 2002) 887.

four ways: draining (promoting urination), aromatically transforming (using pungent, drying substances), cooling to promote fluid metabolism (in cases of Heat), and warming to promote fluid metabolism (in cases of Cold).[18]

To make matters a bit more complicated, there are often other patterns that must be dealt with concurrently. Spleen Qi deficiency is the root of excess Dampness. This is often compounded by Stomach Heat, Qi and Blood stagnation, Qi and Blood deficiency, Kidney deficiency, or Yin deficiency with Heat. In Western terms, this correlates to a build-up of toxins, lack of blood circulation and lymphatic flow, hormonal imbalance, and organ distress attendant with excess weight. Cravings are a sign of deficiency in the body. A desire for sweets indicates Qi and Blood deficiency; a desire for salt, Kidney deficiency. An herbal formula to tonify these deficiencies is necessary so that food cravings do not sabotage weight loss progress.

Western nutrition distills weight loss down to a case of calories taken in versus calories burned. TCM makes a distinction on the qualities of the food consumed. Damp-promoting foods, eaten by those with Phlegm-Damp constitutions, cause weight gain. Appropriate amounts of drying or aromatically transforming foods will actively promote weight loss in those same Phlegm-Damp constitutions. It is not so much the quantity of the foods that make you fat. It is the quality of the foods combined with a constitutional tendency. Eating the Foods That Melt Fat in the following section regularly will transform excess weight.

Lifestyle

1. Break a sweat 3-4 times a week:
Limit intense and cardio workouts to 45 minutes a session. If you enjoy running, do short sprints for 45 seconds interspersed with walking. This transforms Dampness. Do high intensity workouts and use a sauna regularly. Be sure not to exhaust yourself, which will deplete you and undermine your progress. You should feel energized when you finish.

2. Build Muscle:
Lift heavy weights three times a week. Building muscles alone will boost metabolism. Weightlifting requires a great deal of energy and muscles burn calories even at rest. In TCM terms you are making your body hotter (and less prone to Dampness). Lift heavy weights and do compound movements such as squats, pullups, pushups, and deadlifts. Make sure to have a snack before and after exercising to boost the metabolism.

3. Eat Six times a Day:
Eating every three hours is key to boosting the metabolism. It is important to not go hungry, which weakens the Spleen. Every morning take the time to separate out three snack-size portions to eat between bigger meals. These can consist of a protein smoothie,[19] a cup of soup,

18. Henry C. Lu. *Natural Chinese Cures.* (New York: Black Dog and Levanthal Publishers, 1999), 305.

19. Use low glycemic fruits: pineapple, berries, apple, pear, or papaya with vegetables: kale, collard greens, avocado, spinach, etc.

natural protein bar, hard-boiled eggs, vegetables with hummus, a fruit with nuts, a piece of chicken with a stick of celery, or divide a regular meal into smaller portions.

4. Eat Slimming Bisque:
For rapid weight-loss, eat vegetable-based blended soups for 4 of 6 meals daily. Many lose several pounds a week with this method. The high ratio of digestible vegetables powerfully yet gently detoxifies and alkalizes the body. Add lean protein to promote muscle development.

5. Avoid Extreme Dieting:
Unless there is a case of pure excess, extreme dieting is not helpful. It can greatly weaken Qi and Yang leading to further weight gain. A better long-term strategy is to have a diet that supports the Spleen and clears excess Phlegm, Damp, and Heat from the body. Eat 50% vegetables at every meal. Minimize sugar, simple carbohydrates (white bread, fruit juice), excessive salt, and animal fats. Avoid "non-food" items such as diet soda and processed foods. Processed foods contain addictive additives and non-food compounds that can wreak havoc with hormones and health.

6. Eat Bitter:
It is important to incorporate bitter-tasting foods, particularly at the end of the meal, as the bitter taste reduces appetite. (Sweet taste increases appetite and can be eaten at the beginning of meals when low appetite is an issue). Bitter foods include arugula, watercress, broccoli, lettuce, rye, tea, and bitter melon. The average American diet is inundated with sweet taste and sorely lacking in bitter.

7. Drink Ku Ding Cha:
Ku ding cha or "bitter nail tea" is more effective than green tea to clear Dampness and Heat, and promote weight loss. Drink with meals.

8. Get treated:
Acupuncture, massage, endermologie, body wraps all help balance and speed the weight-loss process.

9. Sleep:
Get 8 hours of uninterrupted sleep every night. Be in bed by 10 p.m.

10. Eat Foods That Melt Fat:
Drain Water: red adzuki beans, Yi Yi Ren (Job's tears), asparagus, green tea, ku ding cha, wintermelon, cornsilk, He Ye (lotus leaf).

Aromatic Transforming: Bai Bian Dou (hyacinth bean), Huo Xiang (agastache), Chen Pi (tangerine peel), radish, daikon radish, cardamom.

Heating (if you are always cold): spices, ginger, garlic, chives, cayenne pepper, kidneys, liver, shrimp, mussels.

Cooling (if you are always hot): mint, bitter melon, mung beans, daikon radish.

Formulas:
Slimming Tea, Weightloss Fomula (page 276), take herbs to balance deficiencies.

> **Slimming Tea**
>
> **Ingredients:**
> He Ye (lotus leaf) 10g, Yi Yi Ren (Job's Tears) 24g, Chen Pi (tangerine peel) 5g, Green Tea 5g.
>
> Decoct the herbs (page 330). This simple formula clears Heat in summertime and drains excess Dampness from the body. It is an excellent weight loss tea. Take between meals, long-term.

Types of Obesity

Obesity can further be divided into 2 types:

Excess Type

Symptoms:
There may also be deficiency signs present but excess symptoms predominate:

Hard fat, tissue is tight to the touch. May not have cellulite. Very strong, easily develop muscles, big calves.

Heat symptoms: overheat easily, excessive sweating, get flushed, red skin

Conditions:
Loud, pushy personality.

Approach:
Requires clearing and draining treatment. These individuals are among the few that do well on "detox" diets though they will not be pleasant to be around.

Diet:
1. Bitter foods are key such as ku ding cha and leafy greens. Include at end of every meal to curb appetite.
2. 50-70% vegetables. High percentage raw. Include vegetable juices.
3. 30% lean protein.
4. Minimize carbohydrates.
5. Eat six small meals a day.

Exercise:
Focus on cardio and stimulating movement. (Cardio, spin class, etc.). They need results and instant feedback to stay motivated.

Formulas:
Focus on clearing Heat: Xiang Lian Wan, Huang Lian Su Pian

Combination Deficiency/Excess Type

Symptoms:
Fat is soft. Skin feels loose. Cellulite and varicose veins. Feel cold, tire easily.

Requires harmonizing treatment. Spleen Qi, Blood, and Kidney Yin or Yang deficiency is more pronounced and must be addressed or there will not be any results.

Passive aggressive, repressed personality.

Approach:
Concurrently clear excess and tonify deficiency. Use harmonizing approach. Balance hormones. Avoid extremes.

Diet:
1. Include some bitter. Drink green tea with meals.
2. 50% vegetables. Mostly cooked.
3. 25% lean protein.
4. 25% complex carbohydrates.
5. Eat 6 small meals a day.

Exercise:
Lift weights, heavier for fewer reps. More gentle cardio. Steam room/sauna/hot tub, but not to exhaustion.

Formulas:
Tonify deficiencies to curb cravings:

Weightloss Formula (page 276) + Bu Zhong Yi Qi Tang or Si Wu Tang

PRACTITIONER SECTION: WEIGHTLOSS FORMULA

General Formula – for Spleen and Kidney Deficiency with Phlegm Damp and Blood Stagnation. This formula also lowers cholesterol and high bood pressure:

Dan Shen (salvia) 30g, Jue Ming Zi (cassia seed) 9g, Huang Qi (astragalus)15-30g, Bai Zhu (white atractylodes) 10g, Chuan Xiong (ligusticum) 10g, He Shou Wu (polygonum) 15g, Ze Xie (alisma) 6g, Yin Chen Hao (artemesia) 9g, Yin Yang Huo (epimedium) 10g, Shi Chang Pu (acorus) 9g, Yu Jin (curcuma) 9g, Mai Men Dong (ophiopogonis) 9g.

For constipation, add Da Huang (rhubarb) 1-9g. If there is low stomach acid add Shan Zha (hawthorn berry) 10g.

Be sure to use ear acupressure/acupuncture: Stomach, Shen Men, Mouth, Throat, and Appetite Control. This helps curb addictive eating.

Rapid Weightloss Plan

Table 6.3. Rapid Weightloss Plan

Before Breakfast	Drink 1 cup of warm water with lemon or lime juice or 1 tsp apple cider vinegar
Breakfast	1. Purèed vegetable soup 2. Salad, steamed or stir-fried vegetables – greens, mushrooms, broccoli, turnips, celery, carrots 3. Drink ku ding cha with meals 4. Lean protein
Snack	Purèed vegetable soup
Between Meals	Optional: Slimming Tea or Weight-loss Formula (page 276)
Lunch	1. Purèed vegetable soup 2. Salad, steamed or stir-fried vegetables – greens, mushrooms, broccoli, turnips, celery, carrots 3. Drink ku ding cha with meals 4. Lean protein
Snack	Celery sticks with hummus, apple slices with almond butter, or protein smoothie
Between Meals	Optional: Slimming Tea or Weight-loss Formula
Dinner	1. Purèed vegetable soup 2. Salad, steamed or stir-fried vegetables – greens, mushrooms, broccoli, turnips, celery, carrots 3. Drink ku ding cha with meals 4. Lean protein

Special Considerations (in chronic cases, take formulas for 3-6 months)

Spleen Weakness, Chronic Digestive Issues

Formulas:
Take a Spleen Qi tonic with meals:

- Xiang Sha Liu Jun Zi Tang – general
- Jian Pi Pian – loose stools
- Mu Xiang Shun Qi Pian – constipation and bloating

Chronic Yeast Infection (Dampness with Heat Toxin)

Formulas:
Xiang Sha Yang Wei Wan, Anti-Candida Formula (page 124)

Chronic Sinusitis, Allergies:

Formulas:
Te Xiao Bi Min Gan

Gallstones:

Formulas:

1. Take Gallstone Dissolving Formula (page 267) for 10-20 days prior to flush.
2. At the end of the detox perform Gallstone Purge (page 268).

Excess Weight (Phlegm-Damp):

Formulas:
Eat every 3 hours.
Weightloss formula.

Detox as Spiritual Purification

Ethical Eating

Growing up, my family always kept vegetable gardens. I remember one particular day as a little girl pulling up a carrot and feeling its life force go. It was the moment of realization that in order for me to live, something else had to die. (And with all I ate in a day, quite a bit had to die.) I vaguely remember not eating for a long time (perhaps 12 hours) until I gave up. Everything in this world has consciousness. A plant will cringe when you approach it with garden shears and you can feel the spirit of a lettuce leave when you tear it from the ground. It is a harsh reality that to live we must consume the life of our earthen brothers and sisters. This is the issue for which we must find an acceptable solution.

In the West much is made of the innate selfishness and greed of humanity. However, there is also an innate compassion and need for connection, which are, I believe, stronger. This is because selfishness is born of a lie of separation, while compassion is born of the memory of union that we all carry. Therefore, there can be no lingering happiness until humanity has learned to eat compassionately.

Daoism pragmatically espouses what will optimize health. I do believe, for example, that men can gain strength and vitality from using thousands of women sexually. However, the karmic ramifications would be tremendous. In a society that saw women and the poor as expendable at the time, this was as acceptable as it is now to say black-boned chicken is good for the Blood. Every person must weigh personal benefits with the affect on the whole.

Over the years I tried vegetarianism, veganism, and a raw food diet, all of which were too clearing for my constitution; and none of which cleared my conscience. The conclusion I came to is to eat consciously, graciously, and with as much kindness for all involved as possible. For example, I always ask permission before I take a part of a plant for food or medicine and I always say a prayer of gratitude for every plant or animal killed for my meal and for the labor required to make it. I also choose to eat less meat and augment my diet with herbal Blood tonics.

Spiritual Fasting

From a physical standpoint, fasting is not good for the Spleen Qi and will weaken digestion. There are, however, spiritual reasons to fast. Absolute fasting is only appropriate for strong constitutions. Fasting, either absolutely or on light foods, is helpful for excess constitutions who lack sensitivity to subtle energies. Deficient constitutions are already sensitive and require building and grounding foods (such as whole grains, root vegetables, and protein) to maintain focus during meditation and spiritual exercises.

For spiritual purposes, simple foods are best. Some traditions caution against onions, garlic, and stimulants (coffee, tea, alcohol, chocolate). Excesses in taste or temperature, or too many flavors together are said to increase earthly desire, and thus should be avoided. The safer approach for spiritual detox is to eat simple bland meals and to eat consciously. It will have the same effect of not stimulating the senses and distracting from spirit. Weak Spleen Qi and Phlegm-Damp formation are not conducive to optimal mental functioning.

Starving for Health

Many food sensitivies[20] are surfacing in areas with genetically modified foods, pesticides, and other "modern" methods of farming. Spleen deficient individuals are the most reactive. The answer is not to restrict the diet, but to strengthen the Spleen, take digestive herbs, and only eat the most naturally grown foods available. Otherwise, the increasing restrictions will weaken the Spleen further.

Escapism & Eating Disorders

Not eating or eating light foods makes us less grounded. For those of us who are too dense, this is ideal. Used excessively, it can give a feeling of not being present. I believe there are spiritually evolved beings that have lessened their attachments to their physical bodies. However, superficially imposing this ideal by severely limiting basic human needs of food, comfort, affection, sexuality, etc. is often more unbalancing than helpful. Some use spiritual pursuit as a form of escapism and neglect their bodies as a means to detach from the world around them. Fasting and extreme diets can also become a form of anorexia. Many see restrictive diets such as Raw Veganism as a way of staying thin.

20. For example, there is an increasing number of people with gluten sensitivity and celiac disease due to the way wheat has been modified in the last century. van den Broeck, de Jong, and Salentijn, "Presence of celiac disease epitopes in modern and old hexaploid wheat varieties: wheat breeding may have contributed to increased prevalence of celiac disease," Theor Appl Genet. 2010 Nov; 121(8):1527-39. doi: 10.1007/s00122-010-1408-4. Epub 2010 Jul 28. (http://www.ncbi.nlm.nih.gov/pubmed/20664999?dopt=Abstract).

Chapter 7

Age 49

7 x 7 , The Ren channel is empty, the Chong channel depleted, the dew of Heaven dries up, the Earth Passage (uterus) is not open, so weakness and infertility set in.

七七，任脉虚，太冲脉衰少，天癸竭，地道不通，故形坏而无子也。（49岁）

The 7th Cycle

Seven x 7 years begins the 7th Cycle in a woman's life. Between the ages of 49 to 55, women enter the Water Phase. The Water Phase is characterized by depth, wisdom, and surrender.

The 7th Cycle brings a depletion in Kidney Jing. This causes a decline in activity in the uterus and ovaries, ceasing of monthly bleeding, and the end to reproduction. Most menopausal issues, however, are caused by Liver imbalance. When menopausal symptoms arise, the focus is still to treat the Liver. After menopause, the focus shifts to strengthening the Spleen.

The passage from the Yellow Emperor above cautions what can happen if we do not take care of ourselves. Some women, even with a suboptimal lifestyle, menstruate until they are 60. While menstruation and fertility will eventually cease, vitality does not have to. We have an opportunity at this time to boost the Jing (hormones). This chapter covers how to reverse menopausal symptoms and issues that affect all of us when we are under stress and not taking proper care of ourselves.

Menopause; Second Spring

In this phase, the Kidney Jing, our reserves of creative energy, declines and we no longer have extra Qi to give to a new life. In Western terms, the ovaries decrease their production of estrogen and shrink.[1] Menstruation will cease around age 50 for many women, though others continue menstruating until 60, and some women stop as early as 45. A woman officially reaches menopause when she ceases menstruating for one year. The most salient symptoms in a healthy woman are vaginal dryness and minor hot flashes. The eyes may begin to recede and there will be changes in skin texture, otherwise it should be uneventful. This, however, runs contrary to the experience of many women in modern times. Just like abnormalities with our menstruation, the pathology has become the norm because we were never taught what "normal" was or how to properly care for ourselves. The decade prior to menopause is a crucial time to lay the foundation for an easy transition.

Menopausal Karma

What has come to be considered "normal menopause" is akin to a complete breakdown of the body. In the common scenario, we push ourselves to the limit for years, perhaps decades; much like constantly withdrawing from our checking account and never putting money in. Eventually our reserves of Jing run dry. We can no longer sustain a suboptimal lifestyle, and years of accumulations and deficiencies surface. Menopause provides both a challenge and an opportunity to change the state of our health. Like menstrual issues, menopausal symptoms are clear indicators of where we are imbalanced. This makes menopause the 3rd Golden Opportunity to change our constitution.

A decline in Kidney Jing means that both Kidney Yin and Yang become more deficient during menopause. Most women exhibit proportionately more Kidney Yin deficiency with Heat symptoms. Women who are more Yang deficient (i.e. cold, no heat signs) do not need to avoid hot-natured foods and drink.[2] Additionally Liver imbalances, Spleen Qi deficiency, and Heart issues may surface. The decline in Jing and concurrent Blood and Qi deficiency creates increased sensitivity (emotionally and physically).

If the Liver is imbalanced, menopause feels like a never-ending premenstrual time manifesting with anger, depression, and a constant unsettled feeling. Typical menopausal imbalance symptoms include hot flashes, 5 Hearts Heat (heat in the head, palms, and soles of the feet), irritability, insomnia, aches and pains, fatigue, itchiness, and memory loss. This chapter addresses optimizing health during menopause, as well as healing the root of menopausal symptoms. The guidance in this chapter applies to overworked (and Yin deficient) women of any age.

---

1. The Ovarian Massage (page 142) stimulates the ovaries to stay active and producing hormones. The ovaries produce hormones even if you are no longer menstruating.

2. With monthly bleeding, childbearing, and caretaking, women tend to become Blood deficient, which leads to more Yin deficiency. Men tend to become more Qi deficient, which leads to more Yang deficiency. Though this is not always the case

Diet and Lifestyle Rules During Menopause

During menopause there are some additional rules to prevent overheating the Liver and weakening the Kidneys:

1. Avoid Yang drinks such as coffee, alcohol (especially red wine), and even in some cases, tea.[3] These increase Heat in the body.
2. Avoid spicy foods, lamb, and excess animal protein (above 25% of the diet). Be sure to get adequate protein each day or sugar cravings will increase.
3. No smoking. Cigarettes and marijuana consume Yin and generate Heat in the body, exacerbating the primary pathology during menopause. It also leeches Vitamin C from the skin, accelerating skin aging.[4]
4. Avoid sugar. Excess sweets in the diet create Dampness and weaken the Spleen leading to illness and excess weight later on. The drop in hormones will often trigger sugar cravings in the body's attempt to rapidly increase Qi in the body. Treat this with Qi, Blood, and Kidney tonics (and low doses of bioidentical hormones if necessary). This is key to avoiding weight gain during menopause.
5. Eat Jing-tonifying foods and herbs (see below and "Menopausal Recipes" on page 374).
6. Perform rejuvenation qigong and Dao-Yin to maintain joint health and mobility (see below).

Top 10 Jing Tonics

Women in their late 40s onwards should take Jing tonics regularly to maintain brain functioning, promote joint health, and to increase overall vitality and youthfulness. Women with constitutional Jing weakness (slow development, infertility) or high stress lifestyles should begin taking these tonics earlier.

1. **Dong Chong Xia Cao** (cordyceps) – Is the fungus of a special caterpillar and a powerful longevity tonic. It nourishes the Jing and Kidney Yang. It also tonifies the Lungs, stops bleeding, and dissolves Phlegm. Cordyceps is the premiere herb to restore energy and to boost the immune system. It is often used in the treatment of cancer (particularly of the lungs), hyperlipidemia, and hypertension. It can be used in cooking or powdered; alone or added to other formulas. Cordyceps is one of the most expensive herbs. The cultivated variety is more reasonable. Standard dosage is 5-10g of the raw herb daily.

2. **Lu Rong** (deer antler) – Is a powerful herb for Kidney Jing and Yang deficiency for conditions such as infertility, underdevelopment in children, and weakness of tendons and

3. Green tea is most cooling and usually well tolerated during menopause.

4. Dr. Richard Huber.

bones.[5] Lu Rong nourishes the Ren (sea of Yin) and Chong (sea of Blood) channels to treat severe anemia.[6] It is more expensive and stronger in action than the gelatin (Lu Jiao Jiao) or deer horn fragments (Lu Jiao Shuang) that can be used as substitutes. Standard dosage is 5-10g of the raw herb daily.

3. **Zi He Che** (placenta) – Is considered a premiere Jing tonic since it is the product of the Jing of the parents. Placenta supports the development of and guards against atrophy of the reproductive organs. It is especially effective postpartum for general recovery and for insufficient lactation. Other than postpartum, when women can use their own placenta, pig or cow placenta are commonly used. Standard dosage is 3-9g of the raw herb daily.

4. H**uang Jing** (King Solomon's seal rhizome) – Nourishes the Yin of the Kidneys and Lungs, tonifies Spleen Qi, and tonifies the Jing. It is ideal for cases of Yin deficiency with Spleen Qi deficiency. It can be too clawing (moistening) for cases of Dampness. Huang Jing also regulates blood pressure, removes fat from the blood, and lowers blood cholesterol. It can be taken in formula or used in Food Therapy. Standard dosage is 10-15g of the raw herb daily.

5. **Rou Cong Rong** (cistanche) – Is a mild and non-clawing herb that tonifies Blood, Kidney Yang, and Jing. It lubricates the bowels to promote bowel movement. Rou Cong Rong can be paired with Yin Yang Huo (epimedium) to boost libido. It is one of the better tasting herbs and lends itself for use in Food Therapy. Standard dose is 10-20g of the raw herb daily.

6. **Yin Yang Huo** (epimedium) – Is a widely used and safe libido enhancer for for both men and women. It strengthens both Kidney Yin and Yang, though more so Yang. Ten-15g of the raw herb can be added to the appropriate formula to boost libido. Yin Yang Huo also expels Wind Cold Damp conditions (alleviates joint pain). Yi Yang Huo should be taken with caution in Yin deficient individuals.[7]

7. **Bone Marrow** – Is an important Jing nourishing food. It nourishes the bones, skin, hair, and nails. It rejuvenates the joints by strengthening tendons, cartilage, and connective tissue. Bone marrow also directly builds marrow and supports brain functioning. Use long bones cut in cross sections along with a small amount of vinegar to make soup stocks. This will extract the marrow and minerals from the bones and deliver them in a form that is easy to assimilate. Bone marrow stock can be used at any age, and is especially important

5. Lu Rong promotes healing of broken bones.
6. The Ren and Chong channels are deeply tied to hormonal functioning in women.
7. Do not take long-term or else pair with moistening herbs.

during menopause and beyond at which time it should be used several times a week as the base for soups.

8. **Hai Shen** (sea cucumber) – Tonifies Kidney Yang and Jing. It is used almost exclusively in food, and not in herbal formulas. Standard dosage is 30-60g.

9. **Hu Tao Ren** (walnut) – Is a mild herb/food that is very effective when used frequently in food or teas. It tonifies the Kidneys and Jing, stops wheezing, and lubricates the bowels to promote bowel movement. It also strengthens the bones and restores luster to the hair. Walnuts can be combined with He Shou Wu (polygonum) for thinning hair. Standard dosage is 10-30g.

10. **Chestnuts** – Are also a mild herb/food that can be eaten daily during winter time, in congees, stews, or baking. They strengthen Jing and Kidney Yang, tonify the Spleen, move the Blood, and dispel Wind Damp (joint pain). Chestnuts are used for pain in legs and lower back, frequent urination, poor memory, and other signs of Kidney decline.

Longevity Exercises

These are short exercises that can be incorporated into other health routines.

Exercise 7.1. Dropping the Heels

It is said in TCM that trouble starts in the feet as we age. Stand hip width apart. Stand on your toes then quickly drop your heels to the ground. Do this 10-20 times, every day.

Exercise 7.2. Keeping the Spine Supple (Figure 7.1)

Be sure to bend your spine in every direction and hang upside down daily. Perform a form of back bend, bend forward, and twist daily. The specific exercise can vary based on your ability, flexibility, and comfort level. Performing a form of inversion (such as a head or handstand) daily is excellent for anti-aging.

Hanging upside down provides the added benefit of decompressing the spine. There are machines made specifically to hang upside down. You can also use the back extension machine at the gym. Stay in the start position with your head and arms hanging. Breathe deeply and relax. Start with 1 min. and work up to 5. Get up very slowly and hold onto the machine until you have recovered your balance.

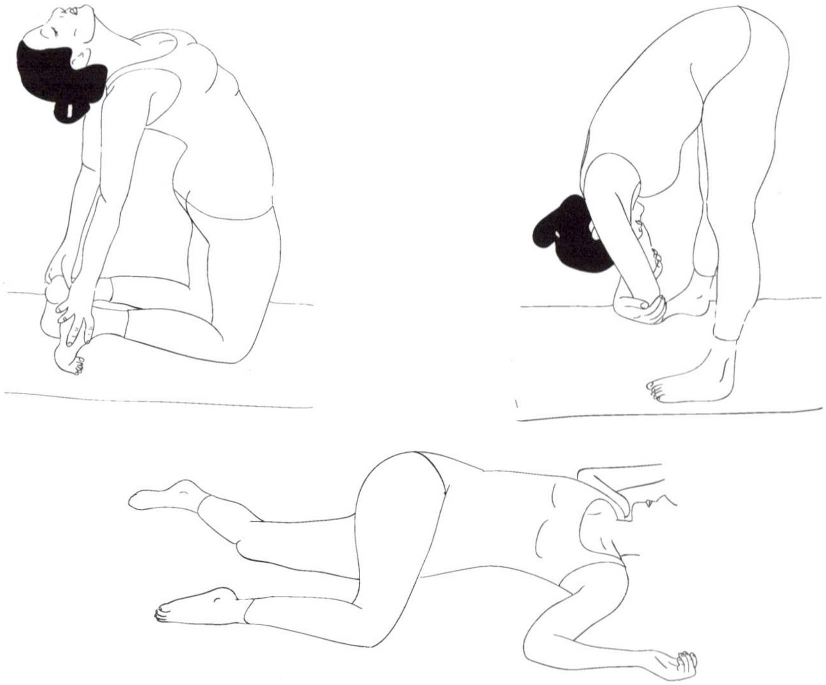

Figure 7.1. Spine Stretches

Exercise 7.3. Perineum Breathing[8] (Figure 7.2)

This can be used as a daily longevity exercise or for problems in the genital region: yeast infections, low libido, UTI, menstrual issues, and prostate inflammation. Do not perform this exercise right before or after sex.

Sit on the edge of a chair. Focus your attention on your perineum[9] and keep it there for the whole exercise.

Inhale. Pull the perineum up into the body (imagine a center line from your perineum to the top of your head). Hold for 2 seconds.

Exhale and relax completely.

Women should perform the exercise for 24 breaths (men for 36).

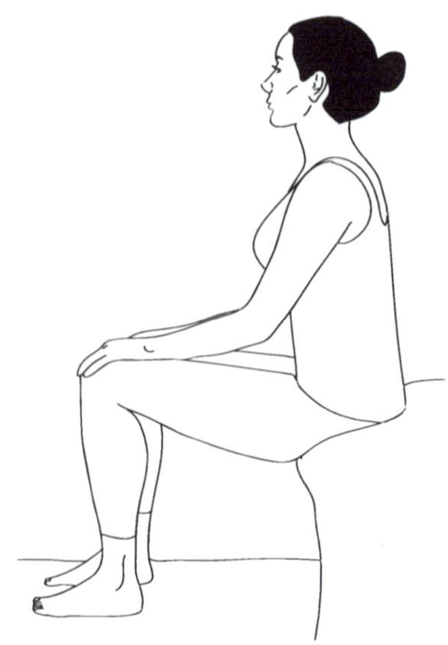

Figure 7.2. Perineum Breathing

8. Modified from Merle Morgan-Drennan. "Medical Qigong I" (lecture, Yo San University, Los Angeles, October 31, 2001). (student of Master Hong Liu)

9. Located between the genitals and anus.

Exercise 7.4. Warming the Kidneys (Figure 7.3)

Perform nightly before bed to tonify the Kidneys. This is a great exercise for those without much time.

Sit on your bed or chair. Rub your hands vigorously until they are warm.

Rub the Kidneys up and down 36 times. The Kidneys are located on the back of the body, under the bottom ribs.

Hold your palms over your Kidneys and feel the warmth penetrating into them. I like to visualize a Golden light warming and strengthening my Kidneys.

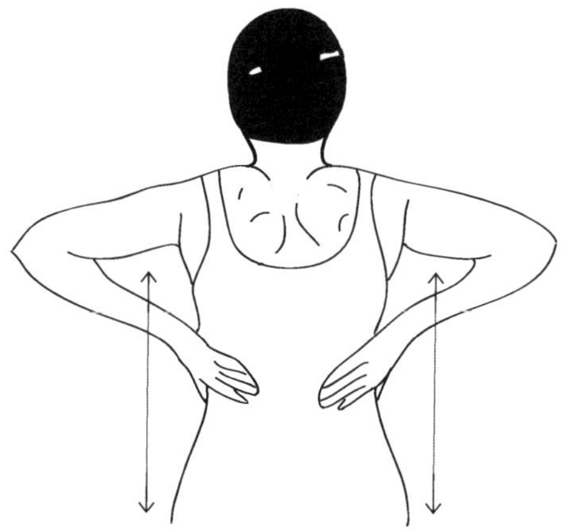

Figure 7.3. Warming the Kidneys

Key Menopausal Patterns

Heart and Kidney Disharmony

This pattern is the most common dysfunction of menopause, though it can occur at any age. It refers to a deficiency of Heart and Kidney Yin with Excess Fire. It is often caused by emotional stress, overwork, heartbreak, blood loss, and/or decline in Jing.

Symptoms:
Mental restlessness, insomnia, poor memory, palpitations, soreness and weakness of the low back, dream-disturbed sleep, dizziness, tinnitus, dry mouth, night sweats, 5 Hearts Heat, hot flashes, mouth sores, and menstrual irregularities.

Excess Above, Deficiency Below

The majority of menopausal symptoms originate from a mixed pattern. The decline of Kidney energy is compounded with the accumulations of years of a modern lifestyle. This means that during perimenopause, both excesses and deficiencies surface. This manifests as combination deficiency and excess symptoms such as weak low back and knees with upper back tension, lack of energy with insomnia, hot and cold conditions, night sweats with obesity.

PRACTITIONER SECTION:

During perimenopause and with combination excess and deficiency conditions, there is often Gallbladder deficiency. Palpate the Gallbladder channel for tender points.

Addressing Menopausal Symptoms

Dryness

Internal Dryness will create a withered complexion and thin the healthy padding under the skin. Always maintain enough Yin to plump up the skin. The ancient Chinese texts advocated keeping an inch reserve layer of fat in case of illness or famine. A little layer of fat will also make the skin look taught. This is the same reasoning behind injectable fillers used in cosmetic procedures.

Vaginal Dryness

Vaginal dryness is a hallmark symptom of menopause, even in healthy women, and is a symptom of Yin deficiency. In biomedical terms it is a sign of estrogen deficiency.

Moisturizing Diet

Diet Plan:
Eat soups and congees.

Sip water throughout the day. Drinking large quantities of water at once taxes the Kidneys and passes through the body quickly.

Beneficial Foods:
Bai Mu Err (white cloud fungus), Shan Yao (Chinese Yam), sesame seeds, nuts, tofu, winter squash, pumpkin, pears, mulberries, seaweed, millet, wheat, and good quality mineralized salt.

Increase Lubrication Formula[1]

This simple, effective formula contains just two herbs. Maintaining balanced vaginal lubrication is not only a sexual issue, it is also a health issue. Lack of vaginal secretions make the vagina more susceptible to infections (UTI, yeast, etc.), and makes the delicate skin prone to tears.

Xu Duan (dipsacus) 9-12g, Nu Zhen Zi (privet fruit) 30g

1. Jiang Zheng. "TCM Gynecology" (lecture, Pacific College of Oriental Medicine, San Diego, February 18, 2007).

General Menopausal Formula

Zhi Mu (anemarrhena), Huang Bai (phellodendron), Yin Yang Huo (epimedium), Huang Lian (coptis), Ge Gen (kudzu), Dan Shen (salvia), Gou Qi Zi (go ji berries), Shan Zha (hawthorn berry), Ju Hua (chrysanthemum), green tea

Treats general menopausal symptoms: hot flashes, insomnia, 5 Hearts Heat, low back weakness and soreness, irritability.

Minimize:
Red adzuki beans, coffee, tea, raw Yi Yi Ren, cornsilk, and mung beans. Take particular care during weightloss ventures; for a weightloss plan to be effective it must dry Dampness. Eat plenty of moistening foods and avoid overheating the body with excessive cardio (more than 45 min, 3 times a week).

Lifestyle:
1. Avoid excessive sweating: sauna, hot room yoga, too much cardio.
2. Acupuncture and massage.

Formula:
Liu Wei Di Huang Wan modifications

Excess Heat

Hot Flashes and Night Sweats

Like vaginal dryness, these are classic menopause signs. In a healthy woman, hot flashes and night sweats will still occur but will not be severe or as frequent. In many women, however, these symptoms are incapacitating. Hot flashes and night sweats are attributed to Kidney Yin deficiency with Heat. In clinical practice, it also relates to Liver excess.[10] The more "Livery"[11] the woman, the worse the hot flashes and night sweats, the more angry she is about them, and the more combative she is about keeping the ambient temperature cool.

PRACTITIONER SECTION: NIGHT SWEAT FORMULA[1]

Chai Hu (bupleurum) 6g, Huang Qin (scutellaria) 6g, Gui Zhi (cinnamon twig) 6g, Ban Xia (pinellia) 9g, Bai Shao (white peony root) 9g, Dang Gui (Chinese angelica) 12g, Gou Teng (gambir vine) 9g, Wu Wei Zi (shizandra berries) 6g, Huai Xiao Mai (wheat) 12g, Gan Cao (licorise root) 6g, Duan Mu Li (calcined oyster shell) 15g, Yin Yang Huo (epimedium) 9g, Huang Bai (phellodendron) 9g.

1. Modified from Shaoting Jing. "TCM Gynecology." (lecture, Yo San University, Los Angeles, June 19, 2004).

Cooling Diet

Diet Plan:
1. Include raw foods in your diet.[12]
2. Eat 50% vegetables.
3. Take milk thistle tincture daily.

10. Huabing Wen. "Acupuncture Anatomy & Therapeutics" (lecture, Yo San University, Los Angeles, September 10, 2001).

11. A "Livery" person is someone who exhibits Liver Qi stagnation and Liver Heat. There are typically attendant control, irritability, and boundary issues as well as physical symptoms.

12. Do not become extreme, however, as an excessive raw diet, especially with liberal garlic intake, will create severe Yin deficiency with Heat over time.

Beneficial Foods:
Summer squash, sprouts, seaweed, wheat grass juice, algae, lettuce, cucumber, spinach, eggplant, millet, wheat, white rice, and calcium.

Minimize:
Avoid spicy food, coffee, garlic, and red wine. Absolutely no smoking. No stimulants. Limit other alcohol and tea. Green tea is best tolerated. Make sure hot flashes and night sweats are not side effects of medication.

Lifestyle:
1. Avoid excessive sweating: sauna, hot room yoga, too much cardio.
2. Acupuncture and massage.
3. Practice daily relaxation.

Formulas:
Jiao Wei Xiao Yan San + Gan Ma Da Zao Tang + Long Gu (fossilized bone), Mu Li (oyster shell)
or
Zhi Bai Di Huang Wan + Gan Mai Da Zao Tang

Steaming Bone Disorder

Steaming bone disorder is a symptom of severe Yin deficiency with Heat. Women describe it as feeling like heat is radiating from their bones but their skin is cool to the touch. Follow a cooling, moistening diet as described above.

Formulas:
Zhi Bai Di Huang Wan + Gui Ban (tortoise shell)

Migraine Headaches

Migraine headaches can occur at any age, but tend to flare up during times of hormonal upheaval. Women often experience migraines premenstrually and during perimenopause. Migraines are due to ascendant Liver Yang, either to pure excess or mixed with Kidney Yin deficiency.

Symptoms:
Severe headache, often one-sided, often near the eye, worse with activity, worse with exposure to light and sound, may include nausea or vomiting, can last for hours or days.

Diet Plan:
1. Include soups and congees in your diet.
2. Eat 50% vegetables.
3. Take milk thistle tincture daily.

Beneficial Foods:
Summer squash, sprouts, seaweed, wheat grass juice, algae, black sesame seeds, mulberries, Gou Qi Zi (go ji berries), lettuce, cucumber, spinach, eggplant, millet, wheat, white rice, and calcium.

Minimize:
Sugar, alcohol, cigarettes, and processed foods. Avoid stimulants such as coffee, tea, chocolate, and other caffeinated foods, though they can offer temporary relief during a migraine attack. Chemical additives, food allergies, and pesticides also may be a contributing factor.

PRACTITIONER SECTION: TREATING MIGRAINES

LV 5 is very effective to relieve migraines. Long-term treatment consists of clearing Liver excess (de-stressing and detoxifying), releasing tension in the upper back and neck, and nourishing Yin.

Lifestyle:
Soak your feet in hot water at first sign of a migraine. Acupuncture and massage, especially 1-2 weeks before menses.

Practice relaxation. Avoid excessive sweating: sauna, hot room yoga, too much cardio. Acupuncture and massage.

Formulas:
At first signs of a migraine, take a double dosage of Long Dan Xie Gan Tang. Take Tian Ma Gou Teng Yin long-term.

High Blood Pressure

Many women who have low blood pressure all of their lives develop high blood pressure around menopause. This is due to Yin deficiency. Combine Tian Ma Gou Teng Yin with Zhi Bai Di Huang Wan. Taking fish oil daily is effective for some women.

Sleep Disorders

Insomnia

After noon, Yin energy slowly grows and the body naturally begins to wind down and draw inward. Following the natural rhythm, one should retire by 10 p.m. At midnight, Yang begins to rise again, and by 6 or 7 a.m. the body naturally wakes up. When the Yin energy is weak or the Yang is excess (as in Heat or Stagnation), it is difficult to settle down and sleep at night.

Good sleep is defined as falling asleep soon after going to bed, sleeping soundly through the night, and waking up feeling rested. Anything less is considered insomnia, which includes: difficulty falling asleep, waking up frequently during the night, staying awake all night, tossing and turning, or dream-disturbed sleep. Insomnia can be an issue at any time in life. With hormonal changes, insomnia can become a serious issue during menopause. The relative decline in Yin can make it difficult for women to settle down, especially at night.

Practices for Good Sleep

Sleep is a habit. Creating a soothing ritual around bedtime can be very helpful in establishing good sleep habits. The goal is to ground over-activity in the brain down to the feet and reduce external stimulation. Choose from the following and see which ones are most effective for you.

1. Start slowing down by 8 or 9 p.m. Shut down lights and sounds gradually to mimic what happens outdoors. Perhaps do your bedtime routine by candlelight with soft music. Be in bed ready to sleep by 10 p.m.
2. Avoid TV, work, internet, or strong mental stimulation an hour before bed. This will keep the mind active and unable to shut off.
3. Daily quiet time is necessary for most people to stay healthy and sane. Before bed is an excellent time to do a relaxing stretching routine, qigong, chanting, prayer, affirmations, or simply sitting in stillness.
4. Make sure to eat your final meal by 6:30 or 7 p.m. This should be the smallest, simplest meal of the day. A full stomach can interrupt a full night's sleep. Those with unstable blood sugar can have some protein before bed.[13] Carbohydrates before bed can be very unsettling.
5. Have acupuncture 3-4 hours before bedtime. (Si Shen Cong, HT 7, SP 6, KD 1, Pc 8, are all very helpful).
6. Shen calming herbs should be taken before going to bed. (See formulas and Insomnia Patterns below).
7. Soak feet in hot water. A traditional formula is to add Chinese rice wine, strong ginger tea, Epsom salts, and hot water to a basin. Make it as hot as you can stand it and keep feet in until it has cooled to room temperature.
8. Massage feet before bed. A simple practice you can do yourself: use the heel of one foot to rub/massage the arch of the other foot. Do so 36 times each foot.Then use the arch of one foot to rub/massage the top of the other foot. Do so 36 times each foot. (Figure 7.4)
9. Use calming scents in your room, on your clothes, or on your body. Scent has a deep effect on the brain. Using calming essential oils and fragrances on a regular basis to create an instant ritual. Try hops, lavender or chamomile.

13. This is especially helpful for children.

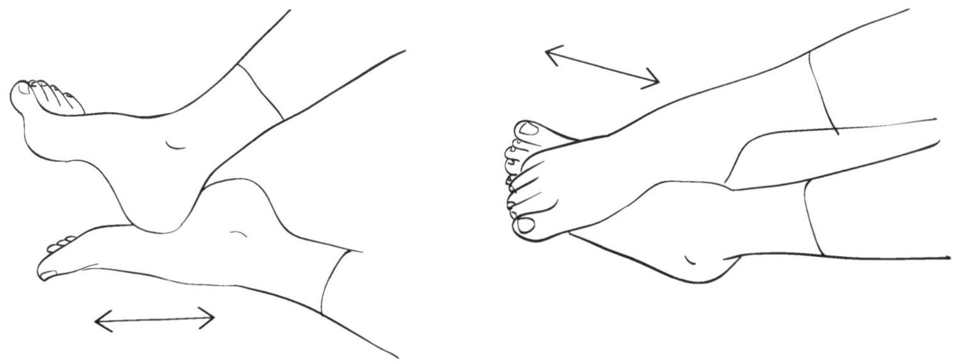

Figure 7.4. Foot Massage

Insomnia Patterns

Heart and Kidney Yin deficiency (Heart and Kidney disharmony)

Symptoms:
Most common perimenopausal pattern. Difficulty falling and staying asleep. Irritable and restless. Tinnitus (ear ringing). 5 Heart Heat.

Remedies:
Tian Wang Bu Xin Dan + Long Gu (fossilized bone), Mu Li (oyster shell)(take 3x a day)

Liver Qi Stagnation with Fire

Symptoms:
Most common pattern for all ages. Can combine with any of the others. Stressed out. Cannot shut the mind off. Hard to fall asleep. Irritated at inability to sleep. Excessive, active or violent dreams. May also have headache, dry mouth, tongue or mouth sores, excess thirst, and dark scanty urine.

Remedies:
Jia Wei Xiao Yao San (take 3 x a day)

Blood Stagnation

Symptoms:
Stubborn case often with chronic, severe depression. History of physical or emotional trauma.

Remedies:
Yunnan Paiyao (take 2 capsules, 3 x a day)

Food Stagnation

Symptoms:
Cannot fall asleep. Eating late at night. Abdominal bloating.

Remedies:
Bao He Wan (with meal). Eat by 7 pm. Eat lightest meal at night.

Simple Sleep Formulas:

Taking Shen (spirit) calming herbs before bed is very helpful for optimal sleep.

Lily Flower Tea:

Place lily flowers (about 1 tbsp of flowers per cup) in a teapot.(1) Bring water to a boil. Pour into teapot and steep for 5-10 min.

Lily flowers (Bai He Hua) clears heat in the Heart (soothes agitation) and calms the Shen (nerves). It is said to increase happiness in the Heart. It can be used in equal parts with He Huan Hua(2) (floss silk flower) for a stronger sedative effect. This combination has the added effect of easing heartbreak. He Huan Hua soothes the Liver and Heart, relaxes the muscles, and eases depression. Other flowers can be added to increase the soothing experience: osmanthus (incredible aroma), rose (moves Liver Qi), and lavender (relaxes the muscles). These flowers also beautify the skin.

Suan Zao Ren (sour jujube seed) Tea:

Crush 20g of Suan Zao Ren (sour jujube seed) with a mortar and pestle. Put in a pot with 2 cups of water and bring to a boil. Simmer for 20 min. Suan Zao Ren astringes Liver Yin and calms the Shen (nerves).

Herbal Paste:

A paste of herbs can be applied to KD 1 area (Figure 7.5) and a Band-Aid placed over it before bed. KD 1 is the most grounding point on the body. It strongly anchors an overactive mind as well as manic conditions

Formula 1: Grind Suan Zao Ren (sour jujube seed), Mu Li (oyster shell), and Long Gu (fossilized bone) in equal parts and mix with vinegar to form a thick paste.

Formula 2: Grind Huang Lian (coptis) and Rou Gui (cinnamon bark) in equal parts and mix with vinegar to form a thick paste.

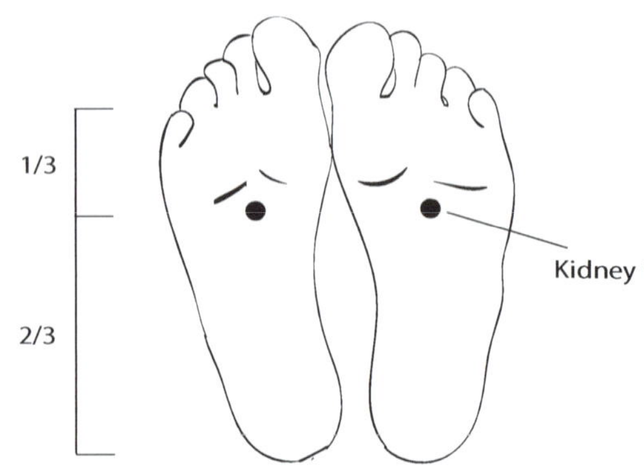

Figure 7.5. Kidney 1

1. Flower teas are traditionally steeped in a little glass teapot so that you can enjoy their beauty. This is not necessary for medicinal reasons, but I prefer this as it adds to the ritual of staying present and slowing down.
2. There are two flowers commonly sold by the name He Huan Hua. Officially it is the Floss Silk Tree Flower. A type of magnolia flower is often used under the same name. I find this magnolia flower to be more relaxing on the muscles.

Heart Blood and Spleen Qi Deficiency

Symptoms:
Common with studen[illegible] overwork. Lots of dreams. Wakes up easily. Poor memory. Fatigue. Poor appetit[illegible]

Remedies:
Gui Pi Tang (take[illegible]

Heart and Gallbl[illegible]

Symptoms:
Light sleeper[illegible]g the night. May wake suddenly. Easily startled. Scared at night. Timid. [illegible]

Remedies:
An Shen Ding Zhi Wan + Suan Zao Ren Tang (big dose at night)*

Liver Blood and/or Yin deficiency

Symptoms:
Trouble falling or staying asleep. Irritability. Forgetfulness. Impatience. Night sweats. Poor eyesight. Dizziness. Palpitations.

Remedies:
Suan Zao Ren Tang + Gan Mai Da Zao Tang (big dose at night)*

* Take a large dose of pills two hours before bed. If larger pills, take 10 pills. If small tea pills take 30 pills at once. If taking a decoction take a larger dose two hours before bed.

Fatigue

Movement and energy are Qi and Yang functions of the body. When the Yang energy is weak or the Yin (Phlegm-Damp) is in excess, it is difficult to wake up in the morning. If Spleen Qi is weak, or Liver Qi is stagnant, energy levels will not be consistent.

A little trick to wake yourself up is to stimulate the tip of your nose with a pen or your finger nail. (Figure 7.6).

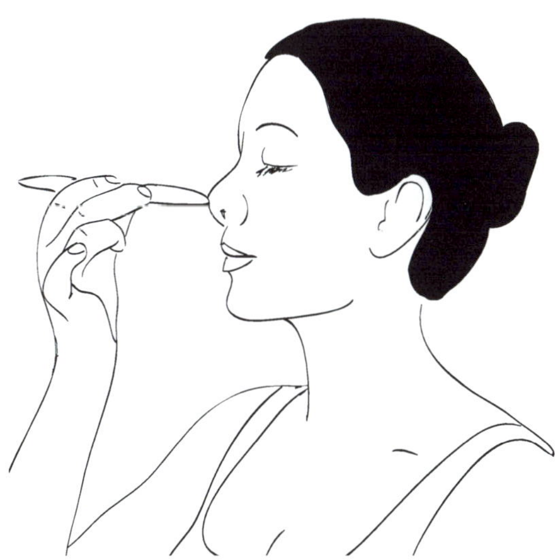

Figure 7.6. Stimulate Tip of Nose

Patterns of Fatigue

Spleen Qi deficiency with Dampness

Symptoms:
Difficulty getting up in the morning. Tired after meals. Foggy-headed.

Remedies:
Ping Wei San. Take Damp-drying Congee (page 327) first thing in the morning daily.

Qi and Blood Deficiency

Symptoms:
Tired after meals. Dips in energy throughout the day. Low blood sugar. In severe cases chronic fatigue and fibromyalgia.

Remedies:
Bu Zhong Yi Qi Tang. Gui Pi Tang. Huang Qi Gui Zhi Wu Wu Tang (page 303)

Kidney Deficiency

Symptoms:
General fatigue. Low back and knee pain and weakness.

Remedies:
Energy Booster (page 298).

Liver Qi Stagnation

Symptoms:
Associated with stress and depression. Better with movement or vacation.

Remedies:

Jia Wei Xiao Yao San or Shu Gan Wan

Energy Booster[1]

Chai Hu (bupleurum) 6g, Huang Qi (astragalus) 20g, Gui Zhi (cinnamon twig) 6g, Ban Xia (prunellia) 9g, Bai Shao (white peony root) 9g, Ba Ji Tian (morinda) 9g, Tai Zi Shen (pseudostellaria)9g, Yin Yang Huo (epimedii) 9g, Zhi Gan Cao (prepared licorise root) 6g, Dang Gui (Chinese angelica)12g.

1. Modified from Shaoting Jing. "TCM Gynecology." (lecture, Yo San University, Los Angeles, June 19, 2004).

Aches and Pains

Wind Damp Bi syndrome (joint pain, aches and pains) becomes increasingly common after menopause (and andropause[14] in men) unless we take action to prevent it. Women are more susceptible. A good general remedy is to make Du Zhong Wine (page 374) and take a small cup daily. Formulas containing the 3 Immortals (Yin Yang Huo (epimedium), Ba Ji Tian (morinda root), and Xian Mao (curculigo)) and the Bone Building formulas (page 303) are very effective, since there is always an element of Kidney deficiency. At the beginning of menopause there may be too much Heat in the system for some of these remedies, so use caution.

Dao Yin is a yoga-esque style of qigong specific for maintaining joint mobility and health and preventing joint pain of Wind Damp Bi syndrome. It is highly recommended for everyone, but especially helpful starting at around age 45, to perform these exercises a few times a week or daily.[15]

50s Shoulder

Around 50 years of age, many people develop immobility, stiffness, and pain in one or both of their shoulders. In severe cases the shoulder will actually become frozen. Acupuncture is necessary for treatment along with the following exercises to be performed daily.

Exercise 7.5. Shoulder Rolls (Figure 7.7)

This is taken from the Dao Yin sequence of exercises. Begin with 1-2 reps. Increase by 1-2 reps and work up to 36 times.

1. Perform in a seated position. Place your right hand on your right hip with your elbow angled out to the side. Perform super slow and exaggerated shoulder rolls backwards. You will likely hear a little cracking at first. Perform the movement in a way that you do not experience pain.
2. Repeat on left hand side.

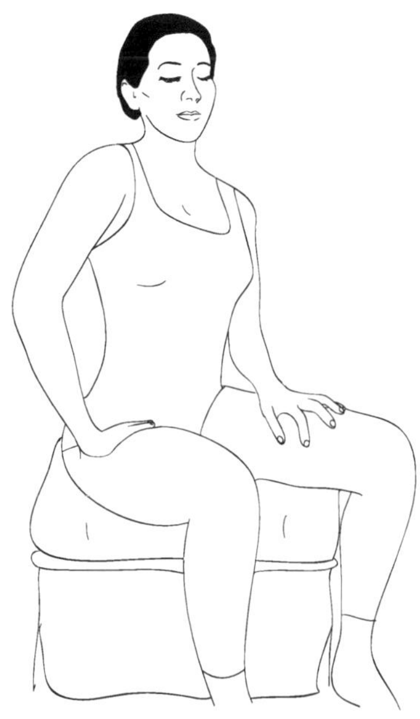

Figure 7.7. Shoulder Rolls

14. Men experience a similar drop in hormones in 40s, 50s, or 60s as women. Reduced testosterone levels are associated with changes in muscle mass, libido, sexual potency, mood, and energy.

15. Huaching Ni. *Attune Your Body With Dao-In.* (Santa Monica: Seven Star Communications, 1989).

se 7.6. *Climbing the Wall* (Figure 7.8)

ı front of a wall and use your fingers (of your restricted shoulder) to climb up the wall to your limitation. Push the limitation a little, but not enough to cause pain. Perform 1 repetition throughout the day when you remember.

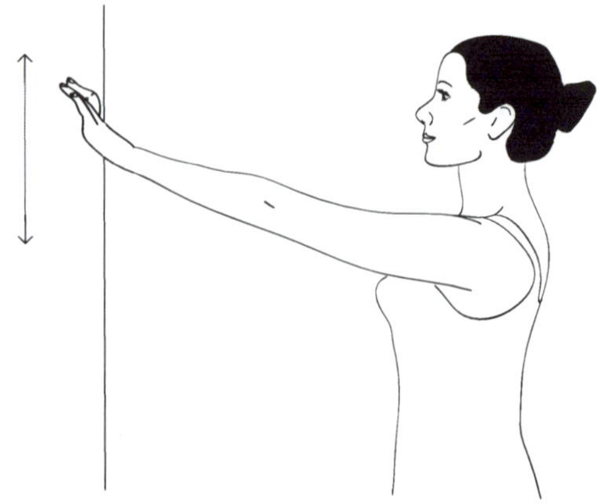

Figure 7.8. Climbing the Wall

Low Back Pain

Low back pain and weakness can happen at any age, but is more common during and after menopause. The knees and low back are connected to the Kidneys.[16] Trauma, aging, constitution, and a rough lifestyle all can weaken the Kidneys, low back, and knees.

The lower back and knees are prone to deficiency and attacks of Cold and Damp. The Kidneys like warmth. Use ice in these areas only after immediate trauma where the skin feels hot to the touch. Applying cold to these areas other than after acute trauma will cause chronic pain, impeded circulation, and stiffness.

Exercise 7. 7. Sacral Opener Qigong

This exercise is a modification of a sandara yoga routine. It gently, yet powerfully, opens up the sacral region and is used to treat a number of gynecological, knee, and Kidney- related maladies such as: sciatica, chronic low back pain or weakness, chronic knee pain or weakness, infertility, emotional trauma lodged in the womb or genitals, prostatitis,[17] chronic bloating, bowel irregularity, and menstrual cramps. The exercises should be performed daily, along with acupuncture treatments, until the condition clears. They can be used daily or once a week as a preventive. This is also a nice relaxing exercise to perform before bed with soft music playing in the background.

1. Integration pose (Figure 7.9): Lie down on your back with your knees and feet elevated at 90 degrees. You can use bolsters, pillows, or furniture. Just make yourself as comfortable as possible. Make sure your buttocks are against the bolsters. When you are in the right position you will feel your sacrum flat

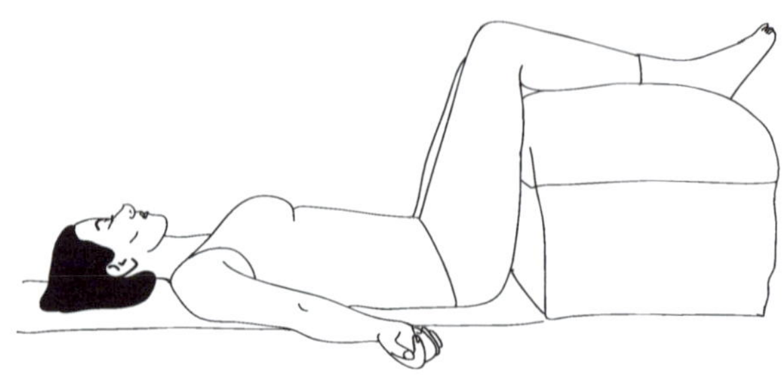

Figure 7.9. Integration Pose

16. The physical Kidney organs are located under the bottom ribs in the back. The entire lower back and sacrum are energetically tied to the Kidneys.

17. Inflammation of the prostate gland causing urinary and sexual dysfunction.

on the floor and your hip bones sit in your hip sockets. Completely relax and let your knees float apart. Do deep belly breathes for 5 min.[18]

2. (Figure 7.10): Bring both knees to the chest. Place hands under the knees and clasp your fingers. Do not strain. Just relax. Breathe deeply for 5 min.
3. Return to Integration Pose for 5 min.
4. (Figure 7.11): Bring your right knee to your chest and clasp your hands under your knee. Hold for 5 min.
5. Return to Integration Pose for 5 min.
6. (Figure 7.11): Repeat with left knee.
7. Return to Integration Pose for 5 min.

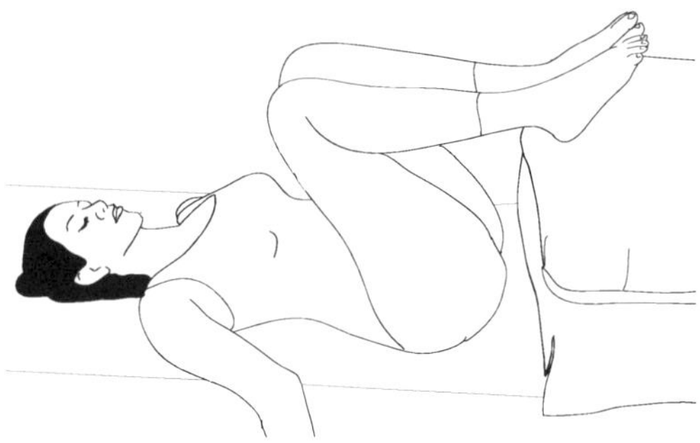

Figure 7.10. Both Knees to Chest

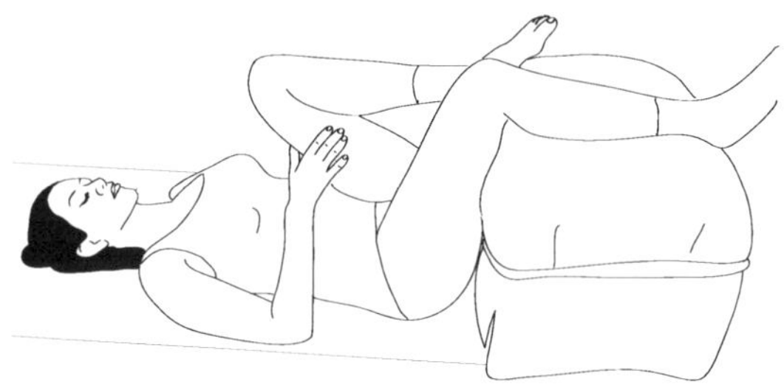

Figure 7.11. Single Knee to Chest

8. (Figure 7.12): Rest your right ankle on your left thigh. With your right hand gently press against your right thigh. Hold for 1 min.
9. (Figure 7.13): Thread your right hand through the triangle created by your legs to hold the back of your left knee. Use both hands to gently pull your left knee towards your chest. Hold for 5 min.
10. Return to Integration Pose for 5 min.

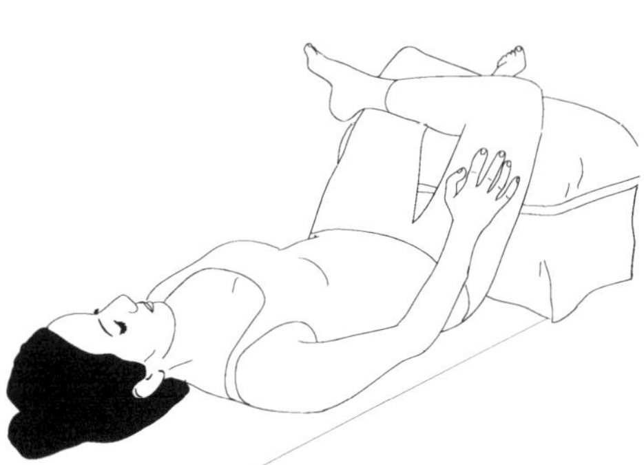

Figure 7.12. Ankle to Thigh

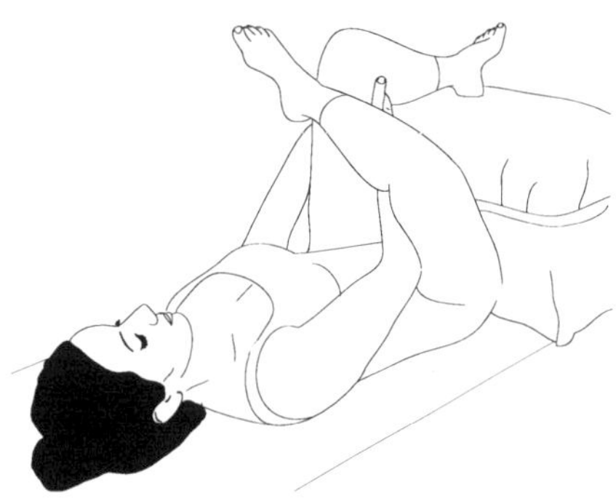

Figure 7.13. Hip Stretch

18. I recommend an interval timer for qigong exercises so you can focus and do not have to watch the clock. Alternately, you can make a sound recording of the exercises.

11. (Figure 7.12 & 7.13): Repeat on other side.
12. Return to Integration Pose for 5 min.
13. (Figure 7.14): Bring right arm out to the side 45 degrees from the body. Bring your knees together and twist to the right, stacking your knees on your right wrist. Turn to the left. Hold for 5 min.
14. Return to Integration Pose for 5 min.
15. (Figure 7.14): Repeat on the left.
16. Return to Integration Pose.
17. Turn your head as far as you can to the right. Very slowly turn your head to the left. Move so slowly that someone watching you wouldn't notice you were moving.
18. Return to Integration Pose.
19. Turn your head as far as you can to the right. Very slowly turn your head to the left. Move so slowly that someone watching you wouldn't notice you were moving.

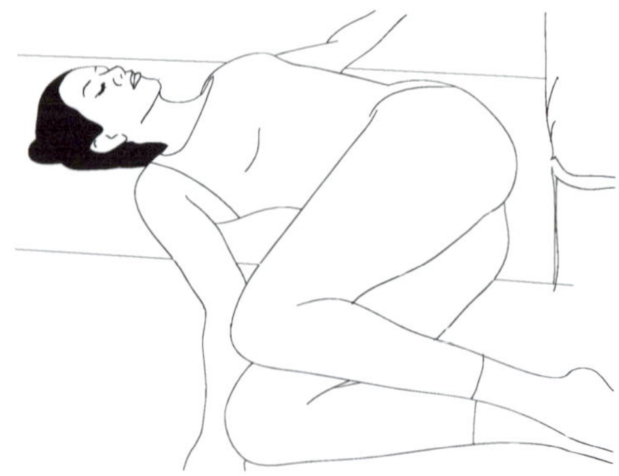

Figure 7.14. Twist

Osteoporosis

As Kidney energy declines, the bones and joints tend to weaken.[19] All women should take preventive measures to keep their bones strong, even when we do not have a genetic tendency. My mom refuses to lose weight as she says she never saw "a fat woman with osteoporosis. They have heart attacks but strong bones."

Steps to Preventing Osteoporosis:

1. Bone loss is more common in thin women. Be sure to eat a nourishing diet and to maintain adequate weight.
2. Incorporate bone broth in the daily diet. Use it as a base for soup or congee.
3. Take a calcium supplement with Vitamin D.
4. It is crucial to lift heavy weights. Heavy weights mean it takes significant mental and muscular control to do five reps of an exercise. The body requires strong stimulus to stay strong. Daoists created various practices of tapping and hitting to stimulate bone health. One of my teachers advised uphill hikes with a heavy backpack.

Fibromyalgia

Fibromyalgia is characterized by widespread pain that is worse with pressure. There is also typically fatigue and sleep disorders. This condition most often affects women who have pushed themselves to exhaustion through overwork, long-term or extreme stress, or emotional turmoil. There are often

19. As an aside, bone spurs in adults, another common bone issue, are due to Liver Blood deficiency.

hormonal deficiencies and many cases are alleviated with bioidentical hormones and taking Jing tonics.

Excessive and Irregular Menstrual Bleeding

Beng lou, or "flooding and trickling," is the TCM disease category for irregular uterine bleeding (metrorrhagia). Beng lou is characterized by periods of excessive uterine bleeding and episodes of spotting, both of which may occur during the regular menses, or may happen abruptly outside normal menses, or else may be continuous. Excessive bleeding exhausts a woman's reserves and

PRACTITIONER SECTION: OSTEOPOROSIS & FIBROMYALGIA

Osteoporosis

To prevent and treat bone loss use herbal formulas long-term (for 3-6 months). These formulas will also stabilize hormones and increase vitality:

Dr. Judith's Beautiful Maiden Formula (modified Young Maiden Formula)

Du Zhong (eucomia) 9g, Bu Gu Zhi (psoralea) 9g, Tao Ren (peach kernel) 2g, Yin Yang Huo (epimedium) 6g, Sheng Di Huang (raw rehmania) 6g, Huai Niu Xi (achyranthes root) 6g, Nu Zhen Zi (privet fruit) 9g, Xu Duan (dipsaci) 6g, Sha Ren (amomi) 3g, Hu Tao Ren (walnut) 6g.

Used for osteoporosis, Bi syndrome (arthritis, joint pain), and general anti-aging.

Bone Building Formula(1)

Chuan Xu Duan (prepared dipsaci), Gui Ban (turtle shell), Sang Ji Sheng (mulberry mistletoe), Shan Zhu Yu (cornus), Zi He Che (placenta), Gu Sui Bu (drynaria), Shu Di Huang (prepared rehmania), Wu Wei Zi (schizandra berries), Lu Jiao Jiao (deer antler gelatin).

This formula is stronger to tonify the Jing. For more Kidney Yin deficiency add Shan Yao (Chinese yam), Huang Jing (polygonatum), Gou Qi Zi (go ji berries). For more Kidney Yang deficiency add Xian Mao (curculigo), Zhi Fu Zi (prepared aconite).

Fibromyalgia

Fibromyalgia involves Qi and Blood deficiency with a latent pathogen. Progress is often slow as these patients are too deficient to handle strong moving treatments. In cases where the Yin is strong enough, use the following formula long-term (for 3-6 months).

Huang Qi Gui Zhi Wu Wu Tang (modified)(2)

Huang Qi (astragulus) 30g, Ghui Zhi (cinammon twig) 3-6g, Bai Shao (white peony root) 30g, Sheng Jiang (fresh ginger), Da Zao (black jujube), Qin Jiao (gentian root), Dang Gui (Chinese Angelica) 18-30g, Ji Xue Teng (millettia) 12g.

1. Modified from Jiling Hu. "TCM Endocrinology". (lecture, Yo San University, Los Angeles, Novemer 7, 2003).
2. Jiang Zheng. "TCM Gynecology". (lecture, Pacific College of Oriental Medicine, San Diego, November 2, 2006).

does not allow for proper recovery. It also can be an indication of serious disease such as cancer or masses. Thus, such symptoms should be taken very seriously.

Beng lou can occur at any age, but becomes increasingly common during perimenopause. This is due in part to a decline in Kidney Jing compounded with additional patterns. It can be challenging to treat and requires that women follow proper menstrual care, diet, sleep, and exercise habits. Modern Western practice is often to use birth control pills to stop menses until menopause is over. Though this alleviates the symptom, it creates additional Liver Qi stagnation.

Patterns of Irregular or Excessive Menstrual Bleeding

Kidney Yin Deficiency

Symptoms:
Hot flashes, red cheeks, night sweats, weak and sore low back and knees, unsettled, fatigue, and tinnitus. Bleeding is red, alternates between light and profuse and is irregular. Most common menopausal pattern.

Important Herbs:
Du Zhong (eucommia), Xu Duan (dipsacus), Han Lian Cao (eclipta), Nu Zhen Zi (privet), E Jiao (gelatin)

Qi Deficiency

Symptoms:
Fatigue, pallor, loose stools, feel wiped out by menses. Bleeding is pale and watery, excessive in the beginning, then spotting long after period should have ended.

Important Herbs:
Huang Qi (astragalus), Dang Gui (Chinese angelica), E Jiao (gelatin)

Kidney Yang Deficiency

Symptoms:
Weak and sore low back and knees, feels cold, fatigue, nocturia. Menses is delayed, pale in color, with spotting long after period should have ended.

Important Herbs:
Du Zhong (eucommia), Xu Duan (dipsacus), Ai Ye (mugwort)

Heat in the Blood

Symptoms:
Red face, feels hot, constipation, unsettled, bleeding is bright red, bleeding comes abruptly and irregularly and is profuse.

Important Herbs:
Zhi Zi (gardenia), Chi Shao (red peony), Mu Dan Pi (tree peony bark), Di Yu (garden burnet root)

Blood Stagnation

Symptoms:
Maybe a dark complexion or dark circles under the eyes. Menstrual cramps, dark blood with clots. Bleeding alternates between light and profuse and is irregular.

Important Herbs:
Yunnan Paiyao (San Qi), Di Yu (garden burnet root)

Damp-Heat

Symptoms:
Generalized heaviness, irritability, abdominal distention, excessive vaginal discharge. Bleeding is dark and sticky, alternates between light and profuse and is irregular. Mid-cycle bleeding.

Important Herbs:
Huang Qin (scutellaria), Huang Lian (coptis), Huang Bai (phellodendron), Di Yu (garden burnet root)

Mental and Emotional Function

"I feel like I could kill someone and I would have no remorse"

--anonymous menopausal woman.

Memory Loss

Deficiency of Jing, Kidney Yin or Yang, Spleen Qi, and Heart Blood or Phlegm Damp excess can all cause a decline in cognitive functioning. It is crucial to constantly keep the mind active through intellectual stimulation and social interaction. Also, frequently take brain tonifying formulas and recipes such as Brain Tonic Soup (page 374).

Restless Organ Disorder

This refers to a combination of Heart Yin deficiency, Liver Qi stagnation, and Spleen Qi deficiency. It is characterized by mostly emotional symptoms: sudden and uncontrollable weeping, depression, manic episodes, uncharacteristic behavior, restless sleep, feeling out of control of one's behavior. It is called restless organ syndrome because the Shen (spirit) literally does not have a home and is trying to find a place to settle. Restless organ disorder can occur at any age, though it is commonly seen during menopause. It can be caused by emotional stress or trauma, or chronic or severe blood loss.

Gan Mai Da Zao Tang

Fu Xiao Mai (wheat), Da Zao (black jujube), Gan Cao (licorice), Long Gu (fossilized bone), Mu Li (oyster shell).

This classic formula is a simple and effective remedy for weepiness and uncontrollable emotionality caused by deficiency, at any age. It is also used for night sweats. It can be easily combined with other formulas.

Sensuality

Healthy sensuality and sexuality are markers of good health. As with everything else in Traditional Chinese Medicine, there can be "too little" and "too much." Low libido, along with feelings of unattractiveness and lack of sexual confidence, is associated with Qi, Blood, Yang deficiencies or Liver Qi stagnation. Excess libido, which may be accompanied by manic or compulsive behavior, is associated with excess Fire or Yin deficiency.

Various Daoist texts offer specific guidelines on how often men should ejaculate and engage sexually. There is no such formula for women's sexual behavior and each woman will have to figure it out for herself. I view libido as being akin to appetite levels: 1.) it depends on your constitution and lifestyle, and 2.) you know it is unbalanced by how you feel and look. A healthy libido has a playful sensuality that is integrated within the personality. It is neither repressed nor does it define you. It enhances rather than interrupts your life and adds a healthy dose of passion.

As women age, our sensuality reaches its full development. Sexuality under the Water Element becomes deeper, more spiritual, and more sensual in orientation. Sexuality at this time is associated with empowerment, acceptance of the self, healing of wounds, and connection with the Divine. This can be stunted by a variety of factors such as unfulfilling relationships and unbalanced hormone levels. Some women do well with lifestyle, herbs, and acupuncture to maintain their sexual health through menopause. Others need to add low doses of bioidentical hormones to optimize their health.

Increasing Libido

Low libido (or repressed libido) arises when your energy is either weak or stagnated. There will be a lack of creativity and freedom. Lack of libido as a disease pattern is distinct from learning to transmute sexual desire. With many spiritual celibates, sexual energy is still present, only it is harnessed and directed towards spiritual evolution. An example of this was Mother Teresa.

Pathological lack of libido is associated with deficiency and/or stagnation of energy, both of which are common with the hormonal fluctuations of menopause. Low libido is associated with depression, fatigue/exhaustion, poor self-image, low back and knee weakness and pain, poor digestion, and social withdrawal.

In such cases it is critical to reduce stress, overwork, and caretaking. Be sure to get adequate rest and take appropriate tonics for three to six months. Low libido can also occur when women feel shut down emotionally to their partner. It is healthy for women to not feel sexual when they do not feel safe or appreciated and such situations should not be forced.

Formula for Increasing Desire

This formula boosts Kidney Yin and Yang in the body: Ying Yang Huo (epimedium), Ba Ji Tian (morinda), Du Zhong (eucommia), Nu Zhen Zi (privet), Han Lian Cao (eclipta), Sheng Di Huang (raw rehmania), Sha Ren (amomi), Ren Shen (ginseng), Wu Wei Zi (schizandra), Mai Men Dong (ophiopogonis), Xiang Fu (cyperus).

Calm Libido Formula

This formula quells excess Fire. Zhi Mu (anemarrhena), Huang Bai (phellodendron), Long Gu (fossilized bone), Mu Li (oyster shell), Gan Cao (licorice), Dang Shen (codonopsis), Sheng Di Huang (raw rehmannia), Shan Zhu Yu (cornus), Fu Ling (poria), Shan Yao (Chinese yam), Mu Dan PI (tree peony bark), Ze Xie (alisma), Sha Ren (amomi).

Calming Excess Libido

This may not seem like a concern as women are capable of much more frequent sexual activity than men without detriment to our health. However, there are signs when it has become too much. Excessive sexual appetite destabilizes the Shen and weakens the Kidneys. Excessive sex brings out Kidney Fire, which can be injurious to the Yin, already depleted in menopause. Such cases may develop mania, agitation, compulsivity, addictive behavior, an excessive need for attention, and restlessness. Over time this is accompanied by an apparent loss of vitality presenting as tinnitus, insomnia, vaginal discharge, night sweats, and low back weakness and soreness. In such cases women should focus on a meditation practice and reduce sexual cultivation. Take a formula to sedate Fire and nourish Yin for three to six months.

PRACTITIONER SECTION: UNSETTLED EMOTIONS

If a person exhibits more aggression, then a Liver sedating formula will be more effective. If someone is manic and truly dangerous, this is Phlegm Fire Misting the Heart and involves stronger herbs and strict diet. Unfortunately, in cases of more severe emotional impairment, individuals are not functional enough to keep up with a regimen of treatment, diet, and herbs and may require medication. In these cases, have the patient take medications while concurrently treating until they can start stepping down their dosage under doctor supervision, without symptoms flaring up.

The Choice of Bioidentical Hormone Replacement[20]

My experience is that some women do best with bioidentical hormones and some are better off without them. Regardless of this choice, bioidenticals are not a replacement for self-cultivation and proper lifestyle. Your body has to be balanced in order to stay young. Bioidenticals simply enhance what you already are doing.

Use lifestyle, diet, practices, herbs, and acupuncture to sustain Jing, then add bioidentical hormones at low dosages if you still need them. Be sure to take each hormone separately in order to adjust each one independently. Approaching bioidenticals in this way allows for individualized dosaging and prevents some of the aging effects such as loss of skin tone, muscle loss, etc. I highly recommend Dr. Uzzi Reiss's approach.[21] His system details how to balance hormone levels based on symptoms rather than solely relying on blood tests.

A word of caution: though proponents of bioidentical hormone replacement claim far fewer risks than chemical hormone replacement, it is still a good idea to have a mammogram and pap smear each year. It is best to supplement with hormones in low dosages to minimize your risk.

When using hormones, whether it be birth control pills or hormone replacement, take milk thistle extract or other Liver detoxifier daily. The Liver must function optimally as it is responsible for metabolizing the hormones you take in. Some signs that your Liver is not handling the hormones well are: irritability, irregularity in menses or bowel movements, or depression.

20. Proponents of bioidentical hormones claim decreased risks and greater health benefits than with chemical hormones. Bioidenticals are also prescribed and adjusted for the individual woman.

21. Uzzi Reiss. *Natural Hormone Balance For Women.* (New York: Pocket Books, 2001).

Gifts of the Water Element

"There is magnificence to aging, because aging, and a Deficiency of Qi as we age, supports surrender to Divine Grace and to the Truth of Life, and the Dao."

--Felice Dumas

The Gift of Death

Ancestor worship plays a central part in Confucianism and the culture that produced Traditional Chinese Medicine. The ritual remembrance of those who have passed on embraces death as part of the life cycle. It gives those who participate in it eternal life in a tangible sense. With an honorary position awaiting us after death, we grow in esteem as we grow older.

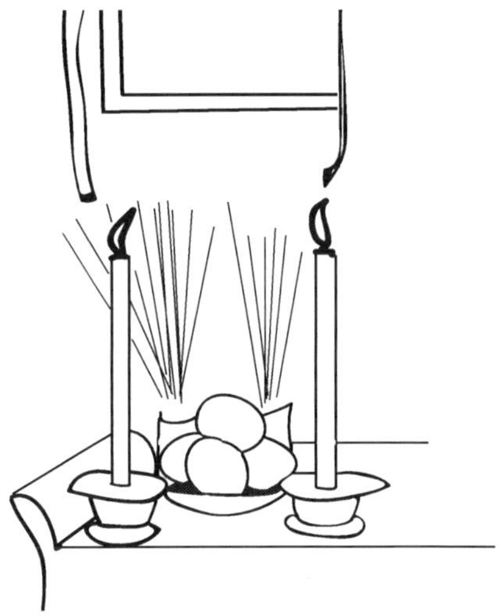

Figure 7.15 Offering to Ancestors

Modern culture does not quite know what to do with death. With no ancestor worship, death takes on a finality rather than a transition. Since we cease to exist and lose significance after death, we matter less and less as we get older. Modern culture seeks to erase every sign of mortality. It erroneously clings to a superficial parody of youth rather than cultivating wisdom. This cultural attitude makes menopause and aging unnecessarily unpleasant.

The death of the reproductive years is also the birth of deeper spiritual development. No longer saddled with children or subsistence work, women are free to devote themselves to their passions. We are free to apply our wisdom for the greater good. It was at the age of 50, after raising two children and a successful business career, that my mom became an acupuncturist. She now lives her purpose and expands her learning daily. Now over 60, she has grown in her intuitive knowledge tremendously.

Stillness

One of my teachers said "To know your purpose you must be as still and quiet as your bones. Only then can you really listen." The secret of our true selves is hidden in the Water Element. To get there we must be still and present in the face of all fears. To reach this still place means journeying into the underworld of the shadow. It means facing the death and chaos of our deepest fears. After this we can experience peaceful stillness.

Truth

Water's quest is for Truth. This is the deepest, naked truth. The pelvic bones act like a cauldron to hold it, and these bones act like a great singing bowl that through its resonance manifests into being. In the Water Phase women transcend biological reproduction into alchemical manifestation.

The Truth means the veils of illusion have to fall. The dark side within ourselves and the world around us: addictions, faults, weaknesses, lies, predators, are all unveiled. The Truth of the situation comes out into the Light. With sight comes the gift of discernment to see plainly beyond the facade of society.

This transition can happen much earlier, however, there are many illusions in youth to distract us. It usually requires a hardship to shatter the illusion of reality in younger people, as I did with my illness as a teenager. What has not been faced before will rise to the surface during menopause. This is a hard time for those who have not faced their Truth, for those who are still looking outside themselves for the answers, and for those who refuse to see below the surface.

Wisdom

With the process of uncovering Truth comes Wisdom. This is the greatest gift of Water. Once the Truth is found within ourselves, the wisdom we gain has the power to transform all of the Elements in ourselves and the world around us.

Each of us must experience the challenges of each Element before transcending them. We experience fear (Water) that is covered up with anger or depression (Wood) in an effort to protect ourselves. We seek to distract ourselves through novel stimulus, extreme experiences, addictions, and constant noise (Fire). We worry and ruminate over problems in our minds because deep down we do not have faith they will be resolved; and what is worse, we do not believe in ourselves (Earth). We grieve for the injustice, suffering, and loss of this world (Metal). This leads to more fear.

Transcendence happens when we face our scariest truths and dispel our illusions. The gift of Water is stillness, silence, peace, and wisdom. It becomes the new womb. This new space naturally, effortlessly heals and transmutes. It is all powerful in its gentleness. Fear cannot exist in its Presence.

Once we are no longer afraid or disempowered, anger is the next to dissipate. This breeds compassion and true forgiveness. We empathize with the mistakes of others rather than become annoyed. We step in appropriately to protect the weak. When we encounter those who are intentionally evil we feel sadness for their smallness. We see that one who leaves chaos and pain in his/her wake is a miserable being, no matter what their facade. We can feel these things because we know we are protected.

We feel light and so we are filled with joy. Not manic joy, but rather a peaceful bliss. It is the happiness of true connection. We feel connected to everyone and everything. No longer do we have fears or resentments to block this. Rather than fear intimacy and stillness, we thrive on it. From a place deep within we know we are loved and we cannot help but share it with everyone.

It is difficult to worry about anything in this state. Rather a deep trust develops in our own discernment and ability to handle what life brings us. We trust in a greater power that works through us. We develop true, unshakeable faith.

From this vantage point we naturally behave with integrity, for it would hurt us deeply not to. We see the natural order at work in the world. Justice begins to act in our lives without us having to struggle for it. All scores are settled.

Exercise 7. 8. 5 Cloud Meditation (Figure 7.16)[22]

The 5 Cloud Meditation is one version of many ancient Daoist alchemical meditations to transmute negative emotions into positive ones. It refines and balances the 5 Elements and is a foundational practice to change your inner landscape. Healing sounds can be added to discharge excess energy.

1. Inhale and exhale into your Heart. Imagine a radiant red cloud of energy there. Feel your Heart energy. Do you notice any scattered, frantic, or contracted energy? Allow your breath to dissolve any negative energy here into unconditional love. Continue until your Heart is radiating love in all directions. On your next exhale send your intention down to your Spleen (located under your left lower ribs).
2. Inhale and exhale into your Spleen. Imagine a warm golden-yellow cloud of energy there. Feel your Spleen energy. Do you notice any worry, guilt, or ungrounded feelings? Allow your breath to dissolve any negative energy here. Continue until your Spleen feels grounded and solid in internal Faith. On your next exhale send your intention up to your Lungs.
3. Inhale and exhale into your Lungs. Imagine the most angelic white cloud of energy there. Feel your Lung energy. Do you notice any sinking, lonely, or grieving energy there? Is there pain and contraction? Allow your breath to transmute any negative energy here. Continue until your Lungs are buoyant in their Purity. On your next exhale, send the cloud down to your Kidneys (located under your lowest ribs on your back).
4. Inhale and exhale into your Kidneys. Imagine a black cloud of energy there, as expansive as the night sky. Feel your Kidney energy. Do you notice any fearful, unsettled, or empty feeling? Allow your breath to dissolve any negative energy here. Continue until your Kidneys are strong, still, and wise. On your next exhale send your intention to your Liver (located under your right ribs).
5. Inhale and exhale into your Liver. Imagine a strong blue/green cloud of energy there.

22. Based on the 5 Cloud Meditation from John Barber. "Daoist Meditation". (qigong class, Yo San University, Los Angeles, January 5, 2003).

Feel your Liver energy. Do you notice any anger or constriction? Allow your breath to transmute any negative energy here. Continue until your Liver relaxes into compassion.

6. On your next exhale begin the cycle again. Linger only 1 breath in each organ. Repeat until you feel complete.

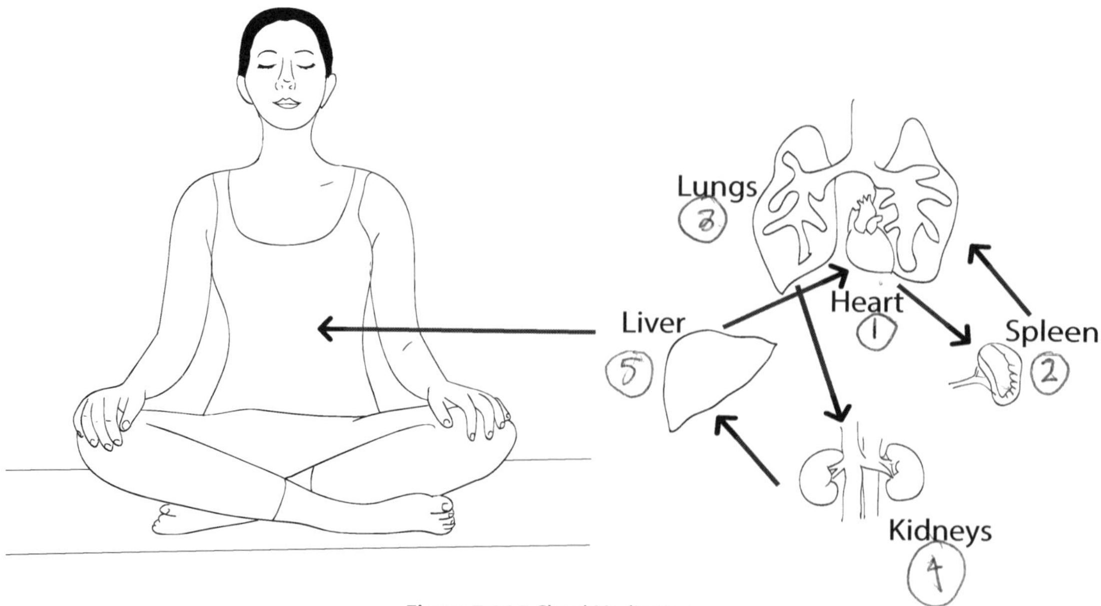

Figure 7.16 5 Cloud Meditation

Table 7.4. Alchemical Transformations for Each Element

Element	Challenge -> Gift
Water (Kidneys)	Fear -> Wisdom
Wood (Liver)	Anger -> Compassion
Fire (Heart)	Overstimulation -> Peaceful Bliss
Earth (Spleen)	Worry -> Faith
Metal (Lungs)	Grief -> Divine Justice

Epilogue

Second Spring

The immortals kept their mental energies focused and refined, and harmonized their bodies with their environment. Thus, they did not show conventional signs of aging and were able to live beyond biological limitations.[1]

After Age 56

If you are picking up this book for the first time and you have already reached menopause, do not despair. You have not missed your chance at achieving vitality or spiritual advancement. Life is cyclical, and the spiral of life has brought you through a sort of reverse puberty. Only now you get to bring the gifts and wisdom you acquired through your life with you. This is a time of coming into your true power.

You are now in your Second Spring, which is the Traditional Chinese Medicine term for when menstruation ceases. The 5 Element Cycles begin anew, on their own schedule. The reproductive years for many women are a time of bondage. It is all about caretaking, sacrificing for a career, putting the needs of others first, and never having the time to do what you really want. Now is the time to invest in your own cultivation and in making positive change in the world around you. This is a time for rejuvenation and spirituality. Practice the Inner Alchemy exercises in Chapter 3. Use the herbs and practices in Chapter 5 to rejuvenate. The beauty you radiate now is different than in youth. It is the kind of beauty that only occurs with time such as in a mature tree.

This is also a time for expansion. As we age, we make a choice. Will we allow our life's experiences to beat us down until we are a cranky, contracted old person? Or do we surrender into acceptance and allow life to make us expansive and free? This is a daily choice.

1. Maoshing Ni, trans. *The Yellow Emperor's Classic of Medicine.* (Shambala: Boston, 1995), 3-4.

Post Menopause

The period before and during menopause often requires harmonizing treatments. During the post menopausal period the focus shifts to tonification, particularly of the Spleen and Kidney Jing. As soon as menopausal symptoms have settled, tonic herbs and foods should be taken daily, warming treatments can be resumed, and daily health promoting exercise performed.

Diet

After menopause, the body cools as excessive Liver energies subside and Spleen and Kidney Yang deficiency becomes more prominent. Warming foods, alcohol, coffee, and tea can be taken again. Small amounts of medicinal wine are particularly helpful to warm the channels and move the Blood. Du Zhong Wine (page 374) is a medicinal wine with the added benefits of guarding against arthritis, preventing aches and pains, beautifying the skin, and calming the mind. Consume longevity foods several times a week (page 374) to strengthen the Spleen Qi and Kidney Jing.

Practice moderation with diet. Due to increasing Spleen weakness as we age, frequent small meals are usually best tolerated. Do not get full or go hungry, and do not sleep on a full stomach. It is helpful to take a 10 min. nap after meals.

Exercise

Aging begins in the joints. Since youth, joint mobility, stretching, and neuromuscular connections should be developed equally with power and tension exercises. All of these are factors in optimizing strength and athleticism, as well as longevity. Unfortunately, most people focus only on tension training. This unbalanced approach avoids some aspects of aging, while accelerating others. Bone density may be retained, however, there is loss of joint mobility and poor movement patterns. These eventually lead to limited activity and strength loss.

A youthful body is elastic and supple. Fortunately, the human body is forgiving, and you can develop these qualities at any age with the right routine. Perform restorative exercises for the joints such as Dao-Yin and Yin Yoga. Swimming is excellent to promote fluidity in the body. Additionally, include weight-bearing exercises and cardio, such as hiking, in the routine.

Rest

Insomnia can increasingly become an issue with age. Soak your feet in hot water every night before bed to settle the mind and relax the body. Be sure to take Kidney tonics with astringent herbs such as Wu Wei Zi (schizandra), Shan Zhu Yu (cornus), or Bu Gu Zhi (psoralea) to prevent night urination.

Purpose

Find a purpose. Retirement means an opportunity to pursue a passion. If a life-long career is a passion, do not give it up. Life requires purpose and deeper meaning. It also keeps us on center stage as we get older. All people need to be seen, honored, and loved. Traditionally, this phase of life was seen as a time to develop the spirit and to make changes in our world from a place of wisdom.

Keep the mind active. Socializing, learning new things, and creating new habits are key. Put yourself in new situations and interact with people of all different ages, walks of life, and cultures. This exercises new parts of your brain. The day you get too comfortable is the day your brain becomes old. Take brain tonics such as Bu Nao Wan.

Creating Your Cycles

The menstrual cycle provided specific phases for correcting excesses and deficiencies in the body. During the Second Spring, women can alternate herbs and therapies that strengthen Yin with those that strengthen Yang. A rotation that works for many women is to tonify Yin for two weeks, then Yang for two weeks. Some women will be more Yin or Yang deficient and require more of one or the other. (This strategy is the same in men who want to strengthen their Kidneys.)

Be sure to always consider the Spleen (your digestion) first. Include herbs to strengthen the Spleen (digestion), that aromatically transform, and that increase digestibility of other herbs. This can mean taking Si Jun Zi Tang or Jian Pi Pian with meals.

Health Issues

The following health issues can occur at any age, though they are increasingly common with age. After menopause, the Spleen becomes more deficient, mimicking the condition of childhood. This leaves women vulnerable to opportunistic pathogens and dietary issues.

Eye Care

The eyes are connected to the Liver, and to a lesser extent Kidney, health.

Steps to Proper Eye care:

1. Massage eyes daily. The eyes benefit from local stimuli.
2. Eat a handful of Gou Qi Zi (go ji berries) daily.
3. Limit TV watching to 30-45 min. at a stretch.
4. Limit computer use to 30-45 min. at a stretch. Use computer glasses to protect against glare. These can be made with prescription lenses if you wear reading glasses.

Common Eye Diseases:
Near Sightedness is caused by Qi deficiency in the eye. Needle LV 3 and GB 37. Use ginger moxa around hair line.[2]

Cataracts are due to Liver and Kidney Yin deficiency. Protect your eyes from sun damage by wearing dark glasses. At the first signs of cataracts, begin taking Ming Mu Di Huang Wan long-term to slow progression.

Loss of vision from the center is Kidney Yin deficiency, while loss of vision from the periphery indicates Kidney Yang deficiency. **Macular Degeneration** creates loss of vision from the center. It is due to Kidney Yin deficiency with Blood stagnation. Use Ming Mu Di Huang Wan with Yunnan Paiyao. **Retinitis Pigmentosa** is caused by Liver Heat.

Psoriasis

Psoriasis is a chronic skin condition caused most commonly by Heat, Phlegm, and Blood stagnation. It is characterized by papules (red bumps) covered by layers of silvery-white scaling that is itchy. The main treatment principles are clearing Heat Toxin with cooling herbs, resolving Phlegm, and moving the Blood. When the body is weakened by stress, in the very young or the elderly, it is easier for Heat Toxin to take over. In addition to addressing psoriasis symptoms, it is important to calm the emotions and strengthen Spleen Qi. There is no cure for psoriasis, but with regular treatment it can be kept in remission for long periods of time.

Recipe E.1. Psoriasis Formula [3]

Tu Fu Ling (smilax) 30g, Bai Hua She She Cao (hedyotis) 20g, Pu Gong Ying (dandelion)15g, She Mei (Indian strawberry) 20g, Long Kui (solanum nigrum) 15g, Ban Zhi Lian (skullcap) 15g, E Zhu (zedoaria) 9g, Sheng Di Huang (raw rehmannia) 30g, Dan Shen (salvia root) 20g, Sha Shen (glehnia root)20g, Da Qing Ye (isatis leaf) 15g, Sheng Shi Gao (gypsum) 30g, Sang Ye (mulberry leaf)10g

Recipe E.2. Topical Formula: Qing Lian Gao[4]

Powdered herbs: Dang Gui (Chinese angelica) 30g, Zi Cao (groomwell) 10g, Da Huang (rhubarb) 5g

Melt together over low heat with 500g Sesame oil and 160g beeswax. Pour into containers to cool and store.

2. Alex Tiberi. "TCM Pediatrics" (lecture, Pacific College of Oriental Medicine, San Diego, February 28, 2008).
3. Alex Tiberi. "TCM Pediatrics" (lecture, Pacific College of Oriental Medicine, San Diego, February 28 2008).
4. Yueying Li, "TCM Dermatology" (lecture, San Diego, CA, September 18, 2011).

Shingles (Herpes Zoster)

After the initial bout of Chicken Pox (varicela zoster) often experienced in childhood, the virus remains dormant in the body as a latent Heat toxin. The virus is opportunistic. When the immune system is weakened, as in times of great stress or a decline in health, the virus resurfaces in the form of Shingles. Shingles can flare up at any age, but is more common in older age and also tends to linger in seniors as they tend to have more Qi deficiency with Blood stagnation. However, it can even affect children. It is characterized by intense nerve pain, often on the torso, followed by an itchy lesion with fluid-filled vesicles. My experience is that it can crisscross the spine (though literature claims it is unilateral), and can affect the body anywhere from the feet to the head and eyes. Jiao Gu Lan (gynostemma) is a particularly effective adaptogenic herb for herpes simplex and zoster, and can be taken daily long-term to keep the immune system strong.

PRACTITIONER SECTION: SHINGLES

The sooner shingles is treated with acupuncture and herbs, the quicker it can be resolved. TCM treatment can be applied whether or not the patient elects to use prescribed antivirals (keep in mind that if the patient takes Aciclovir, you may also need to treat side effects that arise, such as UTI).

As soon as shingles symptoms arise, use a seven-star needle to bleed the line of nerve pain. Follow immediately with stationary cupping. There will be more blood than is typical with bleeding. There is a great deal of local heat, so be prepared by wearing gloves and have gauze handy. This treatment immediately takes the edge off the pain. If the lesion has surfaced, lancet the lesion to open it and follow with stationary cupping to pull out the toxins. Immediately apply the topical solutions given below. This will clear the lesions quickly or avoid them altogether.

Follow this with an acupuncture treatment. Esoteric Acupuncture, Shao Yin or Celestial patterns are excellent to address the emotional aspect.[1] Add needling and microcurrent to the local area of pain. Needle Sp 6, LI 11, ST 36, GB 34, GB 40, and SJ 5.

Herbal Medicine

Powder the following herbs: Bing Pian (borneol), Huang Lian (coptis), Dang Gui (Chinese angelica), Huang Bai (phellodendron), Duan Shi Gao (calcined gypsum).

If the lesion is wet, sprinkle the powder. If the lesion is dry use Zi Cao Oil first then sprinkle powdered Bing Pian (borneol) and Duan Shi Gao (calcined gypsum).

An internal formula is also necessary to clear the acute phase and avoid postherpetic neuralgia, where the nerve pain can linger for years after the initial lesion has gone. In acute attack on excess patients a modification of Long Dan Xie Gan Tang with a hefty dose of Yunnan Paiyao can be very effective. As soon as the acute phase is over, i.e. the intense pain has subsided, begin tonifying Qi and Blood and soothing the Liver. For example, modify Gui Pi Tang with Yu Jin (curcuma), Mu Dan Pi (tree peony bark), Zhi Zi (gardenia fruit), Jiao Gu Lan (gynostemma), Di Long (lumbricus), and Zi Su Geng (perilla root). Continue taking Yunnan Paiyao for several months.

1. Dr. Judith Andrews discovered that Mikio Sankey's Esoteric Protocols work best. Mikio Sankey. Sea of Life-Cosmic Fire; Esoteric Acupuncture Volume IV. (Inglewood: Mountain Castle Publishing; 2006), 257.

Heart Disease

Heart disease becomes increasingly common in women after menopause, but can occur in women much younger. Most cases involve a combination of these disease patterns: Phlegm, Blood stagnation, and Heart Qi deficiency, all of which tend to become prevalent with age. High cholesterol and arterial plague relate to Phlegm. Anyone with high cholesterol and women after menopause, should take the Date and Wood Ear Tea (page 372) at least once a week. It can be taken monthly as a preventative. Regularly consuming herbs such as He Shou Wu (polygonum), Hong Zao (red dates), Ge Gen (kudzu), Shan Zha (hawthorn berry), Jue Ming Zi (cassia seed), and Ju Hua (chrusanthemum) with oolong tea will lower cholesterol naturally. It is important to cut down on sugar, simple carbohydrates, fatty foods, and other Phlegm-Damp producing foods. Shi Chang Pu (acorus) reduces arterial plaque.

Blood stagnation shows itself as a purple-tinged tongue, dark engorged sublingual veins, purple veins, dark circles under the eyes, blue nails and lips, and most apparently as a sharp-fixed pain. Blood stagnation is the main pattern indicated in heart attacks. All of us tend to get Blood stagnation as we get older unless we actively guard against it. Moving our bodies daily and reducing stress are key to maintaining healthy circulation, but is not enough. Exercise does not directly affect the microcirculation which is more affected by hormonal fluctutations, and the strength of our Qi and Blood. Regular acupuncture, massage, qigong, and yoga affect the Qi directly to move the Blood. Additionally, Blood moving herbs should be taken on a daily basis to prevent stagnation from accumulating. An example of this is to take a low dosage of Yunnan Paiyao (1-2 capsules) daily with longevity tonics.[5]

Heart Qi deficiency manifests as palpitations, spontaneous sweating, shortness of breath, and fatigue, all worsened upon exertion. To strengthen the Heart Qi you want to increase the general Qi in the body by take Qi tonics regularly such as Ren Shen (ginseng) and Huang Qi (astragalus).

PRACTITIONER SECTION: STRENGTHENING THE HEART

Most of the cases of heart disease U.S. practitioners see can be treated with a modification of Bu Qi Yin. This formula will lower cholesterol, reduce heart pain, strengthen Qi and Blood, and disperse Blood stagnation. It should be taken for several months.

Heart Strengtheing Formula

Dan Shen (salvia) 30g, Sheng Di Huang (raw rehmannia) 30g, Mai Men Dong (ophiopogon) 30g, Chao Suan Zao Ren (roasted jujube seed) 30g, Dang Shen (codonopsis) 20g, Ge Gen (kudu) 24g, Tan Xiang (sandalwood) 10g, Shi Chang Pu (acorus) 12g, Xia Ku Cao (prunella) 10g, Jue Ming Zi (cassia seed) 10g, Sha Ren (amomi) 6g, Zhi Gan Cao (honeyed licorice) 6g.

5. Blood moving herbs are contraindicated with Coumadin and other blood thinning medications. Blood moving herbs are likely contraindicated with other heart medications.

Rebirth

The ego fears death. We fear growing old. We fear being alone. We fear not having the money to support ourselves. We fear becoming irrelevant. In a superficial society made of sound bites rather than wisdom, where is our place?

Underlying these fears is the death of our own illusions. Perhaps it was the little perks that our physical beauty gave us. Now we must develop true beauty and true power. Maybe we felt our worth was in the man we could attract. Now we have to know our true worth, with or without a lover. One by one, the lies we have believed fall away. The more we resist, the more painful it is. What we do not realize just yet is that on the other side is all the peace and bliss we could ever want.

The death of illusion gives birth to who we really are: pure consciousness, part of the Dao, part of God, or whatever words you choose. The death of our fears gives birth to our real selves. We are able to manifest Heaven on Earth, integrating the two. At this point we live a spiritual life while walking the Earth. When we arrive at this state, whatever our age may be, we are at our most relevant. As more spiritual, empowered women show up in this world, our collective reality changes for the better. What is called for is our presence.

The death of the physical body is the death of the last illusion before we return to pure consciousness. Once you have become conscious, even physical death becomes a peaceful and conscious process. One where you decide it is time to leave after you have done what you came here to do. In this way, our presence lives on after the physical body, through our works and those we have touched.

Conclusion

Most women, barring fatal illness or injury, will live to be 7 Times a Woman, much of which is unique to the female existence. Each Cycle contains a mystery and a rite of passage. When we do not have a tradition or sisterhood to guide women and girls through each Cycle of life what is a gift can become scary or traumatic. When we cannot put what is happening in the greater context, it loses its meaning.

When we do not understand that a girl is still developing her Spleen and Kidneys until 6 and 14 years, respectively, we may not appropriately protect and nurture her. When we have this wisdom we can raise girls with a solid, strong foundation. When we do not understand our menstruation, our sacred creative power becomes a "curse." We can learn that the reality is the opposite. The menstrual cycle attunes us to the Earth's rhythms and is a prime opportunity to balance our health. When we are ignorant of our sacred power as women we may become prey to predators, drugs, abuse, and sexuality that is dishonoring to us. When we become aware, our sexuality, creativity, and freedom are gifts we share with the world, and the world is no longer a scary place. In ignorance, pregnancy and childbirth can be devastating to our bodies. In wisdom, and with support, they become the second prime opportunity to improve our health, as well as of the next generation. When we do not understand Jing, it is something that runs out of us leaving us spent. When we understand how to cultivate and circulate our Jing, our beauty transforms and deepens with age. When we do not understand how to rid ourselves of accumulations our systems become overburdened with toxins or else we use harsh methods that deplete us. With understanding we are able to maintain a balance of cleansing and building that is right for us as individuals. Unaware, menopause catches us off guard, rather like being blind-sided by a train. With foreknowledge we prepare ourselves well in advance to coast through menopause, which is transformed into yet another prime opportunity to increase our vitality. Far from insignificant, we reach the state of the wise crone, who guides the younger generations on how to live a harmonious life.

Rather than enter each Cycle with trepidation or loathing, we as women should embrace and address the challenges, changes and opportunities presented to us. With this wisdom we cease to be cursed, and to be a woman becomes the greatest blessing.

Recipes

Foundational Recipes

The recipes in this section form the basis of a healthy diet. Proper diet is discussed in Chapter 1 ("Diet; Chinese Food Therapy" on page 70) and optimizing intestinal health in Chapter 6 (page 246).

Congee

Congee (zhou) is the traditional Chinese breakfast. It is a gruel or thin soup made out of rice with 5 to 6 times the amount of water cooked for several hours. Congee opens the digestion and helps regulate the intestines. It tonifies Qi and Blood, soothes the mucous membranes, is cooling, and is easily digestible. It is intentionally bland, as the bland taste tonifies the Spleen. Other ingredients may be added which enhance the therapeutic value of the congee. Grain-based soups are popular cross-culturally and similarly help open the digestion in the morning. They predate the current cold cereal fad that has the opposite effect of shocking the stomach.

Breakfast should be the largest and most complex meal of the day, consisting of protein, grains, and vegetables. This follows the natural cycle, as Yang energy and digestive functioning peak in the morning. Begin with a small bowl of congee, followed by a well-rounded meal of vegetables, protein, and complex carbohydrates. In cases where there is not any time for an elaborate breakfast, make a more substantial congee with vegetables and protein. I list a few congee recipes with their therapeutic values. All grains are Qi tonics. In addition they have the following properties.

Table 8.1. Properties of Grains

Type of Grain	Property
White (all types)	Harmonizes the Spleen and Stomach. Cooler and easier to digest than brown rice. Best for digestive weakness, convalescence, and Heat conditions.
Brown Rice (all types)	More warming and difficult to digest. Calms the Shen. Presoak (like beans) overnight prior to cooking.
Basmati Rice	Most aromatic and best for Damp conditions. The texture is a bit off in congee and it makes a sour rice wine.
Sweet Rice (glutinous rice, sticky rice)	Warming. Stronger action to tonify Qi and Blood (has more protein and fat). Avoid in excess conditions as it can increase Phlegm-Damp. Contains gluten. Can cause Stomach Heat (acid reflux).
Black Sweet Rice (black glutinous rice, black sticky rice)	Most tonifying of all types of rice. Used as base for tonifying rice wines and in 8 Treasure Rice.
Amaranth	Dries Dampness.
Buckwheat	Dries Dampness. Strengthens blood vessels. Warming.
Millet	Moistening. Cooling. Nourishes Yin. Bland taste. Anti-fungal.
Oats	Calms the Shen. Warming. Lowers cholesterol.
Quinoa	High protein content. Warming.
Rye	Dries Dampness. Balances Liver and Gallbladder.
Wheat	Moistening. Calms the Shen (nerves). Can create Dampness.

Basic Congee Recipe

Ingredients:

½ – ¾ cup of rice (or other grain)

4-6 cups of water

Preparation:

1. Prepare before bed at night. Rinse rice.[1]
2. Place ingredients in rice cooker and set to porridge. Or, place in crock pot and set to medium.

Method of Administration:

Eat first thing in the morning.

1. Always rinse rice and herbs prior to cooking.

Congee Recipes for Different Conditions

Forbidden Congee (general tonification):
Gou Qi Zi (go ji berries) ¼ cup, Lian Zi (lotus nuts) 5 pieces, Long Yan Rou (longan berries) 5 pieces, Fu Ling (poria) 2 pieces, Yi Yi Ren (coix seed) ¼ cup, Chen Pi (tangerine peel) 1 tsp ground, black glutinous rice (forbidden rice) ½ -3/4 cup.

Astringe the Kidneys Congee (for frequent urination/ polyuria due to deficiency):
Bu Gu Zhi (psoralea fruit) ¼ cup ground, white rice ½ – ¾ cup.

Clear Skin Congee #1 (excess heat):
Yi Yi Ren (coix seed, half raw, half roasted) ¼ cup, mung beans ¼ cup, fresh ginger 3 pieces, white rice ½ – ¾ cup.

Clear Skin Congee #2 (heat with deficiency):
black beans ¼ cup, Yi Yi Ren (coix seed, half raw, half roasted) ¼ cup, Long Yan Rou (longan berries) 5 pieces, brown or white rice ½ – ¾ cup.

Chicken Congee (sick or recovering from illness):
8 ounces chicken, 1 bunch scallions, ½ cup white rice, 2 stalks celery chopped, 1 tbsp. fresh ginger, 1 carrot chopped, 2 inch piece daikon radish chopped. Sauté chicken over high heat until seared in a frying pan before adding to crock pot.

No Appetite in the Morning Congee:
Huang Qi (astragulus) 3 pieces, Cang Zhu (atractylodes) 1 tbsp. powdered, Yi Yi Ren (coix seed) ¼ cup , white rice ½ cup, Chen Pi (tangerine peel) 1 tbsp. powdered, Long Yan Rou (longan berries) 5 pieces, Fu Ling (poria) 2 pieces, white rice ½ – ¾ cup.

Dampness Drying Congee:
Cang Zhu (atractylodes) 1 tbsp. powdered, Yi Yi Ren (coix seed) ¼ cup, ½ cup white rice. Eat daily.

Qi & Yin Tonifying Congee:
Fresh Shan Yao (Chinese yam) ½ cup chopped, Gou Qi Zi (go ji berries) ¼ cup, Hei Zhi Ma (black sesame seed) 1 tbsp., Yi Yi Ren (coix seed, raw and dry-fried) ¼ cup, Long Yan Rou (longan berries) 5 pieces, brown or white rice ½ – ¾ cup. Good for endurance athletes, loss of fluids, dry skin, overwork, and skin rejuvenation.

Spleen Qi Deficiency with Damp Congee:
Yi Yi Ren (coix seed, raw and dry-fried) ¼ cup, Bai Bian Dou (hyacinth bean) ¼ cup, Fu Ling (poria) 2 pieces, Qian Shi (foxnut) ¼ cup, Lian Zi (lotus nut) 5 pieces, ½ cup white rice.

Yin-Nourishing Congee:
White cloud fungus, Shan Yao (Chinese yam), black sesame seed, Chen Pi (tangerine peel), ½ cup white rice.

Brain Tonifying Congee:
Walnuts ¼ cup, chestnuts 5 pieces boiled and shelled, Shan Yao (Chinese yam) ½ cup chopped fresh or 9g dried, Long Yan Rou (longan berries) 5 pieces, white rice ½ cup.

Bone Broth

Bone broth extracts the Jing, or essence, from food. It is a slow, gentle process to procure the deepest, most guarded parts of the bones and vegetables. It is worth the effort in improved nutrition, as well as the taste, of food. Making bone broth is a simple process that takes time to master. It is worth the effort as good bone broth will both make a recipe and build the Kidneys and immunity. Rinse bones first and blanch to remove dirt and blood.

Table 8.2. Properties of Stock Ingredients.

Stock Ingredients	Qualities
Bones	Nourishs Jing Essence. Adds calcium and minerals. **Neutral:** Pork – nourishes Yin, increases fluids. Fish – moisten Dryness, dry Damp. **Warming:** Beef – builds Blood, tonifies Qi. Chicken – Qi tonic, aids digestion. Lamb – builds Blood, tonifies Qi.
Chicken feet, pig's feet (trotters)	Add collagen. Thicken stock. Benefit joints. Rejuvenate skin.
Carrots, winter squash, pumpkin	Tonify Qi
Beets, carrots, greens, turnips	Blood Building
Seaweeds, tomatoes, use culinary green herbs, avoid spices	Nourish Yin
Cooking spices (clove, cinnamon), garlic	Tonify Yang
Cabbage, beets, ginger, turmeric, pepper, mushrooms, turnips, onions	Blood Moving
Daikon radish, celery, seaweeds, mushrooms, parsnips, turnips, onion family, most culinary herbs and spices	Phlegm-Damp Resolving
Cabbage, celery, carrot, onion, burdock root, parsley, seaweeds, beets, greens	Liver Cleansing
Parsley, beets	Kidney Cleansing

Stock Ingredients	Qualities
Garlic, ginger, scallion, pepper, daikon radish	Exterior resolving

Basic Rules of Broth:[2]

1. Rinse bones first and blanch to remove dirt and blood.
2. Roast bones in the oven for 1-2 hours to greatly increases flavor.
3. Use a combination of long bones, tendons, feet, and odds and ends.
4. Cook stock at low, continuous temperature.
5. Cook animal parts 6 or more hours. Add vegetables during the final 45 minutes of cooking.
6. At the end of cooking, gently strain the stock to make it transparent.
7. Begin with an approximate ratio.
   Bone broth: 1 lb. bones and bits : 1 qt. cold water : ½ cup vegetables
   Vegetable Broth: 1 cup vegetables : 1 qt. cold water

Example Bone Broth Recipe

Ingredients:
5 lbs. Split bones, knuckles, tendons, etc.
6 chicken feet or 2 pig's feet
5qt. cold water
2 ½ cups vegetables of your choice
1 tbsp. each: star anise, tangerine peel, fennel seed, cinnamon bark, ginger

Preparation:
1. Preheat oven to 425 degrees F.
2. Bring pot of water to a boil. Rinse bones, chicken feet, and/or trotters and place in boiling water for 2 minutes. Remove.
3. Put bones (not chicken feet or trotters) in oven to roast for 1 hour until nicely browned.
4. Put bones, chicken feet/trotters in cold water over low heat. Skim bubbles and scum as they emerge. Once the water is clear add spices.
5. After the broth has cooked for 4-5 hours add vegetables. Cook an additional 1-2 hours. To strain, ladle slowly out of pot and through a fine colander. Take care not to agitate the broth. This is to avoid disturbing the sediment at the bottom of the pot.

Method of Administration:
Once cooled, divide stock into airtight containers. Refrigerated stock will keep for a few days. The rest can be frozen.

2. Adapted from Thomas Keller. *The French Laundry Cookbook.* (New York: Artisan, 1999).

Evening Soups

The last meal of the day should be simple, small, and easily digestible. Yin is growing at this time and digestive fire naturally weakens. Eat dinner by 7pm. This improves digestion and helps sleep. Dinner should be vegetable-based. A good combination is a soup and salad. Replace the salad with steamed vegetables in cold weather, during convalescence, a weak Spleen Qi (digestion), or a Cold constitution. Eat a cooled soup in hot weather or in case of Heat conditions.

Student's Soup

Tonifies Heart Blood and Spleen Qi. Benefits memory, boosts mental focus, and calms disturbed sleep. Excellent if forced to do late night cramming for a test or work on projects.

Ingredients:
6 pieces Long Yan Rou (longan berries)
1/4 cup Gou Qi Zi (go ji berries)
2 sticks Huang Qi (astragalus)
3 pieces Fu Ling (poria)
2-3 cups soup stock
1 cup carrots, celery, and daikon radish, chopped
½ cup of rice
leftover chicken or protein
small bunch of parsley

Preparation:
1. Place ingredients in pot. Bring to a boil and simmer for 1 hour.
2. Remove from heat and serve.

Method of Administration:
Eat 1 bowl for evening meal.

Herbal Decoctions

To make an herbal decoction, cook the herbs 2-3 times, straining the tea from each cooking and combining them at the end. First rinse and soak the herbs for 30 minutes. Cover with water and simmer the herbs for 45 minutes to extract the Yang. Strain. Add more water. Simmer for 45 minutes to extract the Yin. Strain. If a third cooking is desired, add more water. Simmer for 45 minutes to extract the Jing. Strain and combine with the other two decoctions.

Homemade Ferments

Fermentation is an enigmatic, chaotic, messy process that is central to every traditional culture; as a preservative, community-building ritual, and to provide vital nourishment. When modern conveniences removed fermentation from daily life, it weakened our natural vitality. Fermentation increases the bioavailability of nutrients, and provides enzymes and probiotics. Additionally, the process of fermentation connects us to an innate aspect of our humanity; the alchemical process. Fermented foods and/or drinks should be taken daily. If you suffer from digestive weakness, fungal infections, low immunity, or allergies, try to take a little fermented food with every meal.

Do not be intimidated by fermentation. It is a simple, natural process that requires minimal equipment. All you will need are a medium, a fermenting agent, and a clean container. There are endless foods and liquids that can provide a medium for fermentation: cabbage, milk, dough, sugar water, juice, tea, etc.

In terms of fermenting agents, there are two choices: buying a fermenting agent, such as kefir grains or sourdough starter, or capturing a wild ferment. Using a known fermenting agent produces more predictable results. These are readily available online (see Resources, page 392). Capturing wild ferments involves preparing an ideal medium and allowing whatever is in the air or lingering in the ingredients to ferment. This has added risk of molds and other undesirable elements taking over, but potentially introduces an exciting new flavor.

The final component is a clean container. Fermenting containers and the preparation area for ingredients should be as sterile as possible. I prefer using an airlock (Figure 8.1) for most fermentations; from sauerkraut to rice wine. Airlocks can be used on bottles or jars. They keep molds and airborne agents from invading the ferment and are relatively cheap. Endless recipes can be found in books and online. Here are some basic recipes to get you started.

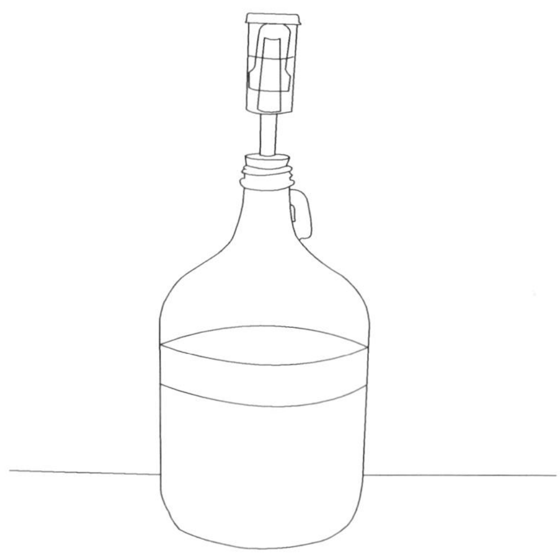

Figure 8.1. Airlock Fermentation

Milk Kefir

Indications:

Milk kefir is virtually fool-proof. It populates the digestive tract will beneficial bacteria, providing probiotics and digestive enzymes. Cow's milk or goat's milk can be used. Goat's milk is a Yang tonic, with a warming thermal property, and better tolerated by some. Low fat or full fat milk can be used, however, the milk must be organic and as natural as possible. Kefir grains are an excellent indicator of the quality of milk, as they do not proliferate in the presence of antibiotics and chemicals. Do not let metal utensils come in contact with kefir grains. Use plastic or wooden spoons and a plastic strainer. Note: Kefir grains proliferate after repeated fermentations so you will want to share them with others.

Ingredients:
1 ½ cups organic milk
1 tbsp. kefir grains

Procedure:
1. Place ingredients in a glass. Cover with paper towel or cheesecloth and a rubber band.
2. Let sit 12-24 hours. Less time is required in warmer temperatures, more in colder.
3. Strain with a plastic colander. Place grains in new milk. Drink the strained kefir milk.

Method of Administration:
Use kefir milk in smoothies or in small doses with meals. Kefir grains can be stored in milk in the refrigerator up to one week. If not used regularly, it can be dehydrated and frozen for long-term storage.

Coconut Water Kefir

Indications:
To reduce dairy intake, use coconut water instead of milk. Milk kefir grains can be adapted or else use water kefir grains.

Ingredients:
1 ½ cups coconut water
1 tbsp. milk or water kefir grains

Procedure:
1. Place ingredients in a glass. Cover with paper towel or cheesecloth and a rubber band.
2. Let sit 12-24 hours. Less time is required in warmer temperatures, more in colder.
3. Strain with plastic colander. Place grains in coconut water. Drink the strained kefir water.

Method of Administration:
Drink ¼ cup of kefir coconut water with meal.

Sauerkraut

Indications:
If you want to ferment vegetables, cabbage is the best one to start with. It readily turns into sauerkraut under extreme circumstances and builds confidence. Sauerkraut is high in Vitamin C, enzymes, probiotics, and promotes Blood circulation. Any vegetable can be fermented in a similar manner only some vegetables are trickier than others, notably cucumbers. Sauerkraut does not require a fermenting agent, though a vegetable ferment can be purchased online for more predictable results.

Ingredients:
1 head of Cabbage
Salt to taste
Dill or other herbs
Vegetable ferment or whey (optional)

Procedure:
1. Conserve two or three outer leaves of cabbage.
2. Finely chop the rest of the cabbage by hand or in a food processor. Mix with dill.
3. Place a layer of cabbage in a clean glass container. Salt the layer.
4. Add another layer of cabbage and salt. Continue until there is no more cabbage. The salt will make the cabbage weep.
5. Place the outer leaves of cabbage on top of the layers. Place a clean weight on top of the leaves so as to thoroughly submerge the cabbage in its own juice.
6. Close with an airlock lid or cheesecloth. Fermentation time varies widely based on climate and individual taste. It should sit anywhere from 5 days to several weeks.
7. Place in glass containers and refrigerate.

Method of Administration:
Eat ¼ cup of sauerkraut with meals as a digestive tonic.

Beet Kvass

Indications:
This is another amiable vegetable-based ferment. Beets nourish and move the Blood, and help balance the hormones. Additionally, beet kvass contains probiotics and digestive enzymes. Again, a vegetable fermenting agent may be used for predictability.

Ingredients:
2 beets
Salt to taste
3 cups water
Vegetable ferment or whey (optional)

Procedure:
1. Place ingredients in a glass jar with an airlock or other fermenting container.
2. Let sit 2-4 days. Less time is required in warmer temperatures, more in colder.
3. Strain and discard the dregs. Refrigerate the kvass.

Method of Administration:
Drink 1/4 cup of beet kvass with meals.

Chinese Rice Wine

Chinese rice wine has a complex, sherry-like taste that gets better with age. Rice wine was traditionally made in every household and is easy to make. It is not a true "wine" in that wines are made from fruit and beers from grains. Fruits contain available sugars and simply require a yeast to create alcohol. Grains, unlike fruit, do not have ready sugars available for fermentation. To make alcohol, grains are first sprouted (malted). This produces enzymes that convert starches into sugars to fuel the sprouts' rapid growth. The sprouted grains are then cooked to 170 degrees Fahrenheit and the liquid (now containing free sugars) is strained. Herbs are often added at this time along with yeast and flavorings and left to ferment. Fermenting grains in this manner is called beer.

Sprouted barley has the highest concentration of these starch-converting enzymes, hence its extensive use in beer. Rice has the least, meaning additional fermentation methods had to be developed. There are two other methods employed to convert starches into sugar for fermentation. These are 1) chewing the grains allowing enzymes present in saliva to convert the starches, or 2) using a mold to convert the starches into sugars. The latter method was used throughout Asia to make rice-based alcohol.(3)

Originally, ginger was dried, ground, and mixed with rice flour. These cakes were allowed to ferment the naturally occurring molds on the ginger.(4) The fermented cakes were mixed with cooked rice and allowed to ferment indefinitely. There are now commercially available wine cakes containing various yeasts and molds. White sweet rice is most often used. Through personal experimentation, basmati rice produces a sour wine and brown rice can be problematic. Short grain white rice and black sticky rice ferment well and provide distinct flavors.

Rice Wine can be used as a basic cooking wine, for drinking, or for making herbal tinctures and liniments. Red Rice Wine is preferred in some regions for postpartum and menstrual care recipes. Note: Sake cannot be used as a substitute for Chinese rice wine. It has a different taste and properties. Though it is made with rice as well, it undergoes a process more similar to beermaking.

Wine Cakes and Ferments:

Wine cakes come in two basic types, though there are numerous brands. Xiao qū (小麴, 小曲, found as 甜酒饼 in Vien Dong Vietnamese Market) translates as "small ferment." They are sold as dime-size cakes. They contain 2 active molds: one of the Mucor genus and the other of the Rhizopus genus, with the addition of a yeast. These are probably closest to the original profile of the fermented ginger cakes. They are more common in warmer parts of China and southeast Asia as they are slower to ferment and produce less heat.

The second type is called dà qū 大曲 or maì qū 麦曲, which translates as "big ferment" or "wheat ferment." As the name indicates, wheat rather than rice is cultured with Aspergillus oryzae, also

3. Stephen Harrod Buhner. Sacred and Herbal Healing Beers: The Secrets of Ancient Fermentation. (Boulder: Brewers Publications, 1998), 118.

4. Buhner, Sacred and Healing Beers, 118-119.

known as koji-kin in Japan, and other molds and yeasts. They likely evolved from the same process as the ginger rice cakes, only using wheat, the staple crop in colder parts of China. These are sold in bigger cakes. They provide more aggressive fermentation and are more popular.

A third ferment is sometimes used. Hóng qū (红曲) or "red yeast [rice]" does not come in cake form, but rather as dark red rice grains. This is rice that has been cultured with Monascus purpureus (hóng qū jùn, 紅曲菌). Red yeast rice is used as a natural colorant in food, as a ferment, and as an herb in TCM. It is used in TCM to treat Food Stagnation, Strengthen the Spleen and Stomach, and Invigorate the Blood. Traditionally, it is used in the postpartum period in the form of Red Rice Wine to treat Blood Stagnation and strengthen digestion. It is also used to treat trauma.

Basic Chinese Rice Wine

Indications:
Clay jars are traditionally used to brew rice wine. I use a glass jug with a plastic airlock top. This allows gases to escape while keeping potential contaminants out. Note: do not use a sealed container during any fermentation process or it will explode. You will only make this mistake once. Thankfully my grandfather made it for me in a notorious sauerkraut incident.
Ingredients:
1 kg (2.2 lb) of white sweet rice (4 cups)
8 cups of water
wine cake: xiao qu or da qu (according to package directions, usually 10-12 dime-sized cakes or 1 big cake) a bowl of water.

Procedure:
1. Soak rice overnight.
2. Cook rice: Put rice and 8 cups of water into a large saucepan. Bring to a boil. Lower heat and simmer until water has been absorbed and rice is cooked; usually 20 min. (Or follow directions on rice cooker).
3. Allow to stand and cool to room temperature; usually about 3 hours.
4. Grind or pound wine cake(s) into powder. Get a clean fermenting jug or vessel ready.
5. **Traditional way:** Set out three bowls: 1 bowl with the cooled cooked rice, 1 bowl with the powdered wine cake, and 1 bowl with water. Take a handful of rice, dip it in the powdered wine cake. Remove it from the bowl and thoroughly mix the powder with the rice in your hands. Drop it in the fermenting pot. Wet your hands in the bowl of water and repeat until all the ingredients have been used. At the end, use the water to rinse any last bit of powder into the fermenting container. The mixture should be moist.
6. **Modern way:** Use an electric mixer to gently mix the ingredients with the addition of a little water. Pour into fermenting jug or vessel.
   - Wait 30 days.
   - Strain the brew through a colander into a pitcher. The leftover fermented rice grains can be saved and used to make traditional recipes.

- Strain the brew a second time, this time through cheese cloth or other fine sieve into wine jugs for storing. These should be firmly closed. The wine can be used after nine months or can be allowed to age indefinitely, refining its flavor.

Method of Administration:
Use homemade rice wine to drink or in recipes and tinctures.

Red Yeast Wine

Indications:
Red Rice Wine is preferred in some regions for postpartum and menstrual care recipes. It has the added benefit of improving digestion and lowering cholesterol. Recently, red yeast rice has become popular in the U.S. for lowering cholesterol. This is attributed to its naturally occurring lovastatin, however the herb as a whole works is more effective than the isolated compounds.(5) Though red yeast rice does not contain the same level of lovastatin as synthetic statin drugs, it is still contraindicated in those with liver disease. The most common side effects of excessive statin use are muscle pain and liver and kidney dysfunction. The process for making Red Yeast Wine is identical to that of basic Rice Wine, only with the addition of the red yeast rice.

Ingredients:
1 kg (2.2 lb) of white rice (4 cups)
8 cups of water
wine cake: xiao qu or da qu (according to package directions, usually 10-12 little cakes or 1 big cake)
40g red yeast rice
bowl of water

Procedure:
Follow steps 1-10 of the Sweet Rice Wine recipe above. Only, grind the red yeast rice together with the wine cake.

Method of Administration:
Use in all Postpartum recipes and Menstrual recovery recipes as desired. Red yeast wine is also used to lower cholesterol and move the Blood.

5. "The therapeutic dose of Hong Qu delivers approximately 7.2 mg of lovastatin, while the synthetic drug lovastatin (Mevacor) contains 10 to 40 mg of lovastatin. Yet, despite the lower dose of the supposed active component, the hypolipidemic effects of Hong Qu are much greater than the synthetic drug lovastatin. Thus it is clear that lovastatin is not the only active component, and more research needs to be done on Hong Qu as an herbal medicine, not just on lovastatin as a single herb." Chen, *Chinese Medical Herbology*, 528.

Black Glutinous Rice Wine Recipe

Indications:
For tonification purposes, rice wine made with black glutinous rice is preferred. The taste is decidedly more complex and smoky. Tonic herbs can be added after the initial fermentation and allowed to age together.

Ingredients:
1 kg (2.2 lb) of black glutinous rice (4 cups)
8 cups of water
wine cake: xiao qu or da qu (according to package directions, usually 10-12 little cakes or 1 big cake)
bowl of water

Preparation:
Follow steps 1-10 of the Sweet Rice Wine recipe above.

Method of Administration:
Medicinal wines are heating and usually reserved for times of convalescence (postpartum or menses) or after menopause.

Immunity Recipes

These home remedies are effective for the beginnings of a cold. Take them, bundle up, and go to bed to sweat out the cold. Be sure to stay warm after taking the remedy and repeat every four hours. These are not strong remedies, but if the cold is caught early enough it can be enough push them out of the body before they can take hold. Once a cold has settled, it will require a more complex herbal formula.

Ginger Scallion Tea

Indications:
Take at the first sign of a cold.

Ingredients:
½ inch piece of fresh ginger, grated
1 scallion, finely chopped
1-2 tsp honey
1 ½ cups water

Procedure:
1. Put ginger, scallions, and water into a small saucepan over med-high heat. Bring to a boil, then simmer for 10 min.
2. Strain. Add honey and serve.

Method of Administration:
Bundle up right after taking to sweat out the cold.

Garlic Tea

Indications:
My great-grandfather swore by this remedy, though the rest of the family was not so fond of it. Best for cold weather or Cold constitutions.

Ingredients:
1-2 cloves of garlic
1 cup water honey to taste

Procedure:
Mash garlic and place in a cup. Add boiling water and honey to taste. Serve hot.

Method of Administration:
Bundle up right after taking to sweat out the cold.

Steamed Asian Pears

Indications:
This is a wellknown Chinese remedy to clear Phlegm from the Lungs and nourish Lung Yin. Excellent to strengthen the Lungs, for persistent dry cough, and to recover from colds. Preventive eaten in Fall and Winter months.

Ingredients:
1 Asian Pear (regular pear can be used)
10g Chuan Bei Mu (fritillaria), powdered

Preparation:
1. Core the pear and put powdered herbs inside.
2. Steam for 15 min. Serve.

Method of Administration:
Can be eaten daily for dry cough.

Menstruation & Postpartum Recipes

Recipes and care are similar during Menstrual Recovery and Postpartum Recovery. The main distinction is that Postpartum Recovery has longer stages and uses rice wine in most recipes. The addition of rice wine is optional during menses and should be omitted in cases of Heat or Damp-Heat. The plan presented here adheres to Shuqi Zhuang's[(6)] basic outline. I was influenced by my two TCM gynecology teachers, Dr. Shaoting Jing and Dr. Jiang Zheng. I also have added my experiences.

Stage 1: Cleansing the Uterus

Recipes for Menstrual Recovery Days 1-2, Postpartum Recovery Week

General Recipes

Sheng Hua Tang – 3 x a day

Indications:
Sheng Hua Tang is the most widely used postpartum formula and is commonly used during menses. It was first listed in Fu Qing Zhu's Gynecology (early Qing dynasty). Fu Qing-zhu advocated giving Sheng Hua Tang to all women for 2 weeks after giving birth and with modifications to treat several post-birth diseases. It both nourishes and invigorates the Blood. Sheng Hua Tang cleans out the contents of the uterus and helps to shrink it back to normal size. Taken for 1-2 days it raises antibodies and physical strength. It is very important that the lochia (postpartum) and uterine lining (during menses) be completely discharged in order to avoid health problems, such as fibroids, cancer, and painful periods.[(7)] Ideally, use with Red Yeast Wine or other Chinese Rice Wine.

Ingredients (1 day's dosage):
Whole Dang Gui (Chinese angelica) 24g, Chuan Xiong (ligusticum) 18g, Tao Ren (peach kernel, remove core) 1.5g, Pao Gan Jiang (fresh ginger, stir fry ginger in pan until browned on both sides) 1.5g, Zhi Gan Cao (honey fried licorice) 1.5g.
Water 4 ½ cups with Rice Wine ½ -1 cup or Yue Zi Water 5 ½ cups

Preparation:
1. Rinse medicinal herbs in a colander with hot water.
2. Pour 3 cups of liquid into a large non-aluminum pot. Add medicinal herbs, cover, and

6. A wellknown Taiwanese TCM doctor who specializes in postpartum and menstrual care.

7. Shuqi Zhuang. *Postpartum Recovery Program; a Manual of Rules and Recipes for the Postpartum Woman.* (Taiwan: Guang He Chu Ban She, 2005). ISBN 9578807015

bring to a boil. Simmer over low heat for 45 min. The liquid should reduce to a little less than a cup. Pour out and strain decoction. Reserve both herbs and decoction.
3. Add 2 ½ cups of liquid into the pot with the reserved herbs. Bring to a boil and allow to simmer until the liquid is reduced to a littele less than a cup. Strain decoction and throw out the excess herbs.
4. Combine first and second decoctions.

Method of Administration:
Divide into 3 doses and take before meals, about 1/2 cup each time. Warm before drinking.

Postpartum Recovery Tea:(8)

Indications:
This tea hydrates the body while still promoting water metabolism. Traditionalists are adamant that consuming water and other beverages (especially cold drinks) can have a harmful effect on the metabolism. The Postpartum Recovery Tea is a traditional way to quench your thirst and stay hydrated. It is made with rice wine with the addition of appropriate amounts of Shan Zha (hawthorn berry), Li Zhi Pi (lychee shell), Long Yan Rou (longan berries), or Guan Yin (clerodendri) and always taken warm. A modern modification is to make it with water with a smaller amount of rice wine or with Yue Zi Water. If you choose to forgo the rice wine altogether, make sure you still only drink warm fluids. Warm fluids conserve the Qi and help promote proper water metabolism. I also recommend using smaller amounts of Shan Zha (hawthorn berry) to avoid hyperacidity in the Stomach.

Ingredients (10 day supply):
Shan Zha (hawthorn berries), Li Zhi Pi (lychee shell), Long Yan Rou (longan berries)and/or Guan Yin (clerodendri) together 600g
brown sugar to taste (optional)
1 ½ gallons water with rice wine or Yue Zi Water

Preparation:
1. Rinse herbs and put them in a pot with liquid.
2. Place pot over high heat, cover. Bring to a boil and reduce to low heat. Simmer for1 hour.
3. Strain. Store decoction and discard herbs.

Method of Administration:
Drink warm throughout the day in place of water to hydrate the body.

Liver (1-2 servings a day)

Liver is the ideal food during menses and postpartum as it strongly tonifies Blood while moving and

8. Modified from Shuqi Zhuang. *Postpartum Recovery Program; a Manual of Rules and Recipes for the Postpartum Woman.* (Taiwan: Guang He Chu Ban She, 2005). ISBN 9578807015

detoxifying at the same time. Pork liver is traditionally used. It has a neutral thermal temperature, is more bitter than other types of liver, has the added benefit of reducing edema, and I suspect is preferred because pig's are genetically closer to us. In the U.S., this may be difficult to procure. It is most important that the liver be organic and humanely raised. In my opinion, pork liver is the least palatable and beef liver is the best tasting of the livers. Chicken liver is hot in nature and best suited to those with cold and Yang deficiency. Beef liver is neutral and benefits the eyes.[9] Choose liver that is soft, elastic, and thick. Eating liver will be the biggest hurdle for most women, and yet it is the best food to both build your Blood and move old Blood out of the body.

Cooking:
To remove strong taste, soak liver in water with citrus juice (lemon, lime, orange, calamondin) or vinegar for 30 min prior to cooking. This is necessary for pork liver. I prefer liver in larger "steaks," about 1 ½ inches thick, with the outside seared and the middle still pink. This removes much of the texture issues, creating a crunchy/creamy experience. The nice seared crust is achieved by a combination of first warming the black sesame oil to high heat before adding the liver to the pan. Dusting the liver first with cornstarch or arrowroot powder mixture prior to frying makes it even better. You may prefer to cut the liver into tiny pieces that disappear into the seasoning. The following is a basic liver recipe to get you started. Feel free to experiement with the key ingredients: liver, ginger, black sesame oil, and Chinese rice wine.

Ginger:
Use fresh mature ginger as you would find in most supermarkets. Dried ginger is very warming and goes to the Kidneys. Fresh ginger releases the exterior and harmonizes the Spleen and Stomach. When charred, ginger helps stop bleeding. When browned (not blackened) it has a specific function as a guiding herb to the uterus and helps to move stagnant Blood there. To brown ginger, slice thinly and fry on each side until it crinkles and browns. It will become more fragrant. This is an important detail.

Chinese Rice Wine:
Alcohol is warming and helps move the Blood. The use of rice wine is more important postpartum. Take care not to add alcohol to your diet during the Menstrual Renewal Program if you run hot or have Liver issues.

Basic Stir-Fried Liver

Indications:
Breaks up Blood stagnation in the uterus and helps discharge lochia. Begin eating this recipe the first day postpartum or the first day of menstrual bleeding to nourish and transform the blood. It is crucial to clean out the uterus and encourage it to contract back to its normal state. Otherwise this can lead to chronic Blood stagnation and mass accumulations in the long run.

9. Pitchford, *Healing with Whole Foods*

Ingredients (1 day's dosage):
17-25 ounces, 1-1.5 lbs. organic liver
citrus juice or vinegar to cover the liver
40 g fresh ginger
1 tsp. black sesame oil
2 1/2 cups water with rice wine or Yue Zi water (optional during menses)
seasoning (cumin, tarragon, thyme, and turmeric are a good combination)

Preparation:
1. Clean liver, cut into ½ inch steaks or small pieces. Soak in citrus juice or vinegar.
2. Clean ginger and cut into thin pieces.
3. Pour sesame oil into wok or frying pan and put over high heat.
4. Add ginger and cook until browned.
5. Add liver and sauté until it changes color. It is done when it is seared on the outside but is still soft when pressed with a fork.
6. Add rice wine and quickly bring to a boil, eat while still warm.

Method of Administration:
Divide into 2 dosages. Eat the first bowl at breakfast and the second at lunch as the main dish. It can be paired with rice or congee.

Red Adzuki Beans (2 servings per day)

Edema is typical in the final stage of pregnancy, the month postpartum, and during menstruation. These excess fluids must be discharged from the body or they will quickly transform into fat. Red adzuki beans have a strong diuretic effect and benefit the heart. They also move the Blood and drain Dampness. It is an indispensable food for postpartum and menstruating women. The daily dosage is 60g or 1/3 cup of the dried beans divided in two dosages. Eating excess red adzuki beans causes gas, therefore limit intake to two bowls a day. Brown sugar is used postpartum as it is warming.

Red Adzuki Bean Drink

Indications:
This is the easiest way to include red adzuki beans in the diet.

Ingredients (1 day's dosage):
1/3 cup red adzuki beans
1 bay leaf
2 cups water or Yue Zi Water
dash of rice wine (postpartum)
add seasoning (such as coriander) or sweetener (dates, brown sugar, etc.)

Procedure:

1. Soak beans 8 hours or overnight.
2. Place beans, bay leaf, and water in saucepan. Bring to a boil and skim off bubbles. Simmer for 1 hour or until beans are thoroughly cooked.
3. Add seasoning or sweetener and blend in a blender. Skim off any bubbles.

Method of Administration:
Divide and drink throughout the day. Recipe can be doubled or tripled to last a few days.

Water Reducing Congee

Indications:
This recipe combines several key postpartum ingredients: red adzuki beans, Yi Yi Ren, rice, and ginger.

Ingredients:
1/3 cup red adzuki beans
¼ cup Yi Yi Ren (Job's tears)
¼ cup of white rice (jasmine, or sushi; postpartum use sweet rice)
3 slices of fresh ginger
1 piece of tangerine peel (optional)
5 cups of water (postpartum add 1 cup rice wine or use Yue Zi Water)
add brown sugar to taste (optional)

Preparation:

1. Sauté ginger in saucepan over high heat until browned.
2. Place ingredients in crock pot or rice cooker and cook overnight.

Method of Administration:
Eat 1 bowl first thing in the morning. One bowl equals 1 serving of red adzuki beans and 1 serving of rice.

Rice (2 servings a day)

Eat white rice during Stage 1. Postpartum women can use sweet glutinous rice as it has a stronger action to tonify Qi and Blood and promotes bowel movements. Constipation during the postpartum period can lead to organ prolapsed and must be avoided. In later stages, brown rice can be used, but should be soaked and sprouted before cooking to increase digestibility. If still hungry, supplement with more Yi Yi Ren Rice.

Yi Yi Ren Rice

Indications:
Yi Yi Ren (Job's tears) has several functions that make it an ideal food postpartum and during menses. It strengthens the Spleen, leeches out Dampness (reduces edema), expels Wind-Damp (joint pain), and clears Damp-Heat (balances the tonifying diet). It also has a slightly cool temperature. Raw Yi Yi Ren drains edema and Heat. Roasted, it tonifies the Spleen. Note: Yi Yi Ren is different from pearl barley. It can be ordered from Asian food markets or Chinese herb shops.

Ingredients:
¼ cup Yi Yi Ren (Job's Tears), half raw and half toasted, broken with mortar and pestle
1 cup white rice (postpartum use sweet glutinous rice)
2 cups water (postpartum add rice wine or use Yue Zi Water)

Preparation:
1. Bring all ingredients to a boil in a saucepan. Let simmer 20 min.
2. Turn off heat and let stand 5 min.
3. Alternately can be prepared in rice cooker. (use rice cooker cup and measurement line for proportions)

Method of Administration:
Eat up to two bowls of Yi Yi Ren Rice a day.

Sweet Rice Congee

Indications:
The addition of Longyan Rou (longan berries) strengthens the Qi and Blood tonifying function of the congee. Lian Zi (lotus nut) tonifies the Spleen and black wood ear fungus moves the Blood. If constipation is an issue, add hemp, chia, or sesame seeds to this congee. It is important to eat sweet rice in moderation as it can be difficult to digest and can cause flatulence and indigestion when eaten in excess.

Ingredients:
½ cup sweet (glutinous) rice
½ cup Long Yan Rou (longan berries)
5 pieces Lian Zi (lotus nut)
3-5 pieces Hei Mu Er (black wood ear fungus)
5 cups water (postpartum, with ½ cup rice wine or 5 ½ cups Yue Zi Water)
brown sugar to taste (optional)

Preparation:
1. Soak sweet rice for 8 hours or overnight.

2. Soak herbs for 30 min.
3. Put all ingredients into rice cooker (set on porridge) or crock pot. Cook for 8 hours.On the stovetop, put ingredients into pot. Bring to a boil over high heat, then reduce heat and simmer for 8 hours.
4. Add sweetener if desired and serve.

Administration/Dosage:
Divide the day's dose into two bowls. Take with breakfast and lunch.

Eggs (1 serving a day)

Eggs should be eaten the entire month postpartum as they nourish Yin and Blood, promote lactation, and help recover the body after illness. They are also helpful during and post-menses.

Postpartum Eggs[10]

Ingredients (5 day's dosage):
10 raw eggs
1 bottle of rice vinegar
1 lb. of fresh ginger, chopped
brown sugar to taste[11]

Preparation:
1. Thirty days prior to projected delivery, put all ingredients in a pot (except sugar) and bring to a boil. Simmer for 10 min.
2. Remove from heat and mix in sugar.
3. Cool and refrigerate for 30 days.

Method of Administration:
After delivery, eat 2 eggs a day for 5 days.

Vegetables (2-3 servings a day)

Traditionally, there are no vegetables during the first week postpartum. They are considered excessively cooling and clearing. A modification is to eat cooked red and orange vegetabes (carrots, beets, yams, winter squash) which are more tonifying. During cycle days 1-4 of menstruation eat 2-3 servings of cooked vegetables. Avoid raw salads and raw fruit as they are too cooling.

---

10. Modfied from Shaoting Jing. "TCM Gynecology." (lecture, Yo San University, Los Angeles, May 22, 2003).
11. Brown sugar is often added to recipes postpartum as it is warming. Omit if there are Damp conditions or blood sugar issues.

Fish Soup (1-2 servings a day)

Light, soft fish is eaten as it is easy to digest and helps build the strength of new mothers. Traditionally, postpartum women eat Flathead Mullet fish (Mugil cephalus), Black Larvel, or Yellow Croaker fish (Pseudosciaena crocea and polyactis) for the first two weeks after giving birth, after which they can eat richer fish. During menses any fish may be used and vegetables added to the soup.

Fish Soup

Ingredients:
½ -1 lb. mild fish about
½ inch fresh ginger
1 tsp. black sesame oil
lime
1 bunch parsley or cilantro, chopped
2 cups soup stock dash of rice wine or Yue Zi Water

Preparation:
1. Bring stock to a boil. Allow to simmer while preparing rest of ingredients.
2. Clean fish and ginger and cut into pieces. Marinate fish in lime juice.
3. Add black sesame oil into wok and place over high heat.
4. Add ginger and sauté until browned.
5. Add fish. Sear on both sides. Lower heat and allow to cook a few min. Be sure the fish is still soft when pressing down on it with a fork.
6. Remove fish from heat and add to the stock. Add parsley or cilantro.

Method of Administration:
Eat 1-2 bowls daily.

Special Postpartum Remedies

Uterine Pain

Note: If you are experiencing pain, see a doctor to assess the severity of the condition, even if you choose alternative methods for addressing it. It is important to make informed decisions.

Hawthorn Berry Tea

Shan Zha (hawthorn berry) clears Blood stagnation, dissolves Food stagnation (particularly from protein), and resolves pain. Interestingly, though Fu Qing Zhu advises against the use of Shan Zha, many modern practitioners utilize it during postpartum care.

Ingredients (3 day's dosage):
600g Shan Zha (hawthorn berry)
4 ½ cups liquid (water with a dash of rice wine or Yue Zi Water)
brown sugar (optional)

Preparation:
1. Place Shan Zha and rice wine (or water) in a non-aluminum pot. Bring to a boil over high heat. Cover and reduce to low heat. Simmer for 1 hour.
2. Strain decoction into uncovered pot. Cook over high heat until reduced to about 2 ½ cups.
3. If desired, add sweetener to taste. Mix well and turn off heat. It is ready to serve.

Administration/Dosage:
The daily dosage is about 1 cup. Take small amounts several times throughout the day. Drink for three consecutive days. This will dissolve congealed blood. Note: Shan Zha is very acid and should be avoided in those with Stomach Heat or hyperacidity in the stomach.

C-Section, Miscarriage, or Abortion:

In these cases, drink Bai Du Tang for 3 days postpartum to combat infection. Replace Stir-fried Pork Liver with Liver Congee days 1-3. Drink Red Date Tea throughout the day for one week before and after C-section or abortion to protect the Liver from anesthesia.

Liver Congee with Chinese Herbs[12]

In cases of C-section birth, abortion, or miscarriage, this recipe is indicated as a staple food for the first 3 days postpartum. Liver Congee replenishes nutrients, tonifies Qi, promotes urination, and prevents inflammation.

Ingredients:
1 cup Fresh Shan Yao (Chinese yam) or 12g of dried Shan Yao, chopped
¼ cup Yi Yi Ren (Job's tears)
½ cup white rice
5 pieces of Fu Ling (poria)
6 pieces of Lian Zi (lotus seed)
6 Bai Guo (gingko nuts)
¼ cup Qian Shi (foxnut)
½ lb organic liver, chopped

12. Modified from Shuqi Zhuang. *Postpartum Recovery Program; a Manual of Rules and Recipes for the Postpartum Woman.* (Taiwan: Guang He Chu Ban She, 2005). ISBN 9578807015

lime, orange, or lemon juice
4 cups of water
1 cup rice wine

Preparation:
1. Rinse all dried medicinal herbs with hot water and soak in water for 45 min.
2. Wash liver, cut into cubes, and soak in lime, lemon, or orange juice for 15-30 min.
3. Place all ingredients into a crock pot or rice cooker. Cook for 6 hours or overnight.Eat while still warm.

Administration/Dosage:
Eat 1 bowl, twice a day for the first 3 days postpartum.

Red Date Tea (Yang Gan Tang)[13]

This formula protects and strengthens the Liver. It is indicated 1 week prior and 2 weeks after anesthesia. Possible side effects from anesthesia include: flatulence, hair loss, insomnia, memory loss, constipation, and other symptoms. Since C-sections are not always foreseeable, it is recommended that all expectant mothers begin taking Red Date Tea one week prior to projected delivery. Prior to birth, use water to make a tea. Postpartum women can switch to rice wine.

Ingredients (2 day's dosage):
7 pieces of Hong Zao (red jujube dates), split
2 cups water (postpartum, use water with rice wine or Yue Zi Water)

Preparation:
1. Rinse Hong Zao with hot water. Use a knife to cut open the fruits longitudinally. Soak in water or rice wine for 45 min.
2. Put ingredients into a pot. Bring to a boil and simmer for 1 hour.
3. Strain decoction and serve.

Administration/Dosage:
The daily dose is 1 ¼ cup and can be taken in multiple doses throughout the day. Serve as a tea. During the postpartum period serve warm.

Bai Du Tang[14]

This formula is used in women who have had a C-section birth, abortion, or miscarriage in order to prevent wound inflammation and infection. Take for the first 3 days postpartum.

---

13. Modified from Shuqi Zhuang. *Postpartum Recovery Program; a Manual of Rules and Recipes for the Postpartum Woman.* (Taiwan: Guang He Chu Ban She, 2005). ISBN 9578807015

14. Modified from Shuqi Zhuang. *Postpartum Recovery Program; a Manual of Rules and Recipes for the Postpartum Woman.* (Taiwan: Guang He Chu Ban She, 2005). ISBN 9578807015

Ingredients (1 day's dosage):
Jin Yin Hua (Japanese honeysuckle) 20g, Tian Hua Fen (tricosanthus) 20g, Chuan Xiong (ligusticum) 10g, Yan Hu Suo (corydalis) 7g, Bai Zhi (angelica) 7g, Tu Fu Ling (smilax) 25g, Dang Gui (Chinese angelica) 7g, Guang Chen Pi (tangerine peel) 12g, Gan Cao (licorice) 7g, Jie Geng (platycodi) 15g, Zhe Bei Mu (fritillaria) 20g
4 cups of water or Yue Zi Water

Preparation:
1. Rinse medicinal herbs.
2. Add 2 ½ cups of the water into a large non-aluminum pot. Add medicinal herbs.Soak for 45 min.
3. Bring to a boil and simmer, covered, over low heat for 1 hour. There should be approximately 1 cup of liquid left. Strain decoction and reserve decoction and herbs.
4. Add remaining 1 ½ cups of water to the herbs. Repeat steps for the first decoction. About ½ cup should remain. Strain and reserve decoction. Throw out herbs.
5. Combine first and second decoctions, totaling about 1 ½ cups.

Method of Administration:
Divide into two dosages and drink daily for the first 3 days postpartum.

Stage 2: Contracting the Uterus

Recipes for Menstrual Recovery Days 3-4, Postpartum Recovery Week 2

General Recipes

Continue Sheng Hua Tang and Postpartum Recovery Tea from Stage 1.

Kidneys (2 servings a day)

Eating kidneys is incredible medicine during any period of deficiency. They tonify the Kidneys for issues such as low back pain, low libido, fatigue, etc. They also treat the emotional level: timidity and weak boundaries. These are symptoms of Gallbladder deficiency, which is supported by the Kidney Yang.

Cooking:
Most find kidneys more palatable than liver. Be sure to cut them in half and remove all the white membranous material prior to cooking. If not, there will be a distinct urine smell and taste that renders the kidneys inedible. Many also prefer to soak the kidneys in citrus (lemon,

lime, orange) juice or vinegar. Prepare them with browned ginger, black sesame oil, and rice wine, as the liver above. Be sure to buy organic kidneys. Pork kidneys are preferred by traditionalists due to their neutral thermal temperature. I find them too strong tasting and prefer lamb or beef. Lamb kidneys are the most heating and appropriate for Yang deficiency. Beef kidneys are less warming.

Basic Stir-Fried Kidney

Indications:
Speeds metabolism and helps contract the uterus.

Ingredients (1 day's dosage):
2 organic kidneys
citrus juice or vinegar to cover kidneys
½ inch fresh ginger, grated
1 tsp. black sesame oil
2 ½ cups water with rice wine or Yue Zi water (optional during menses)
seasoning (cumin, tarragon, thyme, and turmeric are a good combination)

Preparation:
1. Rinse the kidneys. Cut in half. Remove the white-colored membranes (urinary glands). Rinse the kidneys again.
2. Soak in citrus juice or vinegar for 30 min. Strain and pat dry.
3. Traditionally the kidneys are scored in two directions so that the kidneys form "flowers" when cooked. You may do this or leave them whole.
4. Add black sesame oil to frying pan and put over high heat,
5. Add ginger, reduce to low heat. Sauté until ginger is browned on both sides.
6. Turn up to high heat again. Add kidneys and sauté until you see a change in color.
7. Add rice wine and bring to a boil. Turn off heat and serve while still warm.

Method of Administration:
Divide into two bowls. It can be paired with a serving of rice.

Red Adzuki Beans (2 servings a day)

Eat 2 servings as in Stage 1.

Rice (2 serving a day)

Eat 1 serving of Yi Yi Ren rice or congees as in Stage 1. Add 1 serving of Stir-Fried Sticky Rice. If still hungry, supplement with more Yi Yi Ren Rice.

Stir-Fried Sticky Rice

Indications:
This recipe is a nice treat.

Ingredients:
¾ cup sweet (glutinous) rice (during menses can choose any rice)
5 pieces dried shitake mushrooms, stem removed
2 pieces black wood ear fungus
1 carrot, chopped
1 clove of garlic, minced
½ inch ginger, grated or chopped
1 tsp black sesame oil
1 ½ cups of water (postpartum, add rice wine or use Yue Zi Water)

Preparation:
1. Wash rice and rinse. Soak rice for 8 hours or overnight. Strain.
2. Soak dried mushrooms and wood ear until soft. Discard stem and chop into small pieces.
3. Add sesame oil to frying plan over med-high heat. Add ginger and garlic. Sauté until browned.
4. Add carrot, mushrooms, and fungus. Sauté until it has some color and remove.
5. Add more sesame oil to frying pan and sauté rice.
6. Add liquid.
7. Place all ingredients into rice cooker and cook.

Method for Administration:
Eat 1-2 small bowls daily.

Eggs (1 serving a day)

Eat an eggs scrambled, poached, or boiled.

Vegetables (2 servings a day)

By the 2nd week postpartum, traditionalists consider it safe to add red and orange vegetables such as beets, carrots, tomatoes, yams, winter squash, red radishes, and red-tinged greens. Vegetables should be prepared with browned ginger and a dash of rice wine, like all postpartum recipes. During cycle days 3-4 of menstruation eat 2-3 servings of any cooked vegetables. Avoid salads and raw fruit as they are too cooling.

Fish Soup (1 serving a day)

Light, soft fish is eaten as it is easy to digest and helps build the strength of new mothers. Add carrots, beets, and/or greens to fish soup recipe from Stage 1. Traditionally, postpartum women eat Flathead Mulletfish (Mugil cephalus), Black Larvel, or Yellow Croaker fish (Pseudosciaena crocea and polyactis) for the first two weeks after giving birth, after which they can eat richer fish. During menses any fish may be used.

Stage 3: Tonification

Recipes for Menstrual Recovery Days 5-7, Postpartum Recovery Weeks 3-4/5

General Recipes

Discontinue Sheng Hua Tang and replace with a stronger Qi and Blood tonifying formula, such as Ba Zhen Tang, Gui Pi Tang, or Gui Shao Di Huang. This is also the time to nourish Yin. If postpartum, continue taking Postpartum Recovery Tea. Supplement the diet with recipes and formulas to increase lactation 3-7 days a week (p.371).

Chicken (2 servings a day)

During Stage 3 it is finally safe to use strong tonics. Chicken is an important Qi and Blood tonic and should be eaten regularly for a full six months after giving birth. Doing so will promote adequate milk production, as well as build good health in both mother and baby.

Dang Gui Chicken Soup (Black Chicken Soup)

Dang Gui Chicken Soup is a key recipe to rebuild the Blood after menstruation has ended. It is too tonifying to eat while still bleeding. It strongly boosts energy and recovers the body. It is an excellent beautifying formula and is high in collagen. It always includes Dang Gui and black (silkie) chicken,[(15)] though there are many versions. This is my version. If there is Heat omit the rice wine. Note: Simmer on low setting of crock pot. If it gets too hot it will turn more bitter.

Ingredients:
1 whole black (silkie) chicken
20g Huang Qi (astragalus)
10g Dang Gui (Chinese angelica)
5 pieces Longyan Rou (longan berries)

15. Black-boned or Silkie chicken is stronger to nourish the Blood. Purchase frozen at Asian markets. Do not remove skin before cooking.

3g Chen Pi (tangerine peel)
fresh ginger
9g Du Zhong (eucomia)
2 cups - 1 bottle of Black Glutinous Rice Wine
water to cover, if necessary

Preparation:
1. Bring a large pot of water to a boil. Blanch chicken for 2 min. Drain and remove chicken from heat.
2. Rinse medicinal herbs.
3. Add all ingredients to crock pot. Add rice wine and water to cover chicken and herbs. Cook for 2-3 hours.
4. Remove Du Zhong (eucomia) and Huang Qi (astragalus) pieces. Shred the chicken and remove bones.
5. Consume the rest of the herbs, de-boned chicken, and decoction as a soup.

Method of Administration:
Divide into doses to be eaten over a three-day period.

Basic Stir-Fried Chicken

Indications:
Postpartum recipe.

Ingredients (1 day's dosage):
chicken (approximately half chicken)
½ inch piece fresh ginger, chopped
1 tsp. black sesame oil
2 1/2 cups water with rice wine or Yue Zi water (optional during menses)

Method of Preparation:
1. Wash chicken, then cut into pieces with a knife.
2. Add black sesame oil to sauce pan over med-high heat.
3. Add ginger and sauté until it browned.
4. Add chicken pieces. Sauté chicken for 7 min.
5. Add rice wine. Cover pot and bring to a boil. Reduce heat and simmer for 15-20 minutes.

Method of Administration:
Divide dosage into two bowls. During the third postpartum week eat one bowl at breakfast and one at lunch each day. This recipe can be paired with rice.

Red Adzuki Beans (1 serving a day)

Cut the amount of daily consumption by half; 30g per day.

Rice (2 servings a day)

Eat congee, Yi Yi Ren Rice, or Stir-Fry recipes from Stages 1 & 2. Eat more servings of Yi Yi Ren Rice if still hungry.

Eggs (1 serving a day)

Eggs may be scrambled, poached, or boiled.

Vegetables (2-3 servings a day)

All vegetables can be eaten during the 3rd week postpartum, provided they are cooked. Ideally they are sautéed in black sesame oil and ginger, but they can also be steamed. One serving of fruit a day is also permitted. Green papaya is a good choice as it aids breast milk.

Fish Soup (1 serving a day)

Other fish can be added, particularly red and black fish. White Perch or Black Sea Bass are especially helpful for recovery from C-section.

Special Remedies

Increasing Lactation

The following are traditional recipes to increase lactation. Food therapy is sufficient in some cases. Other cases require one of the Chinese herbal formulas listed after the recipes. In addition to the pig's trotters and peanuts and the carp and tofu combinations below, chicken, lamb, and green papaya also promote milk production.

Pig's Trotter's Soup

Indications:
This is my rendition of the traditional postpartum formula. It always contains pig's feet and peanuts, often with Chinese herbs. I find it tastes better to drink the herbs separately as a

formula. This recipe not only promotes breast milk production, but its high collagen content makes it also a skin beautifying and joint recovery recipe.

Ingredients (3 day's dosage):
1-2 lbs. pig's trotters (feet, have butcher cut each one into 4 pieces)
1 cup raw peanuts with shells removed
1 inch piece fresh ginger
½ cup dried shitake mushrooms with stems removed
1 tbsp. black sesame oil
2-4 cups water with rice wine or Yue Zi Water
water to cover
3 scallion stalks, finely chopped

Seasoning:
3 pieces star anise
1 tbsp fennel seeds
2 pieces cinnamon bark
¼ tsp nutmeg
2 pieces of Gan Cao (licorice)
1 clove minced garlic (omit in Heat conditions)
2 tbsp soy sauce
2 tsp powdered orange peel
salt and white pepper to taste

Preparation:
1. Soak shitake mushrooms in water until soft. Strain and cut into slices. Reserve.
2. Put peanuts into a pot with water and bring to a boil. Strain and cool slightly. While still warm, peel off the membrane and break into halves.
3. Add black sesame oil into a pot and heat. Add ginger and sauté until browned.
4. Add pig's trotters to the pot and sauté until skin changes color. Remove from pot.
5. Add peanuts to pot and sauté. Return pig's trotters and ginger to the pot. Add shitake mushrooms, seasoning, rice wine, and water to cover ingredients.
6. Cover and bring to a boil. Lower heat and simmer for 2-8 hours. (Can be transferred to crock pot).
7. Remove from heat and stir in scallions.

Method of Administration:
Lactating mothers can eat 1 bowl, 3-7 times a week to promote abundant breast milk and strengthen their bodies. In cases of scanty milk due to deficiency, eat 1 small bowl twice a day for three days in a row. This soup can be eaten anytime for rejuvenation, skin beautification, or joint health.

Carp and Tofu Soup

Indications:
Carp is the preferred fish to promote lactation. It is also called grass carp or white amur, or wan yú 鯶魚 in Chinese. It is traditionally paired with tofu and eaten postpartum. This is my version.

Ingredients:
½ lb. carp (remove skin, bones, and cut into pieces)
½ package of firm tofu (cut into cubes)
½ cup winter squash or pumpkin (cut into cubes)
1 large tomato, diced
1 large carrot, chopped
1 small onion, finely chopped
½ inch fresh ginger, finely chopped
3 cups vegetable broth, with a little rice wine or Yue Zi Water
black sesame oil for sautéing salt and white pepper to taste

Procedure:
1. Add black sesame oil to medium sauce pan over med-high heat. Add ginger and onions. Sauté until browned.
2. Add vegetable broth, tofu, squash, tomato, and carrot to the pan. Bring to a boil and simmer 20-30 min., until squash is tender.
3. Meanwhile, add black sesame oil to a frying pan over med-high heat. Add carp, sautéing until browned on both sides. Add to soup and cook 2-5 min.
4. Add salt and white pepper to taste and serve.

Method of Administration:
Lactating mothers can eat 1-2 bowls, 3-7 times a week to promote abundant breast milk. In cases of scanty milk due to deficiency, eat three days in a row.

Tong Gan Shen Ru Tang(16)

Indications:
This formula is indicated for Liver Qi Stagnation Type, insufficient or absent lactation. Additional symptoms include: breast distention and soreness, abdominal bloating, and irritability.

Ingredients:
Bai Shao (white peony root, wine-fried) 15g, Dang Gui (Chinese angelica, washed in wine) 15g, Bai Zhu 15g, Shu Di Huang (cooked rehmannia) 30g, Sha Ren (amomi) 3g, Mai

16. Modified from Jiang Zheng. "TCM Gynecology." (lecture, Pacific College of Oriental Medicine, San Diego, January 20, 2007).

Men Dong (ophiopogonis, fried with millet) 5g, Tong Cao (rice paper pith)3g, Chai Hu (bupleurum) 3g, Yuan Zhi (senega root) 3g, Gan Cao (licorice) 1g.

Preparation:
1. Rinse herbs.
2. Place in non-aluminum pot and cover with 4 cups of water.
3. Bring to boil and simmer for 45 min. until reduced to 1 cup.
4. Strain, conserving both herbs and tea.
5. Add herbs and 4 cups of water and bring to a boil. Simmer for 45 min. until reduced to 1 cup.
6. Discard herbs. Combine first and second batch of tea.

Method of Administration:
Divide into 3 doses and finish in one day. Repeat for three consecutive days.

Tong Ru Dan

Indications:
This formula is indicated for Qi and Blood Deficiency Type, insufficient or absent lactation. Additional symptoms include: no breast distention, watery milk, sallow complexion, dry skin, poor appetite, and fatigue. Traditionally these herbs are cooked in a soup with peanuts and either two pig's feet or ox tails. For reasons of taste, I prefer the herbal tea separately from soup. **Note:** This is also an excellent formula for sagging breasts as part of a breast rejuvenation protocol and to recover low hormone levels.

Ingredients:
Ren Shen (ginseng) 30g, Huang Qi (astragalus) 30g, Dang Gui (Chinese angelica) 60g, Mai Men Dong (ophiopogonis) 15g, Mu Tong (akebia) 1g, Jie Geng (platycodon) 1g.

Preparation:
1. Rinse herbs.
2. Place in non-aluminum pot and cover with 4 cups of water.
3. Bring to boil and simmer for 45 min. until reduced to 1 cup.
4. Strain, conserving both herbs and tea.
5. Add herbs and 4 cups of water and bring to a boil. Simmer for 45 min. until reduced to 1 cup.
6. Discard herbs. Combine first and second batch of tea.

Method of Administration:
Divide into 3 doses and finish in one day. Repeat for three consecutive days.

Reducing Lactation

Roasted Mai Ya Tea (Sprouted Barley Tea)

Indications:
Stops lactation, eases breast distention, and dissolves Food stagnation.

Ingredients (3 day's dosage):
180g Mai Ya (sprouted barley)
8 cups of water
brown sugar or other sweetener (optional)

Preparation Method
1. If Mai Ya is not already toasted, dry fry it in a frying pan until slightly browned but not burnt.
2. Place Mai Ya and 8 cups of water in a non-aluminum pot and bring to a boil over high heat. Cover. Lower to low heat and simmer for 1 hour.
3. Strain decoction into an uncovered pot. Bring to a boil over high heat and reduce to about 6 cups.
4. Add brown sugar and mix thoroughly. Turn off heat and serve.

Method of Administration:
Divide into six doses; about 1 cup each. For three consecutive days, take two doses per day: the first after breakfast, the second after dinner.

Vegetarian Options

Pregnancy, the postpartum period, and during menses are the most challenging times to be vegetarian. The body requires extra nutrients to replenish the Blood and rebuild hormone levels. Even small amounts of animal product strongly replenish the Blood, particularly when cooked with Blood-building herbs.

Strict vegetarians should supplement their diet with extra protein during these periods. Incorporate soy products and protein powders into the diet. Chinese grocery stores offer fake meat and bean curd skin, made out of soybean and wheat that are both highly nutritious and tasty. They can be prepared with Chinese herbs. I find them easier on the digestion than tofu. Try to eat eggs during these periods. Raw food diets are not advisable during the postpartum month or menstruation.

During the postpartum period, vegetables are very limited. Choose warming, tonifying vegetables such as carrots, winter squash, and beets. Incorporate the following foods in every meal. Add two or three of the food herbs below to soups, congees, and stir fry. Additionally, the seed milks and mochi from the Rejuvenation Recipes can be added.

Removing animal protein makes these recipes less heating and congesting. They are excellent tonic formulas for Heat and Damp constitutions at any time. These recipes can also be eaten by postpartum women who wish to forgo the traditional liver and kidney dishes of the first two weeks.

Vegan Qi and Blood-building foods:
Hong Zao (red jujube date), Da Zao (black jujube date), blackstrap molasses, spirulina and chlorophyll-rich foods, Lian Zi (lotus seeds), leafy greens, Hei Zhi Ma (black sesame seeds), Gou Qi Zi (go ji berries), Long Yan Rou (longan berries), carrots, beets, black beans, chestnuts.

Vegan Blood-moving foods:
Shitake mushrooms, garlic, eggplant, Hei Mu Er (black wood ear fungus), cabbage.

Stir-Fried Tofu

Indications:
Nourishes and moves Qi and Blood.

Ingredients (1 day's serving):
½ of firm tofu cut into cubes
1 clove minced garlic
¼ cup shitake mushrooms, finely chopped
½ carrot, finely chopped
3 slices of fresh ginger
black sesame oil to coat pan
dash of rice wine

Preparation:
1. Add black sesame oil to sauce pan and bring over high heat. Add ginger and garlic and sautèe until begins to brown.
2. Add tofu and sear.
3. Lower heat and add vegetables and rice wine. Cook for 15 min.

Method of Administration:
Use to replace a meat dish.

Date & Squash Soup

Indications:
Nourishes Qi and Blood.

Ingredients:
½ cup winter squash, chopped
½ cup sweet potato, chopped
1 medium tomato, chopped

½ onion, chopped
½ inch piece of ginger, grated
3 Da Zao (black dates), split
3 Hong Zao (red dates), de-pitted
¼ cup Go Qi Zi (go ji berries)
2 tsp. spirulina (optional)
1 tsp. black sesame oil
1 tsp. black sesame oil
3 cups of soup stock
salt and white pepper (omit salt postpartum)
dash of rice wine

Procedure:

1. Rinse the herbs.
2. Put sesame oil in sauce pan over med-high heat. Add ginger and onions. Sauté until browned.

Add soup stock and rest of the ingredients (except for spirulina). Bring to a boil, then simmer 30 min. Remove from heat. Mix in spirulina to serving bowl while soup is still hot.

Method of Administration:
Use to replace fish soup.

8 Treasure Rice

Indications:
This is a traditional tonifying dish of which there are many variations. The 8 herbs vary according to the recipe. White sweet rice is generally used. This recipe uses black sweet rice, as it is more tonifying for the Blood and Kidneys. The recipe is traditionally steamed. I use a rice cooker. This is the easiest method though it doesn't look as pretty as when it is steamed. Sweet rice doesn't cook well in a regular saucepan and sticks to the pot. Coconut milk and sweetener can be added to transform it into a dessert.

Ingredients:
1 cup black glutinous rice
6 Lian Zi (lotus nuts)
6 Long Yan Rou (longan berries)
¼ cup Gou Qi Zi (go ji berries)
¼ cup Hei Zhi Ma (black sesame seeds), crushed
1 tbsp Chen Pi (tangerine peel), crushed
4 pieces Fu Ling (poria), crushed
6 Hong Zao (red dates), de-pitted
¼ cup raisins or other dried fruit
2 cups water (or as directed on rice cooker)

Procedure:
Place ingredients in rice cooker and cook.

Method of Administration:
Eat with meals, as snack, or as dessert.

Pregnancy Recipes

General Wellbeing

Women are Yang during pregnancy and so should follow a mildly cooling diet. A high proportion of vegetables, mostly cooked to strengthen the Spleen, is advised. It is very important for pregnant women to incorporate bone broth into their daily diet. Pregnancy strains the Kidneys and women can experience bone loss.

Bao Chan Wu You San (Protecting Labor Worry Free Powder)

Indications:
This is a traditional formula used to strengthen Qi and Blood and stabilize the womb. It benefits both mother and baby. In modern times many acupuncturists and herbalists avoid giving herbs to pregnant women for legal reasons.

Ingredients:
Dang Gui (Chinese angelica) 12g, Bai Shao (white peony root) 12g, Huang Qi (astragalus) 3g, Hou Po (magnolia bark) 2g, Tu Si Zi (dodder seed) 1g, Zhi Ke (bitter orange) 1g, Ai Ye (mugwort) 1g, Chuan Xiong (ligusticum) 3g, Qiang Huo (notopterygium)1g, Chuan Bei Mu (fritillaria) 3g, Jing Jie (schizonepeta) 2g, Sheng Jiang (fresh ginger) 2 slices.
9 cups water

Procedure:
1. Rinse and soak herbs for 30 min.
2. Place herbs with 5 cups of water in a non-aluminum pot. Bring to a boil, then simmer for 45 min. Reduce liquid to about 1½ cups.
3. Strain, conserving both decoction and herbs.
4. Place herbs with 4 cups of water in the pot. Bring to a boil, then simmer for 45 min.Reduce liquid to about 1½ cups.
5. Strain. Discard herbs. Combine both decoctions.
6. Drink about 1 cup at a time.

Method of Administration:
Traditionally, during pregnancy take 4 bags during 4th month, 5 bags during 5th month, 6 bags during 6th month, 7 bags during 7th month, 8 bags during 8th month, and 9 bags during 9th month.

Kidney Yin Congee

Indications:
This is an example recipe for a breakfast congee pregnant women can eat first thing in the morning. This congee nourishes Kidney Yin and gently promotes bowel movements.

Ingredients:
½ cup brown rice
¼ cup meat, cut into small pieces
¼ cup daikon radish, chopped
¼ cup napa cabbage, chopped
¼ cup celery
12g Shan Yao (Chinese yam)
¼ cup Gou Qi Zi (go ji berries)
2 cups bone broth
3 cups water
salt and white pepper to taste

Procedure:
1. Soak brown rice 6-8 hours. Strain.
2. Place all ingredients in a crock pot or rice cooker. Cook 6 hours or overnight. Serve warm.

Method of Administration:
Eat 1 bowl first thing in the morning.

Asparagus Soup

Indications:
This soup gently reduces edema and promotes bowel movements.

Ingredients:
1 bunch asparagus
1 stalk celery
½ inch piece fresh ginger, sliced with peel
1 tbsp chia seeds salt to taste
2 cups soup broth

Procedure:
1. Place ingredients in saucepan. Bring to a boil and simmer 20 min.
2. Place in a VitaMix or other blender and blend until smooth.
3. Serve.

Method of Administration:
Eat as desired.

Special Conditions During Pregnancy

Edema During Pregnancy

The skins of many vegetables and fruits can brewed into tea or added to soups to clear edema: organic potato skin, ginger peel, tangerine peel, etc. Red adzuki beans are very effective to promote proper water metabolism and reduce swelling. Eat red adzuki bean recipes such as Red Adzuki Bean Drink regularly (page 343).

Red Adzuki Bean with Carp Soup

Indications:
This soup regulates water metabolism. Benefits the heart.

Ingredients:
1 cup red adzuki beans
½ lb. carp or other fish
1 carrot, chopped
2 stalks of celery, chopped
½ onion, chopped
½ inch fresh ginger with peel
1 tsp. Chen Pi (tangerine peel), powdered
salt and white pepper to taste
3 cups soup stock
1 tsp vegetable oil (safflower, grapeseed, or coconut oil)

Procedure:
1. Soak beans for 8 hours. Strain.
2. Add ingredients, except carp and oil, to a pot. Bring to a boil and simmer for 45 minutes or until beans are cooked through.
3. Season fish with salt and white pepper.
4. Add oil to pan over med-high heat. Add carp and sear both sides. Cook 5-7 min.Make sure fish is still soft when pressed with a fork.
5. Add fish to soup and serve.

Method of Administration:
Eat 1 bowl, once or twice a day to reduce swelling and edema.

Cold During Pregnancy

Daikon Radish Soup

Indications:
Clears toxins. Early signs of cold during pregnancy.

Ingredients:
1 large daikon radish, chopped
1 long burdock root, chopped
1 inch fresh ginger, grated
4 cups water

Procedure:
1. Place all ingredients in a pot. Bring to a boil and simmer for 45 min.
2. Strain and serve.

Method of Administration:
Drink throughout the day.

Preparing for Delivery

One week prior to projected delivery, begin taking Red Date Tea (page 349). This protects the body in case of anesthesia. The following are recipes and formulas traditionally taken leading up to delivery to build strength and ease labor.

Slippery Baby Formula (Hua Tai San)[17]

Indications:
This is Fu Qing Zhu's formula to ease delivery. It contains some moving herbs, but focuses on strengthening the mother in preparation for delivery. He recommended taking it throughout the ninth month and particularly the days leading up to delivery.

Ingredients:
Dang Gui (Chinese angelica) 3-5 qian (15-25g), Chuan Xiong (ligusticum) 5-7 qian (25-35g), Du Zhong (eucommia) 2 qian (10g), Shu Di Huang (prepared rehmannia) 3 qian (15g), Zhi Ke (bitter orange) 7 fen (3.5g), Shan Yao (Chinese yam) 2 qian (10g).
9 cups water

---

17. From Yang Shou-zhong, trans. *Fu Qing Zhu's Gynecology*. (Boulder: Blue Poppy Press 1995). This is the earliest book on TCM obstetrics and gynecology. Dating from the early Qing dynasty, it is still used by modern practitioners as a reference. Fu Qing Zhu is a well known TCM doctor, artist, and ideologist (1607 – 1684).

Procedure:

1. Rinse herbs. Soak for 30 min.
2. Place herbs with 5 cups of water in non-aluminum pot. Bring to a boil, then simmerfor 45 min.
3. Strain. Conserve decoction and herbs.
4. Return herbs to pot with 4 cups of water. Bring to a boil and simmer for 45 min.
5. Strain. Discard herbs. Combine the two decoctions.

Method of Administration:
Drink 1 cup warmed decoction, 1-3 times a day.

Slippery Baby Congee

Indications:
These mucilaginous greens ease labor, as well as promote bowel movements, ease urination, reduce swelling, and clear Heat. Choose between Ma Chi Xian (purslane), Kong Xin Cai (ong choy/water spinach), and Dong Xian Cai (hin choy/winter amaranth).

Ingredients:
1 cup greens: purslane, ong choy, or hin choy, chopped
½ cup white rice
4 cups water

Procedure:

1. Add ingredients to crock pot or rice cooker.
2. Cook 6 hours or overnight.

Method of Administration:
Have 1 bowl, three times a day. Begin 1-2 days prior to projected delivery date.

Rejuvenation Recipes

Rejuvenation recipes should be eaten regularly during times of stress and after a woman turns 35.

Black Sesame Seed Milk

Indications:
This milk treats Liver Blood and Kidney Yin deficiency. It beautifies the hair and skin. For a creamier consistency, add 1 tsp. sweet rice flour prior to heating to improve the texture.

Ingredients:
½ cup Hei Zhi Ma (black sesame seeds)
2-2 ½ cups water
sweetener to taste (medjool dates, honey, palm sugar, etc.)
1 tsp. sweet rice flour (optional)

Procedure:
1. Rinse black sesame seeds and soak in water overnight.
2. Add water, seeds, and sweetener to a blender or food processor (VitaMix works very well). Blend.
3. Warm the desired amount until begins to steam. Do not let it reach a boil or it will separate. Drink warm. Refrigerate the rest. Will keep for a 3 days in the refrigerator.

Method of Administration:
Drink daily to nourish Liver and Kidneys. Drink as a snack before bed, as a tea, or add to smoothies.

Walnut and White Sesame Seed Milk

Indications:
This milk improves brain functioning and beautifies the skin. For a creamier consistency, add 1 tsp. sweet rice flour prior to heating to improve the texture.

Ingredients:
½ cup walnuts
½ cup white sesame seeds
2 ½ cups of water
sweetener to taste (medjool dates, honey, cane sugar)
1 tsp. sweet rice flour (optional)

Procedure:
1. Rinse sweet apricot kernels and walnuts. Soak in water overnight.

2. Add water, kernels and walnuts, and sweetener to a blender or food processor (Vi-taMix works very well). Blend.
3. Refrigerate. Will keep for a 3 days.
4. To serve, heat over medium heat, pour, and serve. Do not bring to a full boil as the liquids and solids will separate.

Method of Administration:
Drink daily to beautify the skin and improve memory. Drink as a snack before bed, as a tea, or add to smoothies.

Sweet Apricot Kernel Milk

Indications:
The "almonds" used by Imperial concubines to soften and brighten the skin were actually sweet apricot kernels (south almonds, Nan Xing Ren). These are different from the northern, bitter apricot kernels (Ku Xing Ren) used in medicine. Regular almonds also have a skin beautifying effect and can be substituted.

Note: Using a VitaMix blender will create a creamy texture.

Ingredients:
½ cup Nan Xing Ren (sweet apricot kernels; almonds can be substituted)
1/8 cup Ku Xing Ren (bitter apricot kernels)
1 tbsp. brown rice
1/8 cup Bai Mu Er (white cloud ear fungus) (optional)
2 ½ cups of water
sweetener to taste (medjool dates, honey, cane sugar)

Procedure:
1. Rinse and soak apricot kernels, rice, and cloud ear fungus 2-6 hours.
2. Add sweetener and blend in VitaMix or other blender until smooth.
3. Warm in a saucepan until steaming but do not bring to a rolling boil or it will change the consistency.

Method of Administration:
Drink daily to soften and brighten the skin. Drink as a snack before bed, as a tea, or add to smoothies.

Beautifying Mochi - Baked[18]

Indications:
For Qi and Blood deficiency. Replace Fu Ling powder with Shan Yao powder for Qi and Yin deficiency. Note: the sweet rice makes this recipe warming.

Ingredients:
1 box Sweet Rice Flour (like Mochiko)
2 eggs
2 ½ cups soy milk, rice milk, seed milk, or cow's milk
40g Fu Ling (poria) powder or Shan Yao (Chinese yam) powder
10g Gou Qi Zi (go ji berries)
1 tblsp. Hei Zhi Ma (black sesame seeds), ground
8 medjool dates or 1 cup brown sugar (optional)
1 tsp. baking powder
1 tbsp. vegetable oil (safflower, grapeseed, or coconut)
1 tsp. vanilla extract (optional)

Preparation:
1. Preheat oven to 400 degrees. Lightly grease a 9x13 inch baking pan, then dust with flour..
2. Blend milk and dates in blender.
3. Mix dry ingredients and wet ingredients separately.
4. Pour wet ingredients into dry ingredients. Mix with an electric mixer or whisk. Pour dough inside baking pan.
5. Bake at 400 degrees for 30 min.
6. Cool and serve.

Method of Administration:

Eat as a tonifying dessert or snack.

---

18. Adapted from Yueying Li. "TCM Nutrtion." (lecture, Yo San University, Los Angeles, May 6, 2002).

Detoxification Recipes

Increasing the proportion of vegetables to 50% is an effective and gentle way to detoxify the body. I recommend Shelley Young's vegetable-based recipes and steam-frying cooking method. The following are specific detox recipes.

Bitter Melon Juice

Indications:
Damp-Heat, Liver imbalance with bitter taste in the mouth (use bitter and sour foods), to cut sugar cravings, or detoxification. Honey dew melon cuts the bitterness. Refreshing summer drink.

Ingredients:
½ bitter melon
1/8 slice of honeydew melon

Procedure:
1. Wash bitter melon. Remove seeds and white core. Slice.
2. Remove rind from honeydew melon. Slice.
3. Add bitter melon and honeydew melon to blender with enough water to cover.
4. Blend until smooth and serve.

Method of Administration:
Drink daily as for detoxification, to treat Liver/Gallbladder imbalance, bacterial or fungal infections, or to cool off in hot weather. Drink 2 times a week for prevention.

Slimming Tea

Indications:
Lotus leaf tea is a common tea to cool off in hot weather. It also promotes weightloss. This tea clears Dampness, Heat, and promotes water metabolism.

Ingredients:
15g He Ye (lotus leaf)
24g Yi Yi Ren (Job's Tears)
5g Chen Pi (tangerine peel)
5g green tea
5 cups water

Procedure:
1. Rinse ingredients.

2. Soak for 30 min. in 5 cups of water.
3. Bring to a boil and simmer for 30 min.
4. Strain and refrigerate.

Method of Administration:
Drink 1 cup three times a day to cool off during hot weather or for weightloss.

Mung Bean Detox Soup[19]

Indications:
Clears Damp-Heat and Heat Toxins. This can manifest as inflammatory skin conditions (acne, rosacea, psoriasis, or excema), toxicity (pesticides, heavy metals, drugs), or Liver/Gallbladder disorders.

Ingredients:
½ (60g) cup mung beans
1/3 (30g) cup red adzuki beans
½ (24g) cup Yi Yi Ren (Job's tears, ½ toasted, ½ raw)
5 pieces Long Yan Rou (longan berries), rinsed
½ inch piece fresh ginger, sliced
5 cups of water

Procedure:
1. Rinse first 3 ingredients and soak for 8 hours or overnight.
2. Drain and add to pot with last 3 ingredients.
3. Bring to a boil, then lower heat to simmer for 45 min or until soft.
4. Add seasoning as desired.

Method of Administration:
Eat daily to treat conditions of Damp-Heat or toxicity. Divide into 2 dosages and finish in 1 day for detoxification program. Smaller amount can be eaten weekly for maintenance.

Date and Wood Ear Tea[20]

Indications:
This tea strengthens and detoxifies the Liver, moves the Blood, and reduces Phlegm. Taken regularly, it lowers cholesterol.

Ingredients:
4 Hong Zao (red dates)
4 Da Zao (black dates)

19. Adapted from Dr. Jiling Hu, conversation, May 2002.
20. Modified from Alan Morris. *Healthy Soups to My Beloved Karen.* (China: Culture and Arts Publishing House, 2010),94-95.

2 Chinese honeyed dates (substitute medjool dates)
19g Hei Mu Er (black wood ear fungus)
7 dried shitake mushrooms (stem removed)
4-5 cups of water

Procedure:

1. Put ingredients in a pot over high heat. Bring to a boil, lower heat, and allow to simmer for 2 hours.
2. Remove from heat and serve.

Method of Administration:
To lower cholesterol, drink 1 cup daily. Drink a few times a month as a preventive. The herbs can be eaten with the tea or strained.

Liver-Cleansing Broth

Indications:
This broth gently detoxifies the Liver and Gallbladder systems. It clears Damp-Heat.

Ingredients:
1 cabbage
1 carrot
1 organic potato with skin
2 stalks of celery
2 inch piece daikon radish
2 inch burdock root, peeled
1 onion
1 bunch parsley
1 lime
pinch cayenne pepper (optional)
water to cover

Procedure:

1. Chop ingredients except parsley and lime. Place in pot and cover with water. Bring to a boil. Lower heat and simmer for 45 min.
2. Add parsley. Cook an additional 5 min.
3. Remove from heat and strain. Add lime juice and cayenne pepper and serve.

Method of Administration:
Take 1 cup three times a day as part of a detox program.

Menopausal Recipes

These are more potent rejuvenation recipes. They can be used at any age provided there is sufficient Cold and Kidney deficiency present. Those who do excessive physical or mental work can take Jing tonics at any age.

Du Zhong Wine[21]

Indications:
This recipe uses a common pairing, Du Zhong and Long Yan Rou, to make Du Zhong Wine, though other herbs can be used as well. Du Zhong wine is a gentle wine taken long-term to treat and prevent Bi Syndrome (joint pain, aches and pains), beautify the skin, and for general anti-aging. Alternately, purchase black glutinous rice wine. Add the medicinal herbs, and allow to sit for at least 2 months.

Ingredients:
100g Long Yan Rou (longan berries)
10g Du Zhong (eucommia)
1 bottle black glutinous rice wine

Procedure:
Rinse the medicinal herbs and place in the bottle with the raw wine. Allow to mature for 9 months.

Method of Administration:
Medicinal wines are heating and usually reserved for times of convalescence (postpartum or menses) or after menopause. If menopausal symptoms do not prohibit, Du Zhong wine should be taken daily, a small cup in the evening, starting at age 49. In cold, deficient women it can be started earlier.

Brain Tonic Soup

Indications:
This soup strengthens brain functioning.

Ingredients:
½ lb. beef, cut into pieces
½ cup walnuts
½ cup chestnuts
6 Long Yan Rou (longan berries)
1 carrot, chopped

21. Alan Morris. *Healthy Soups to My Beloved Karen.* (China: Culture and Arts Publishing House, 2010), 84-85.

2 stalks celery, chopped
½ onion
salt and pepper to taste
3 cups soup stock

Procedure:

1. Add ingredients to pot and bring to a boil. Reduce heat and simmer for 30 min.Pour into VitaMix or other blender. Blend until smooth and serve.

Method of Administration:
Eat 1 bowl as evening soup.

Hair Beautifying Drink

Indications:
Tonifies Liver Blood and Kidney Jing. Nourishes the skin and prevents gray hair. Strengthens brain function.

Ingredients:
1/2 cup (100g) walnuts
1/2 cup (100g) Hei Zhi Ma (black sesame seeds)
1/4 cup (50g) He Shou Wu (polygonum)
honey to taste

Procedure:

1. Grind all ingredients into powder. Store in sealed jar.
2. To serve, add 2 tbsp. to hot water. Add honey to taste.

Method of Administration:
Take 1 cup daily to rejuvenate the hair.

Dang Gui Lamb Soup

Indications:
This soup is very warming. It is used in cold weather, for Cold constitutions, arthritis, pain exacerbated by cold, and for cold in womb during menses (especially in wintertime).

Ingredients:
12g Dang Gui (Chinese angelica)
¼ lb. lamb
½ inch piece of ginger
10g Du Zhong (eucommia)

5 pieces Long Yan Rou (longan berries)
¼ cup Gou Qi Zi (go ji berries)
1 cup rice wine
1 cup of water

Procedure:
1. Rinse and soak herbs for 30 min.
2. Bring ingredients to simmer and allow to cook for 2 hours.
3. Remove from heat, add salt, and serve.

Method of Administration:
Eat 1 bowl, 3 days in a row to warm the body.

Appendix A - Table of Chinese Herbs

Pin Yin	English Common Name	Botanical Name	Pharmaceutical Name	Chinese Characters
Ài Yè	Mugwort, artemesia argyi, argy wormowwod leaf	*Artemesia argyi*	Folium Artemesiae Argyi	艾叶
Bā Jǐ Tiān	morinda	*Morinda officinalis*	Radix Morindae Officinalis	巴戟天
Bái Biǎn Dòu	dolichos nut	*Dolichos lalab*	Semen Lablab Album	白扁豆
Bái Huā Shé Shé Cǎo	Hedyotis, oldenlandia	*Oldenlandia diffusa*	Herba Oldenlandia	白花蛇舌草
Bài Jiàng Cǎo	thalspi, patrinia	*Patrinia scabisaefolia*	Herba cum Radice Patriniae	败酱草
Bái Mù Ěr	white cloud fungus, wood ear	*Tremella fuciformis*	Fructificatio Tremellae Fuciformis	白木耳
Bái Sháo (Yao)	white peony root	*Paeonia lactiflora*	Radix Paeoniae Alba	白芍
Bái Zhǐ	angelica root	*Angelica dahurica*	Radix Angelicae Dahuricae	白芷
Bái Zhú	white atractylodes	*Atractylodes macrocephala*	Rhizoma Atractylodis Macrocephalae	白术
Bǎn Lán Gēn	isatis root, indigo root	*Isatis tinctoria*	Radix Isatidis	板蓝根
(Jiang) Bàn Xià	(ginger-processed) pinellia	*Pinellia ternata*	Rhizoma Pinelliae	半夏
Bì Xiè	dioscorea root, tokoro	*Dioscorea hypoglauca*	Rhizoma Dioscoreae	萆薢
Bīng Lang	betel nut	*Areca catechu*	Semen Arecae	槟榔
Bīng Piàn	borneol	*Dryobalanops aromatica*	Borneolum Syntheticum	冰片
Bò He	mint	*Mentha haplocalyx*	Herba Menthae	薄荷
Bǔ Gǔ Zhī	psoralea fruit	*Psoralea cordylifolia*	Fructus Psoraleae	补骨脂
Cāng Zhú	atractylodes	*Atractylodes lancea*	Rhizoma Atractylodis	苍术
Cè Bǎi Yè	platycladus leaves	*Platycladus orientalis*	Cacumen Platycladi	侧柏叶
Chái Hú	bupleurum	*Bupleurum chinense*	Radix Bupleuri	柴胡
Chē Qián Zǐ	plantago seed	*Plantago asiatica*	Semen Plantaginis	车前子
Chén Pí	tangerine peel	*Citrus reticulata*	Pericarpium Citri Reticulatae	陈皮

Chì Sháo (Yao)	red peony root	*Paeonia veitchii*	Radix Paeoniae Rubrae	赤芍
Chì Xiǎo Dòu	red adzuki bean	*Phaseolus calcaratus*	Semen Phaseoli	赤小豆
Chuān Bèi Mǔ	fritillaria, Sichuan fritillaria bulb	*Fritillaria cirrhosa*	Fritillariae Cirrhosae Bulbus	川贝母
Chuān Liàn Zǐ	melia	*Melia toosendan*	Fructus Toosendan	川楝子
Chuān Xiōng	cnidium	*Ligusticum chuanxiong*	Rhizoma Ligustici Chuanxiong	川芎
Chūn Gēn Pí	ailanthus bark	*Ailanthus altissima*	Cortex Ailanthi	椿根皮
Cì Wǔ Jiā	Siberian ginseng	*Acanthopanax senticosus*	Radix et Caulis Acanthopanacis Senticosi	刺五加
Dà Fù Pí	betel nut husk	*Areca catechu*	Pericarpium Arecae	大腹皮
Dà Huáng	rhubarb root	*Rheum palmatum*	Radix et Rhizoma Rhei	大黄
Dà Qīng Yè	isatis leaves, indigo leaves	*Isatis tinctoria*	Folium Isatidis	大青叶
Dà Zǎo	black jujube, date	*Ziziphus jujuba*	Fructus Jujubae	大枣
Dān Shēn	salvia root	*Salvia miltiorrhiza*	Radix Salviae Miltiorrhizae	丹参
Dāng Guī	Chinese angelica, dong quai	*Angelica sinensis*	Radicis Angelicae Snensis	当归
Dǎng Shēn	codonopsis root	*Codonopsis pilosula*	Radix Codonopsis	党参
Dì Gǔ Pí	wolfberry root, lycium root	*Lycium barbarum*	Cortex Lycii	地骨皮
Dì Lóng	earthworm	*Pheretima aspergillum*	Pheretima	地龙
Dì Yú	garden burnet root, sanguisorba	*Sanguisorba officinalis*	Radix Sanguisorbae	地榆
Dōng Chóng Xià Cǎo	cordyceps	*Cordyceps sinensis*	Cordyceps	冬虫夏草
Dōng Yáng Shēn	Japanese Ginseng	*Panax ginseng*	Radix Ginseng Japonica	东洋参
Dù Zhòng	eucommia bark	*Eucommia ulmoides*	Cortex Eucommiae	杜仲
Ē Jiāo	gelatin	*Equus asinus*	Colla Corii Asini	阿胶
É Zhú	curcuma zedoaria	*Curcuma zedoaria*	Rhizoma Curcumae	莪术
Fáng Fēng	ledebouriella root	*Saposhnikovia divaricata*	Radix Saposhnikoviae	防风
Fěi Zi	torreya seeds	*Torreya grandis*	Semen Torreyae	榧子
Fú Líng	poria	*Poria cocos*	Poria	茯苓
Fú Xiǎo Mài	light wheat	*Triticum aestivum*	Semen Tritici Aestivi Levis	浮小麦

Fù Zǐ	aconite	*Aconitum carmichaeli*	Radix Aconiti Lateralis	附子
Gān Cǎo	licorice root	*Glycyrrhiza uralensis*	Radix Glycyrrhizae	甘草
Gé Huā	kudzu vine flower	*Pueraria lobata*	Flos Puerariae	葛花
Gōu Qǐ Zǐ	gou ji berries	*Lycium barbarum L.*	Fructus Lycii	枸杞子
Gǔ Suì Bǔ	drynaria	*Drynaria fortunei*	Rhizoma Drynariae	骨碎补
Guā Lóu (Shi)	trichosanthus fruit	*Trichosanthes kirilowii*	Fructus Trichosanthis	瓜蒌
Guan Yin	clerodendri		Radix cum Stem Clerodendri	觀音串
Guī Bǎn	tortoise plastron	*Chinemys reevesii*	Plastrum Testudinis	龟板
Guì Huā	osmanthus flower	*Osmanthus fragrans*		桂花
Hǎi Shēn	sea cucumber	*Strichopus japonicus*	Strichopus Japonicus	海参
Hǎi Jīn Shā	lygodium spore (spore of fern)	*Lygodium japonicum*	Herba Lygodii	海金沙
Hàn Lián Cǎo	eclipta leaf	*Eclipta prostrata*	Herba Ecliptae	旱莲草
Hè Shī	carpesium fruit	*Carpesium abrotanoides*	Fructus Carpesii	鹤虱
Hé Shǒu Wū	polygonum, fo-ti	*Polygonum multiflorum*	Radix Polgoni Multiflori	何首乌
Hé Yè	lotus leaf	*Nelumbo nucifera*	Folium Nelumbinis	荷叶
Hēi Mù Ěr	black wood ear fungus		Auricularia Auricula Fungus	黑木耳
Hēi Zhī Ma	black sesame seed	*Sesamum indicum L.*	Semen Sesami Nigrum	黑芝麻
Hóng Huā	safflower	*Carthamus tinctorius*	Flos Carthami	红花
Hóng Shēn	red ginseng, steamed ginseng root (Korean or Chinese)	*Panax ginseng*	Radix Ginseng	红参
Hóng Téng	sargentodoxa vine	*Sargentodoxa cuneata*	Caulis Sargentodoxae	红藤
Hóng Zǎo	red jujube, date	*Ziziphus jujuba*	Fructus Jujubae	红枣
Hòu Pò	magnolia bark	*Magnolia officinalis*	Cortex Magnoliae officinalis	厚朴
Hú Táo Rén	walnut	*Juglans regia*	Semen Juglandis	胡桃仁
Huā Jiāo	Sichuan pepper	*Zanthoxylum bungeanum*	Pericarpium Zanthoxyli	花椒
Huá Shí	talc		Talcum	滑石
Huà Shí Cǎo	orthosiphon	*Orthosiphon aristatus*	Herba Orthosiphon Aristatus	化石草
Huái Niú Xī	achyranthes root	*Achyranthes bidentata*	Radix Achyranthis Bidentatae	淮牛膝

Huáng Bǎi	phellodendron bark	*Phellodendron amurense*	Cortex Phellodendri	黄柏
Huáng Jīng	polygonatum root, king Solomon's seal rhizome	*Polygonatum kingianum*	Rhizoma Polygonati	黄精
Huáng Lián	coptis	*Coptis chinensis*	Rhizoma Coptidis	黄连
Huáng Qí	Astragalus, Mongolian milkvetch root	*Astragalus membranaceus*	Radix Astragali	黄芪
Huáng Qín	scutellaria	*Scutellaria baicalensis*	Radix Scutellariae	黄芩
Huǒ Má Rén	hemp seed, cannabis seed	*Cannabis sativa*	Cannabis Semen	火麻仁
Huò Xiāng	agastache	*Agastache rugosus*	Herba Agastache	藿香
Jī Nèi Jīn	chicken gizzard	*Gallus gallus domesticus*	Endothelium Corneum Gigeriae Galli	鸡内金
Jī Xuè Téng	spatholobus	*Spatholobus suberectus*	Caulis Spatholobi	雞血藤
Jiāng Cán	silkworm with batrytis	*Bombyx mori*	Bombyx Batryticatus	僵蚕
Jiāng Huáng	turmeric	*Curcuma longa*	Rhizoma Curcumae Longae	姜黄
Jiǎo Gǔ Lán	gynostemma	*Gynostemma pentaphyllum*	Rhizoma seu Herba Gynostemmatis	绞股蓝
Jié Gěng	platycodon	*Platycodon grandiflorum*	Platycodi Radix	桔梗
Jīn Qián Cǎo	lysimachia	*Lysimachia christinae*	Herba Lysimachiae	金钱草
Jīn Yín Huā	honeysuckle flower	*Lonicera japonica*	Flos Lonicerae	金銀花
Jīng Jiè	schizonepeta	*Schizonepeta tenuifolia*	Herba Schizonepetae	荊芥
Jú Huā	chrysanthemum flower	*Chrysanthemum morifolium*	Flos Chrysanthemi	菊花
Jué Míng Zǐ	cassia seed	*Cassia obtusifolia*	Cassiae Semen	決明子
Kǔ Dīng Chá	Bitter Nail Tea	*Ligustrum robustum (loose leaf) or Ilex kudingcha(in nails)*		苦丁茶
Kǔ Liàn Pí	melia bark	*Melia toosendan*	Cortex Meliae	苦楝皮
Kǔ Shēn	sophora root	*Sophora flavescens*	Radix Sophorae Flavescentis	苦参
Kūn Bù	kelp	*Laminaria japonica*	Eckloniae Thallus	昆布
Li Zhi Pi	lychee shell	*Litchi chinensis*	Pericarpium Litchi Chinensis	荔枝殼

Lián Qiáo	forsythia fruit	*Forsythia suspensa*	Fructus Forsythiae	连翘
Lián Zĭ	lotus seed	*Nelumbo nucifera*	Semen Nelumbinis	莲子
Líng Zhī	reishi mushroom, ganoderma	*Ganoderma lucidum*	Ganoderma	靈芝
Liú Huáng	sulfur	*sulfur*	sulfur	硫黄
Lóng Dăn Căo	gentiana	*Gentiana scabra*	Radix Gentianae	龙胆草
Lóng Gŭ	fossilized bone, "dragon" bone		Os Draconis	龙骨
Long Yăn Ròu	longan fruit	*Euphoria longan*	Arillus Longan	龙眼肉
Lǚ Dòu	mung bean	*Phaseolus radiatus*	Semen Phaseoli Radiati	绿豆
Lù Jiăo (Pian)	sliced deer horn	*Cervus nippon*	Cornu Cervi	鹿角
Lù Róng	deer antler	*Cervus nippon*	Cornu Cervi Pantotrichum	鹿茸
Luo Shen Hua	roselle	*Hibiscus sabdariffa*		洛神花
Má Huáng	ephedra	*Ephedra sinica*	Herba Ephedrae	麻黄
Mài Yá	barley sprouts, malt	*Hordeum vulgare*	Fructus Hordei Germinatus	麦芽
Mài Mén Dōng	ophiopogonis	*Ophiopogon japonicus*	Radix Ophiopogonis	麦门冬
Máng Xiāo	sodium sulfate		Natrii Sulfas	芒硝
Méi Gui Huā	rose flower			玫瑰花
Míng Fán	alum	*Alumen*	Alumen	明矾
Mò Li Huā	jasmine flower	*Jasminum sambac*		茉莉花
Mò Yào	myrrh	*Commiphora myrrha*	Myrrha	沒藥
Mŭ Dān Pí	tree peony bark	*Paeonia suffruticosa*	Cortex Moutan	牡丹皮
Mù Guā	papaya	*Chaenomeles lagenaria*	Fructus Chaenomelis	木瓜
Mŭ Lì	oyster shell	*Ostrea gigas*	Concha Ostrae	牡蛎
Mù Jĭn Pí	hibiscus bark			木槿皮
Mù Tōng	akebia	*Akebia trifoliata*	Caulis Akebiae	木通
Mù Xiāng	aucklandia, saussurea	*Aucklandia lappa* *(Saussurea lappa)*	Radix Aucklandiae	木香
Nǚ Zhēn Zĭ	privet fruit, ligustrum	*Ligustrum lucidum*	Fructus Ligustri Lucidi	女贞子
Péng Shā	borax	*Borax*	Borax	硼砂
Pú Gōng Yĭng	dandelion	*Taraxacum mongolicum*	Herba Taraxaci	蒲公英
Qiàn Shí	fox nut, gorgon fruit	*Euryale ferox*	Semen Euryales	芡實

Qiāng Huó	notopterygium	*Notopterygium incisum*	Notopterygii Rhizoma seu Radix	羌活
Qín Jiāo	gentiana macrophylla	*Gentiana macrophylla*	Gentianae macrophyllae Radix	秦艽
Qú Mài	dianthus	*Dianthus superbus*	Herba Dianthi	瞿麦
Rén Shēn	ginseng	*Panax ginseng*	Radix Ginseng	人参
Ròu Cōng Róng	cistanche	*Cistanche salsa*	Herba Cistanches	肉苁容
Ròu Guì	cinnamon bark	*Cinnamomum cassia*	Cortex Cinnamomi	肉桂
Rǔ Xiāng	frankincense, olibanum,mastic	*Boswellia carterii*	Gummi Olibanum	乳香
Sān Léng	sparganium	*Sparganium stoloniferum*	Rhizoma Sparganii	三棱
Sān Qī	Pseudoginseng, notoginseng	*Panax notoginseng*	Radix Notoginseng	三七
Sāng Jì Shēng	taxillus	*Taxillus chinensis*	Herba Taxilli	桑寄生
Sāng Shèn Zǐ	mulberries	*Morus alba L.*	Fructus Mori	桑椹子
Shā Rén	amomum	*Amomum villosum*	Fructus Amomi	砂仁
(Huai) Shān Yào	Chinese yam, dioscorea	*Dioscorea opposita*	Rhizoma Dioscoreae	山药
Shān Zhā	hawthorn berry	*Crataegus cuneata*	Fructus Crataegi	山楂
Shān Zhū Yú	cornus	*Cornus officinalis*	Fructus Corni	山茱萸
Shé Chuáng Zǐ	cnidium fruit	*Cnidium monnieri*	Fructus Cnidii	蛇床子
Shēng Dì Huáng	raw rehmannia	*Rehmannia glutinosa*	Radix Rehmanniae	生地黄
Shēng Jiāng	fresh ginger	*Zinziber officinale*	Rhizoma Zingiberis Recens	生姜
Shēng Má	cimicifuga, black cohosh	*Cimicifuga heracleifolia*	Rhizoma Cimicifugae	升麻
Shí Chāng Pú	acorus	*Acorus gramineus*	Acori tatarinowii Rhizoma	石菖蒲
Shú Dì Huáng	prepared rehmannia	*Rehmannia glutinosa*	Radix Rehmanniae Preparata	熟地黄
Suān Zǎo Rén	sour jujube seed	*Ziziphus spinosa*	Semen Ziziphi Spinosae	酸枣仁
Tài Zi Shēn	Pseudostellaria	*Pseudostellaria heterophylla*	Radix Pseudostellariae	太子参
Tán Xiāng	sandalwood	*Santalum album*	Lignum Santali albi	檀香
Táo Huā	peach flower	*Prunus persica*	Flos Periscae	桃花
Táo Rén	peach kernel	*Prunus persica*	Semen Periscae	桃仁

Tiān Mén Dōng	asparagus root	*Asparagus cochinchinensis*	Radix Asparagi	天门冬
Tōng Cǎo	rice paper pith	*Tetrapanax papyriferus*	Medulla Tetrapanacis	通草
Tù Sī Zǐ	dodder seed, cuscuta	*Cuscuta chinensis*	Semen Cuscutae	菟丝子
Wēi Líng Xiān	clematis	*Clematis chinensis*	Radix Clematidis	威灵仙
Wǔ Wèi Zi	schizandra berry, Chinese magnolia vine fruit	*Schisandra chinensis*	Fructus Schisandrae Chinensis	五味
Wú Zhū Yú	evodia fruit	*Evodia rutaecarpa*	Fructus Evodiae	吴茱萸
Xī Yáng Shēn	American Ginseng	*Panax quinqueflium*	Radix Panacis Quinquefolii	西洋参
Xià Kū Cǎo	prunella	*Prunella vulgaris*	Spica Prunellae	夏枯草
Xiān Máo	curculigo	*Curculigo orchioides*	Rhizoma Curculiginis	仙茅
Xiāng Fù	cyperus root	*Cyperus rotundus*	Rhizoma Cyperi	香附
Xiè Bái	chive bulb	*Allium macrostemom*	Bulbus Allii Macrostemi	薤白
Xióng Huáng	realgar	*realgar*	realgar	雄黄
Xù Duàn	dipsacus	*Dipsacus asper*	Radix Dipsaci	续断
Xuán Fù Huā	inula flower	*Inula japonica*	Flos Inulae	旋覆花
Xuán Shēn	scrophularia	*Scrophularia ningpoensis*	Radix Scrophulariae	玄参
Xūn Yī Cǎo	lavender flower	*Lavandula angustifolia*		薰衣草
Yì Mǔ Cǎo	motherwort	*Leonurus heterophyllus*	Herba Leonuri	益母草
Yì Yǐ Rén	Job's tears, coix seed	*Coix lacryma-jobi*	Semen Coicis	薏苡仁
Yín Yáng Huò	epimedium, horny goat weed	*Epimedium grandiflorum*	Herba Epimedii	淫羊藿
Yù Mǐ Xū	corn silk	*Zea mays*	Stigma Maydis	玉米须
Yán Hú Suǒ	corydalis	*Corydalis turtschaninovii*	Rhizoma Corydalis	延胡索
Yù Jīn	curcuma, aromatic turmeric tuber	*Curcuma aromatica*	Radix Curcumae	郁金
Yuǎn Zhì	senega root, polygala	*Polygala tenuifolia*	Radix Polygalae	遠志
Yuè Jì Huā	Chinese rose	*Rosa chinensis*		月季花
Zào Jiǎo Cì	gleditsia spine	*Gleditsia sinensis*	Spina Gleditsiae	皂角刺
Zé Xiè	alisma	*Alisma orientalis*	Rhizoma Alismatis	泽泻

Zhāng Nǎo	camphor	*Cinnamomum camphora*	Camphora	樟脑
Zhè Bèi Mǔ	Zhejiang fritillaria bulb	*Frutillaria thunbergii*	Bulbus Fritillariae Thunbergii	浙贝母
Zhǐ Jǔ Zǐ	hovenia	*Hovenia dulcis*	Fructus Hoveniae	枳椇子
Zhǐ Ké	bitter orange	*Citrus aurantium*	Fructus Aurantii	枳殻
Zhī Mǔ	anemarrhena	*Anemarrhena asphodeloides*	Radix Anemarrhenae	知母
Zhī Zi	gardenia, cape jasmine fruit	*Gardenia jasminoides*	Fructus Gardeniae	栀子
Zhú Rú	bamboo shavings	*Bambusa breviflora*	Caulis Bambusae in Taenia	竹茹
Zǐ Cǎo (Gēn)	lithospermum root	*Lithospermum erythrorhizon*	Radix Lithospermi	紫草（根）
Zǐ Hé Chē	placenta	*Homo sapiens*	Placenta Hominis	紫河车
Zǐ Sū Gěng	perilla stalk	*Perilla frutescens*	Caulis Perillae	紫苏梗
Zǐ Sū Yè	perilla leaf	*Perilla frutescens*	Folium Perillae	紫苏叶
Zé Lán	lycopus, bugleweed	*Lycopus lucidus*	Herba Lycopi	澤蘭

Appendix B - Glossary of Terminology

5 Elements (五行，wǔxíng) – The 5 Elements are Wood, Fire, Earth, Metal, and Water. During the creation of the universe, there was a split between Yin and Yang. This polarity gave birth to the 5 Elements, also known as the 5 Phases. The 5 Elements can be used to describe interaction on all levels of existence, such as between the organs within the body, aspects of the psyche, interactions between people, and seasonal changes.

Acupuncture (针砭, zhēnbiān, or 针刺, zhēncì) – Refers to inserting tiny needles into specific points in the body called acupuncture points. Acupuncture points are places where energy pools along energy pathways.

(Western) Allopathic Medicine – What is typically referred to as standard or conventional Western medicine. It refers to biomedical interventions, such as pharmaceuticals and surgery, to combat disease. Allopathic medicine defines itself as being evidence-based and distinct from "alternative therapies," though there is mounting scientific evidence for alternative therapies as well. This term is controversial in some circles as it was originally used to distinguish it from homeopathy. It is not intended as a pejorative, rather it is used for lack of a better term to differentiate it from other forms of Western medicine such as osteopathy, naturopathy, and homeopathy.

Blood (血, xuè) – In Traditional Chinese Medicine contains the Qi and houses the Spirit. Blood is the physical manifestation of Qi and is inseparable from it. Qi gives life to the Blood, while Blood gives Qi physical form. Blood is moistening and lubricates the sinews and tendons and nourishes the skin and hair.

Blood Deficiency (血虚, xuèxū) – Lack of Blood refers to a lack of substance, as Blood lubricates the body and houses the Mind and Spirit. Common symptoms are pallor, dry skin, emotional and physical sensitivity, insomnia, blurred vision, timidity, pale and light menstrual bleeding with long cycles. Blood deficiency can be due to constitution or caused by blood loss, digestive weakness, poor eating and lifestyle, overwork (especially on the computer), excessive caretaking, and emotional trauma or loss. Affects the Heart and Liver. Blood deficiency is characterized by a pale, thin tongue and thin pulse.

Blood Stagnation (血淤, xuèyū) – Typical symptoms include stabbing, intense, fixed pain. Anything purple, visible dark veins, or blood clots indicates Blood Stagnation. Blood stagnation occurs due to physical or emotional trauma, longstanding Qi stagnation, or Cold invasion. Emotionally it can present as severe depression or insomnia years after physical or emotional trauma. Blood stagnation produces a purple tongue body or dark sublingual veins and a wiry or choppy pulse.

Cold (寒, hán) – It can either be due to external invasion or due to an internal deficiency of Qi or Yang. Cold is causes constriction and chills and is alleviated by warmth. The tongue will be pale or have a white coating and the pulse will be slow or tight.

Constitution – Refers to the strengths and weaknesses of the body. This is largely influenced by the Jing inherited from the parents and care during infancy and early childhood. Diet and lifestyle continuously influence the constitution. The constitution is slow to change. Understanding the constitution gives the ability to predict the outcome of disease and dictates lifestyle and diet choices.

Dampness (湿气, shīqì) – The terms Phlegm and Dampness refer to the congestion of body fluids in different manifestations. Dampness refers to the Middle and Lower Jiaos where it manifests as mucus and bloating in the digestive tract, copious white vaginal discharge, or cloudy and dribbling urination. Dampness can get lodged in the joints causing joint pain or under the skin causing edema and excess weight. Dampness shows itself on the tongue as a thick, greasy coating and as a slippery pulse.

Damp-Heat (濕熱, shīrè) – Refers to a combination of Dampness and Heat. It is most often a complication of longstanding digestive issues, Heat, or stagnation. Damp-Heat manifests as an inability to digest fats, abdominal bloating, yellow vaginal discharge, anger, resentment, indecisiveness, thirst with inability to drink, and red, itchy, and weepy skin conditions. It affects the Liver, Gallbladder, Urinary Bladder, Lower Jiao, and Large Intestine organ systems. It presents as a red tongue with yellow coating and slippery, rapid pulse.

Food Stagnation (家食, jiāshí) – Occurs when more food is ingested than the digestive system can process; either because food consumption is excessive or inappropriate or digestion is weak. Symptoms include belching, bad breath, abdominal bloating, lack of appetite, foul smelling stools, and insomnia. The tongue will have a thick white or yellow coating and the pulse will be slippery.

Heat (热, rè) – Causes inflammation, redness, agitation, bitter taste in the mouth, sensation of heat, excessive hunger, halitosis, or strong body odor. Symptoms are alleviated by cold. Heat can be due to external invasion, in the form of a pathogen (such as bacterial infection) or internally generated due to Yin deficiency, longstanding stagnation, or constitution. Heat creates a red tongue body or yellow tongue coating and rapid or full pulse.

Hun (Ethereal soul) (魂, hún) – The spirit of the Liver. The Hun is the Yang aspect of the soul; the part of the soul that moves and is insubstantial. The Hun connects the individual to the collective, is responsible for dreams, and is connected to creativity. In cases of Liver Blood deficiency, the Hun is not anchored, leading to insomnia and daydreaming.

Inner Alchemy (内丹, nèidān) – Refers to Daoist doctrines and practices designed to refine the inner landscape by transmuting negative thoughts, bad habits, sabotaging emotions, and other impediments to spiritual growth and physical vitality. There are many schools of Inner Alchemy passed down through various lineages.

Jade Egg (玉蛋, yùdàn) – A traditional tool to develop the vaginal muscles in Inner Alchemy exercises. Traditionally jade was formed into "eggs" and placed inside the vaginal canal. Jade increases Yin and seemed like the appropriate stone for this purpose. Currently eggs are available in a variety of stones.

Jade Gate (玉门, yùmén) – A metaphor for the vulva and vaginal canal.

Jing (Essence) (精, jīng) – The product of what is inherited from the parents and what is taken in from the environment (through eating and breathing). It is stored in the Kidneys but also circulates throughout the body. It is influenced by diet, lifestyle, and herbs. It relates to the individual's constitution which is possible, yet difficult to alter. Kidney Jing guides our maturation, development, and reproduction. It is the slow, fluid movement of the Kidney Jing that is described in the 7 year cycles women experience.

Jing Deficiency (精虚, jīng xū) – is a combination of Yin and Yang deficiency presenting with weak teeth, softening of bones, low back soreness, and hair loss. The natural decline of Jing with age signals the beginning of menopause. In younger people can present as developmental abnormalities, infertility, or constitutional weaknesses. Jing deficiency can be constitutional or due to aging, overwork, or excessive drug use, particularly methamphetamines. The tongue will vary depending if Yin or Yang is weaker and the pulse will be deep and weak.

Meridians (经线, jīngxiàn) – The pathways or circuits of energy flow through the body, also called Channels.

Moxibustion (moxa) (艾炷灸, àizhùjiǔ) – A central therapy in Traditional Chinese Medicine, often used with acupuncture during treatment. The leaves of Ai Ye (mugwort) are dried then formed into cones, sticks, or left loose, after which it is called "moxa." Moxa can be burned directly or indirectly on acupuncture points to warm the meridians and stimulate the flow of Qi.

Phlegm (痰, tán) – The terms Phlegm and Dampness refer to the congestion of body fluids in different manifestations. Phlegm can affect the Upper Jiao (Lungs, nose) causing symptoms such as excess mucus in the lungs, runny nose, and sinus congestion. It can present as Insubstantial Phlegm (also called Invsible or Dry Phlegm) where there may not be visible signs of excess mucus, but rather presents as mental impairment causing foggy thinking, poor cognition, manic depression, and irrational behavior. Phlegm can also manifest in certain channel pathology where there is paralysis and severe obstruction of the channels. Many modern diseases have a component of Phlegm such as high cholesterol and tumor formation. Phlegm produces an enlarged tongue body and a slippery pulse.

Po (Corporeal soul) (魄, pò) – The spirit of the Lungs. The Po is the Yin aspect of the soul; the part of the soul that guides the creation of the physical body. The Po defines the individual as separate, is responsible for instinct, is connected the physical senses. Imbalance in the Lungs and Large Intestine can cause dysfunction in proper boundaries.

Qi (气, qì) – Literally translates as "life force energy" or "vital energy." It is insubstantial. Qi can be felt (and seen by some), but it does not have form. It is what enlivens the body; like electricity that lights up a house. Qi has six functions within the body: transforming, transporting, holding, raising, protecting, and warming.

Qi Deficiency (气虚, qìxū) – Weakness of Qi causes weakness of function with symptoms like fatigue, weak limbs, poor muscle tone, bloating, craving for sweets, low immunity, pale menstrual blood and short menstrual cycles. It can be constitutional or caused by poor eating and sleeping habits, overwork, and stress. Qi deficiency can affect the Spleen, Lung, Heart, and Kidney organ systems. Qi deficiency is characterized by a pale tongue and weak pulse.

Qi Stagnation (气滞, qìzhì) – When Qi flow is impeded or stuck it causes symptoms like depression, stiffness, irritability, irregularity of mood, bowel movement, or menstrual cycles, fatigue, and frequent sighing. Qi stagnation involves the Liver organ system or the local area. It is most often caused by emotional stress or toxins, or local trauma. It can also be due to Qi deficiency.

Qigong (气功, qìgōng) – Qigong literally translates as "Qi exercise." It uses meditation, movement, and breath for healing and optimizing health. There are many styles of qigong. Qigong heals the physical, emotional, and spiritual bodies and can be used for self-healing or healing others.

Red Dragon (红龙, hónglóng) – A metaphor for menstruation in Inner Alchemy.

Shen (神, shén) – The spirit of the Heart and can also be translated as "consciousness." In TCM, the Heart houses the Mind. It also refers to the overarching spirit of the person. The Heart Shen is the part of a person that is conscious of being and integrates the other spirits of the four other spirits: the Hun, Po, Yi, and Zhi. Imbalance in the Heart causes the Shen to scatter, leading to mental and emotional disturbances.

Traditional Chinese Medicine (TCM) (中医, zhōngyī) – Often used to describe the standardized traditional medicine of China created by post-revolutionary China. It is also used to describe the broader traditional medicine that evolved in China and Taiwan. Some propose using a broader term such as Traditional Asian Medicine to include Japanese, Korean, and other evolutions of the medicine. TCM relies on acupuncture, moxibustion, qigong, herbal medicine, cupping, gua sha, and massage. In Asian countries is also includes bonesetting and chiropractic.

Wind (风, fēng) – Internally manifests as headaches, migratory pain, vertigo, seizures, or convulsions. Internal Wind is generated by a deficiency of Blood or Yin and/or an excess of Heat. External Wind refers to pathogenic invasion, as in bacterial and viral infections, which is accompanied by Heat or Cold. External Wind causes a superficial pulse. Internal Wind can cause a rigid and deviated tongue.

Women's Alchemy (女丹, nüdān) – Inner Alchemy specific to women. These include breast massage, ovarian massage, and jade egg practices. They traditionally focus on lessening or stopping menstrual flow and balancing women's reproductive organs for the purpose of spiritual advancement. In modern times they are often used for increasing health, vitality, and sensuality.

Yang (阳, yáng) – Relates to the insubstantial, Qi, the sun, heat, movement, excess, rising, morning, back side of the body.

Yang Deficiency (阳虚, yángxū) – Is a progression of Qi deficiency resulting in more weakness of function with the addition of Cold symptoms. Common signs include low back and knee weakness, soreness, and/or cold, loose stools early in the morning (cock's crow diarrhea), edema in the lower body, copious urination. urinary or fecal incontinence, and nocturia (night urination). Yang deficiency can affect the Spleen, Kidney, and Heart organ systems. It can be constitutional or caused by longstanding Qi Deficiency, Cold damage, physical overwork (includes excessive exercise), exhaustion. Yang deficiency presents as a pale tongue with wet coating and deep, slow pulse.

Yi (意, yì) – The spirit of the Spleen. It governs intellect, intention, and the ability to digest ideas and experiences. A weak Spleen and unbalanced digestion can cause fuzzy thinking, rumination, and impair cognition.

Yin (阴, yīn)– Relates to substantial, Blood and body fluids, the moon, cold, stillness, deficiency, sinking, evening, front side of the body.

Yin Deficiency (阴虚, yīnxū) – Is a progression of Blood deficiency resulting in more loss of substance with the addition of Heat symptoms. Common signs include dryness (dry cough, throat, skin, vagina), dizziness, constipation, poor memory, heat worse at night, night sweats, thirst, flushed cheeks, dark urine, 5 Hearts Heat (in the palms, feet, and head), insomnia, tinnitus, memory loss, excess libido, low back soreness, ache in the bones, and bright red menstrual blood. Yin deficiency can affect the Heart, Lungs, Stomach, and Kidneys. It can be constitutional or due to Heat or Fluid damage, chronic illness, excessive sexual activity, mental overwork, prolonged emotional distress, emotional trauma, or older age. Yin deficiency presents as a small red tongue, with scant or mirrored coating and a thin, rapid pulse.

Zhi (智, zhì) – The spirit of the Kidneys. It governs willpower and deepest purpose. If the Kidneys are weak there may be a lack of determination and follow through.

Resources

Nutrition

Pitchford, Paul. *Healing With Whole Foods; Oriental Traditions and Modern Nutrition.* (Berkeley: North Atlantic Books, 1993).

Ni, Maoshing. *Tao of Nutrition.* (Los Angeles: Tao of Wellness Press, 1987).

Fermentation

Katz, Sandor. *Wild Fermentation: The Flavor, Nutrition, and Craft of Live-Culture Foods.* (Vermont: Chelsea Green Publishing Company, 2003).

Buhner, Stephen Harrod. *Sacred and Herbal Healing Beers: The Secrets of Ancient Fermentation.* (Brewers Publications, 1998).

Cultures for Health: www.culturesforhealth.com. Variety of ferments available for purchase.

Connecting with Plants

Cowan, Eliot. *Plant Spirit Medicine: The Healing Power of Plants.* (Columbus: Swan Raven & Company, 1991).

Buhner, Stephen Harrod. *Sacred Plant Medicine: The Wisdom in Native American Herbalism.* (Rochester: Bear & Company, 1996).

Chinese Herbs

Chinese herbs can be purchased from licensed acupuncturists.

Wing Hop Fung: www.WingHopFung.com (Chinese herbs, teas, and dried foods)

Dragon Herbs: www.DragonHerbs.com (Chinese herbs, acupuncture products)

May Way: www.MayWay.com (acupuncturists only)

Chinese Ingredients

99 Ranch Market: www.99Ranch.com. Stores in California, Nevada, Washington, and Texas.

Mitsuwa Market (Japanese): www.mitsuwa.com/english/index.html. Stores in California, New Jersey and Chicago.

Nijiya Market (Japanese): www.nijiya.com. Stores in California, New York, and Hawaii.

Inner Alchemy & Sexual Cultivation

For an overview of Daoist sexual texts: Wile, Douglas. *Art of the Bedchamber The Chinese Sexual Yoga Classics*. (State University of New York Press, 1992).

Mantak Chia: www.Universal-Tao.com. Offers complete instruction in Daoist Internal Alchemy. His teachings have a sexual focus. See: *Healing Love through the Dao: Cultivating Female Sexual Energy, The Multi-Orgasmic Woman, Bone Marrow Nei Kung, and Fusion of the Five Elements.*

Hsi Lai: Presents breast massage, swimming dragon, and other Women's Alchemy practices in questionable ethical context. Lai, Hsi. *The Sexual Teachings of the White Tigress: Secrets of the Female Taoist Masters*. (Rochester: Destiny Books, 2001).

Daisy Lee: www.RadiantLotusQigong.com. Radiant Qigong for Women DVD offers Women's Alchemy instruction.

Zhang, Tina Chunna. *Earth Qi Gong for Women: Awaken Your Inner Healing Power*. (Berkeley: Blue Snake Books, 2008).

Dr. Liu Yafei: www.MedicalQigongSchool.com. Her DVD is Nu Zi Qigong.

Davis, Deborah. *Women's Qigong for Health and Longevity: a Practical Guide for Women Forty and Over*. (Boston: Shambhala Publications, 2008).

Ferraro, Dominique. *Qigong for Women: Low-impact Exercises for Enhancing Energy and Toning the Body*. (Rochester: Healing Arts Press, 2000).

Fertility

For laypeople: Ni, Daoshing. *The Tao of Fertility: A Healing Chinese Medicine Program to Prepare Body, Mind, and Spirit for New Life*. (New York: Harper Collins Pulishers, 2008).

For acupuncturists: Lyttleton, Jane. *Treatment of Infertility with Chinese Medicine*. (China: Churchill Livingstone, 2004).

Postpartum Care

Jing Mommy: traditional Taiwanese postpartum services including frozen meals. English-speaking. Retail bottled Yue Zi Shui (postpartum water). www.JingMommy.com, 810 N. Nogales St. Walnut, CA 91789 Phone: 626-217-7539

Placenta Encapsulation

Placenta Benefits: www.PlacentaBenefits.info

Placenta Bakery: www.PlacentaBakery.com

Credits

Cover
Book Cover Illustrations:
www.backgrounds.mysitemyway.com
www.shutterstock.com
www.depositphotos.com; © ColorValley #11465725; © nataliia-ku #7038038
www.EvidenceoftheHand.com
Cover Design by Lia Andrews

Interior
Content Editing by Anita Edmonson
Layout Design by Miya Uchida
Chapter Opening Illustrations by Miya Uchida
Figure Illustrations by Lia Andrews

Index

Symbols

A

B

C

D

E

F

G

H

I

J

K

L

M

N

O

P

Q

R

S

Y

Z

About the Author

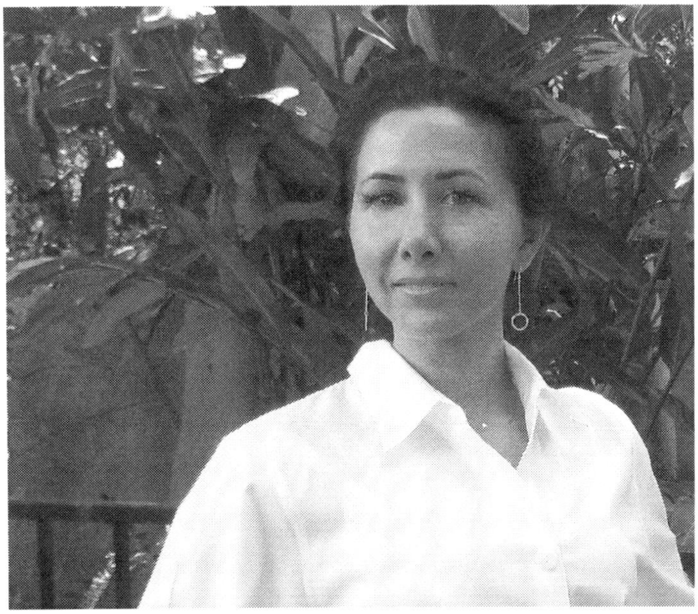

Dr. Lia G. Andrews, DAOM, L.Ac. was born in Norwalk, Connecticut. She attended Bryn Mawr College and the College of William & Mary, where she received her BA in International Studies. She received her Masters in Acupuncture and Traditional Chinese Medicine (MATCM) from Yo San University. Dr. Andrews received her Doctorate of Acupuncture and Oriental Medicine (DAOM) from Pacific College of Oriental Medicine. She is licensed nationally and in the state of California. Also in print is her doctoral capstone on traditional postpartum care: "Partial Translation of 'Postpartum Recovery Program; a Manual of Rules and Recipes for the Postpartum Woman.'" (DAOM capstone, Pacific College of Oriental Medicine, 2013).

Dr. Andrews has traveled to Brazil, Thailand, and China in her study for natural healing. She practices in the clinic she founded with her mother, Dr. Judith Andrews, Cinnabar Acupuncture Clinic & Spa in San Diego, California.

- Dr. Reiss - natural Hormone balance for women
- Clearing negative energy → p 62-64
- Symptoms for types of food to eat. p. 70
- bone broth or stock - good for skin [illegible]

26734492R00246

Made in the USA
Charleston, SC
17 February 2014